Diabetes Associated with Single Gene Defects and Chromosomal Abnormalities

Frontiers in Diabetes

Vol. 25

Series Editors

M. Porta Turin
F.M. Matschinsky Philadelphia, PA

Diabetes Associated with Single Gene Defects and Chromosomal Abnormalities

Volume Editors

Fabrizio Barbetti Rome

Lucia Ghizzoni Turin

Federica Guaraldi Turin

20 figures, 11 in color, and 10 tables, 2017

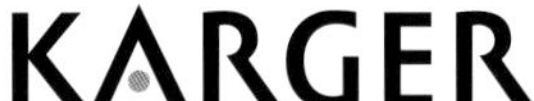

Basel · Freiburg · Paris · London · New York · Chennai · New Delhi · Bangkok · Beijing · Shanghai · Tokyo · Kuala Lumpur · Singapore · Sydney

Frontiers in Diabetes

Founded 1981 by F. Belfiore, Catania

Fabrizio Barbetti, MD, PhD

Department of Experimental Medicine and
Surgery
University of Rome Tor Vergata
Via Montpellier 1
IT–00133 Rome (Italy)
and
Clinical Pathology
San Pietro Hospital – Fatebenefratelli
IT–00189 Rome (Italy)

Lucia Ghizzoni, MD, PhD

Division of Endocrinology, Diabetes and
Metabolism
Department of Medical Sciences
University of Turin
Corso Dogliotti 14
IT–10126 Turin (Italy)

Federica Guaraldi, MD, PhD

Division of Endocrinology, Diabetes and
Metabolism
Department of Medical Sciences
University of Turin
Corso Dogliotti 14
IT–10126 Turin (Italy)

Library of Congress Cataloging-in-Publication Data

Names: Barbetti, Fabrizio, editor. | Ghizzoni, Lucia, editor. | Guaraldi, Federica, editor.
Title: Diabetes associated with single gene defects and chromosomal
  abnormalities / volume editors, Fabrizio Barbetti, Lucia Ghizzoni,
  Federica Guaraldi.
Other titles: Frontiers in diabetes ; v. 25. 0251-5342
Description: Basel ; New York : Karger, 2017. | Series: Frontiers in
  diabetes, ISSN 0251-5342 ; vol. 25 | Includes bibliographical references
  and indexes.
Identifiers: LCCN 2017009939| ISBN 9783318060249 (hard cover : alk. paper) |
  ISBN 9783318060256 (electronic version)
Subjects: | MESH: Diabetes Mellitus--congenital | Diabetes Complications |
  Genetic Diseases, Inborn--complications | Chromosome Aberrations | Insulin
  Resistance
Classification: LCC RC660 | NLM WK 835 | DDC 616.4/62042--dc23
LC record available at https://lccn.loc.gov/2017009939

Bibliographic Indices. This publication is listed in bibliographic services.

© Copyright 2017 by S. Karger AG, P.O. Box, CH–4009 Basel (Switzerland)
www.karger.com
Printed on acid-free and non-aging paper (ISO 9706)
ISSN 0251–5342
e-ISSN 1662–2995
ISBN 978–3–318–06024–9
e-ISBN 978–3–318–06025–6

Contents

VII **Foreword**
Novelli, G. (Rome)

IX **Preface**
Barbetti, F. (Rome); Ghizzoni, L.; Guaraldi, F. (Turin)

Diabetes and Genetic Defects Prevalently Involving the Pancreatic Beta Cells

1 **Neonatal Diabetes: Permanent Neonatal Diabetes and Transient Neonatal Diabetes**
Barbetti, F. (Rome); Mammì, C. (Reggio Calabria); Liu, M. (Tianjin); Grasso, V. (Rome); Arvan, P. (Ann Arbor, MI); Remedi, M.; Nichols, C.G. (St. Louis, MO)

26 **Maturity-Onset Diabetes of the Young: From Genetics to Translational Biology and Personalized Medicine**
Vaxillaire, M. (Lille); Froguel, P. (Lille/London)

49 **Thiamine-Responsive Megaloblastic Anemia Syndrome**
Franzese, A.; Fattorusso, V.; Mozzillo, E. (Naples)

55 **Diabetes Mellitus in Mitochondrial Disease**
Ng, Y.S.; Taylor, R.W.; Schaefer, A.M. (Newcastle upon Tyne)

69 **Diabetes in Wolfram Syndrome: Update of Clinical and Genetic Aspects**
Rigoli, L.C. (Messina); d'Annunzio, G. (Genova)

78 **Type 1 Diabetes Mellitus in Monogenic Autoimmune Diseases**
Bacchetta, R. (Stanford, CA); Maccari, M.E. (Milan)

91 **Genetic and Immunological Features of Insulin-Dependent Diabetes Mellitus as a Clinical Manifestation of Type 1 Autoimmune Polyglandular Syndrome**
Fierabracci, A.; Russo, B. (Rome)

Extreme Insulin Resistance with Diabetes

104 **Syndromes Associated with Mutations in the Insulin Signalling Pathway**
Leiter, S.M.; Semple, R.K. (Cambridge)

119 **Insulin Resistance and Diabetes Associated with Lipodystrophies**
Leiter, S.M.; Semple, R.K. (Cambridge)

Ciliopathies, Obesity, and Glucose Metabolism

134 **Alström Syndrome**
Maffei, P.; Favaretto, F.; Milan, G. (Padua); Marshall, J.D. (Bar Harbor, ME/Mount Desert, ME)

Chromosomal Defects and Diabetes

145 Prader-Willi Syndrome
Grugni, G. (Verbania)

151 47,XXY Klinefelter Syndrome Is Associated with an Increased Risk of Insulin Resistance: The Impact of Hypogonadism and Visceral Obesity
Panimolle, F.; Radicioni, A.F. (Rome)

160 Down Syndrome (Trisomy 21) and Diabetes
Bizzarri, C.; Cappa, M. (Rome)

166 Turner Syndrome and Diabetes
Grossi, A.; Cappa, M. (Rome)

Other Genetic Conditions with Increased Susceptibility to Diabetes

172 Diabetes in Friedreich Ataxia
Ran, S.; Abeti, R.; Giunti, P. (London)

182 Diabetes in Myotonic Dystrophy
Dahlqvist, J.R.; Vissing, J. (Copenhagen)

188 Author Index
189 Subject Index

Foreword

Each generation needs a new music.
Francis Crick

In a rapidly evolving area of modern medicine such as diabetes mellitus and its genetic causes, it is difficult for clinicians to keep up with the latest advances. In this scenario, it is widely accepted that the main types of diabetes mellitus are polygenic forms, called type 1 diabetes and type 2 diabetes, which account for at least 95% of all cases. However, recent etiologic classifications recognize an increasing number of diabetes subtypes linked to mutations of specific genes involved in pancreatic β-cell function or insulin action. Interestingly, in a large number of individuals with a monogenic defect leading to diabetes, a patient's phenotype is not readily distinguishable from those with type 1 or type 2 diabetes.

The goal of *Diabetes Associated with Single Gene Defects and Chromosomal Abnormalities* is to bring the most recent knowledge on specific subtypes of this protean disease to those involved in the etiologic diagnosis of patients with diabetes. To this aim, this book covers not only the monogenic forms of diabetes, but also other genetic conditions and chromosome abnormalities associated with an increased susceptibility to develop diabetes. The new onset of diabetes can be secondary to alterations in one of the hundreds of genes controlling glucose metabolism, or impaired regulation of the immune response, that can lead to autoimmunity. Differently from other conditions (i.e., achondroplasia or Down syndrome) in which a single penetrant mutation or chromosomal aberration is necessary and sufficient to cause the disease, the effect of any individual gene in polygenic syndromes, like diabetes, is dull. The interdependence on environmental variables – diet, age, nutrition, and prenatal exposure – is stronger. The genetic component of the disease acts as a trigger, but is not sufficient per se to cause the illness. All of this variability must be considered when designing treatments addressing polygenic disorders. First of all, patient characteristics have to be taken into account. This approach is commonly referred to as "personalized", or "stratified" or "precision", medicine. Personalized medicine is based on the use of information from the genome and its derivatives (i.e., RNA, proteins, and metabolites) to guide medical decisions about diagnosis, prognosis, and therapy. This goal can be reached only using good biomarkers that should explain either the disease at the molecular level or the response to treatment. The presence or absence of a biomarker can be used to guide treatment choices and to identify targets for drug development. There is a huge demand for the development of new drugs to improve treatment. This demand has arisen due to the gradual change in the nature of therapy in recent years, with the introduction of orphan drugs. As biomarkers begin to embrace genomic tools, the fundamentals of personalized medicine will require the development, standardization, and integration of several important tools into health systems and clinical workflows. These tools include health risk assessment, family health history, and ethnicity. Diseases cannot be studied only individually, as they are clustered in specific ensembles in a given territory at a given time (pathocoenosis). A gene for a particular risk factor for diabetes can be also implicated in the pathogenesis of other diseases. A single risk factor, such as obesity, can be linked to many different diseases. The patients themselves are often clustered in communities, which must also be studied using geographical, territorial, and sociocultural approaches. In this context, basic diabetes management skills are built and diffused to help in preventing the need for emergency care, and the role of the "diabetes educator" is becoming more and more relevant.

Prof. Giuseppe Novelli, University of Rome Tor Vergata, Rome

Preface

In the last decades, rare forms of diabetes secondary to mutations of single genes involved in the regulation of insulin secretion and action have been characterized, together with an increased susceptibility to develop alterations of glycemic control associated with some common chromosomal abnormalities.

This volume provides a comprehensive, authoritative, and updated overview of the current knowledge on the pathophysiology, main clinical features, and treatment of rare forms of diabetes/impaired glycemic control associated with single-gene and chromosomal alterations. Based on the pathophysiological mechanisms responsible for the impairment of glucose metabolism, the volume is divided into 5 main sections. The first section is dedicated to diabetes secondary to genetic alterations mainly involving pancreatic β-cells, i.e., permanent and transient neonatal diabetes; MODY (maturity-onset diabetes of the young); TRMA (thiamine-responsive megaloblastic anemia) diabetes; mitochondrial diabetes; Wolfram or DIDMOAD (diabetes insipidus, diabetes mellitus, optic atrophy, and deafness) syndrome; and monogenic forms of autoimmunity and diabetes, including IPEX (immune dysregulation, polyendocrinopathy, enteropathy, X-linked syndrome) and APS1 (autoimmune polyendocrine syndrome 1). The second section focuses on diabetes associated with extreme insulin resistance, including syndromes associated with mutations of the insulin receptor and lipodystrophies. The third section deals with ciliopathies, obesity, and alteration of glucose metabolism, i.e., Alström syndrome. The fourth section describes chromosomal defects associated with an increased risk of diabetes susceptibility, including Prader-Willi syndrome, Klinefelter syndrome, Down syndrome or trisomy 21, and Turner syndrome. The last section deals with other rare genetic conditions responsible for increased susceptibility to diabetes, i.e., Friedreich ataxia and dystrophia myotonica types 1 and 2. However, although excellent reviews on diabetes associated with cystic fibrosis and Bardet-Biedl syndrome have been recently published, and the association of Huntington disease and diabetes has been suggested in animals but not confirmed in humans, these were not included in this volume.

We truly believe that *Diabetes Associated with Single Gene Defects and Chromosomal Abnormalities* will be an attractive and useful reference bibliographic source for all physicians involved in the care of pediatric and adult diabetes patients.

We sincerely thank all of the contributors who devoted their time and efforts for completing this volume, and the Karger staff who assisted in its production.

Prof. Fabrizio Barbetti, University of Rome Tor Vergata and San Pietro Hospital – Fatebenefratelli, Rome
Prof. Lucia Ghizzoni, University of Turin, Turin
Prof. Federica Guaraldi, University of Turin, Turin

Barbetti F, Ghizzoni L, Guaraldi F (eds): Diabetes Associated with Single Gene Defects and Chromosomal Abnormalities. Front Diabetes. Basel, Karger, 2017, vol 25, pp 1–25 (DOI: 10.1159/000454748)

Neonatal Diabetes: Permanent Neonatal Diabetes and Transient Neonatal Diabetes

Fabrizio Barbetti[a–c] · Corrado Mammì[d] · Ming Liu[e] · Valeria Grasso[b] · Peter Arvan[f] · Maria Remedi[g] · Colin G. Nichols[h]

[a]Department of Experimental Medicine and Surgery, University of Rome Tor Vergata, Rome, [b]Bambino Gesù Children's Hospital, Rome, [c]S. Pietro Hospital – Fatebenefratelli, Rome, and [d]Medical Genetics Unit, BMM Great Metropolitan Hospital, Reggio Calabria, Italy; [e]Division of Endocrinology and Metabolism, Tianjin Medical University General Hospital, Tianjin, China; [f]Division of Metabolism, Endocrinology and Diabetes, University of Michigan, Ann Arbor, MI, and Departments of [g]Medicine and [h]Cell Biology and Physiology, Washington University School of Medicine, St. Louis, MO, USA

Abstract

The concept of monogenic diabetes emerged 25 years ago with a paper reporting the glucokinase locus linkage to maturity-onset diabetes of the young, an autosomal dominant disorder of glucose metabolism. Since then a huge leap forward has been made with the discovery of other clinical forms of monogenic diabetes, such as neonatal diabetes mellitus (NDM), and the identification of literally tens of genes that cause diabetes, either in isolation or syndromic. Of note, NDM genetics not only shed light on several aspects of pancreatic β-cell biology, but revealed new and unexpected therapeutic options for patients carrying mutations in specific genes, such as oral hypoglycemic agents (mutations of KATP genes) or stem cell transplantation (IPEX). In this chapter, we describe the genetic defects leading to neonatal diabetes that recognize dominant, recessive, and X-linked modes of inheritance or the association with incorrect parental origins of chromosomes and disturbances of imprinting. © 2017 S. Karger AG, Basel

Neonatal Diabetes Mellitus: An Introduction

Early reports of single patients with "congenital diabetes" or neonatal diabetes mellitus (NDM) can be found as far back as the mid-19th century, but the first thoroughly described, well-proven, cases of neonates with diabetes were published in the 1950s [1]. Interestingly, the notion that two clinical forms of NDM – permanent and transient – can be distinguished was already established at that time [1], along with the fact that most cases were sporadic. In addition, temporary subcutaneous insulin treatment with long-acting neutral protamine Hagedorn insulin had also been successfully used in patients with transient neonatal diabetes mellitus (TNDM) [1]. Nevertheless, further progress in understanding NDM had to wait another 40 years until the genetic discoveries that paternal uniparental isodisomy (UDP) of chromosome 6 (UDP6) is linked to TNDM [2], whilst homozygous, loss-of-function mutation of insulin promoter factor 1 *(IPF1,* now known as *PDX1)* causes pancreatic agenesis leading to permanent neonatal diabetes mellitus (PNDM) and exocrine pancreas deficiency [3].

Around the same time, the main clinical features of both recognized forms of NDM were (temporarily) established through an extensive review of the literature [4], in which Von Muhlendahl and Herkenhoff proposed the first comprehensive definition of NDM as: "hyperglycemia occurring within the first month of life that lasts for at least two weeks and requires insulin therapy." These authors reported the variability of time between onset and remission of diabetes for patients with the transient form (17–1,914 days), together with the fact that in some TNDM cases, relapse subsequently occurs at a later age (range: 7–20 years) [4]. They also provided a crude estimate of the incidence of NDM in Germany (based on survey of cases with neonatal diabetes between 1977 and 1991) as 1 in 500,000 live births, and in conclusion, put forward the idea that NDM may generally have a genetic origin [4].

In 2000, the gene responsible for Wolcott-Rallison syndrome, a recessive condition that encompasses neonatal (or infancy-onset) diabetes, osteopenia, and liver dysfunction was identified [5], and 1 year later the first 2 cases of PNDM due to homozygous loss-of-function mutations of the glucokinase *(GCK)* gene were reported [6]. Of note, one of the patients described in that paper presented with isolated (i.e., nonsyndromic) diabetes (like all cases with biallelic, inactivating, GCK mutations subsequently reported in the literature), highlighting the key role of glucokinase in coupling glucose to insulin secretion from the pancreatic β-cell [6]. In the same year, the cause of immune dysregulation, polyendocrinopathy, enteropathy, X-linked syndrome (IPEX), presenting with X-linked neonatal autoimmune diabetes mellitus, autoimmune endocrinopathy and enthropathy was linked to mutations of the *FOXP3* gene [7, 8]. Around the same time, Koster et al. [9] reported NDM in mice as a result of ATP-sensitive K^+ (K_{ATP}) channel gain of function (GOF), although it would take another 4 years for the first reports that the same mechanism is the most prominent cause of human NDM (see below).

In 2002, Iafusco et al. [10] showed that patients with permanent diabetes with onset in the first 6 months have different clinical and laboratory features compared with patients with diabetes onset between 6 months and 1 year of life. While individuals belonging to the second group were often positive for type 1a diabetes (T1Da)-associated autoantibodies, and had normal birth weight, those in the first group had low birth weight, rarely carried HLA alleles predisposing to T1Da diabetes, and were almost invariably negative for T1Da autoantibodies. On the basis of these results,

Iafusco et al. suggested that the cause of hyperglycemia in patients with diabetes onset in the first 6 months of birth was probably genetic, thus extending Von Muhlendahl's pathophysiologic hypothesis of NDM well beyond the standard neonatal period of 1 month. This work established the value of systematic assessment of T1D autoantibodies in diabetes of very early onset, and paved the way for a new clinical definition of NDM [10].

In the following 5 years, three genes (*KCNJ11*, *ABCC8*, and *INS*; 2004, 2006, and 2007) were identified as causing most cases of PNDM in developed countries [11–14]. Of note, clinical records showed that patients carrying mutations in these three genes [11–14] typically present with diabetes within 6 months of birth, matching Iafusco's prediction of a genetic origin of hyperglycemia in patients with diabetes onset within 6 months of birth and negative to T1D autoantibodies [10]. Perhaps not surprisingly, retrospective genetic analysis revealed that 19 out of 25 Italian patients with diabetes onset within 6 months of birth included in the original report of Iafusco et al., carry a mutation in either the *KCNJ11, INS, ABCC8,* or *GCK* gene [6, 14–16]. That patients with diabetes onset within 6 months of age do not carry HLA alleles associated with polygenic autoimmune diabetes (i.e., T1Da) was confirmed in 2006 [17]. Further analyses have led to the current diagnostic guidelines for and definition of NDM (i.e., diabetes with onset within 6 months of age instead of 1 month) such that molecular genetic screening is recommended for this condition, with an estimated incidence that is currently calculated at around 1:200,000 live births for the permanent form only [18, 19] and at 1:90,000 for both PNDM and TNDM [19]. This incidence is twice that estimated in previous investigations for Western countries [4, 20], but is lower than the incidence estimate for the Middle East, which is set between 1:48,000 and 1:21,000 [21, 22], due to the high recurrence of recessive forms of NDM.

In the last 10 years, many other genes responsible for very rare, usually syndromic, conditions that include permanent neonatal diabetes have been discovered. Most encode transcription factors important for embryonic development of endocrine pancreas and other organs [23, 24]. The clinical features of each syndromic subtype may be helpful in directing molecular genetic screening, even though with the advent of next-generation sequencing of genomic DNA, a selection based on clinical characteristics need not be an absolute requirement [25].

In this chapter we will place emphasis on the major genetic determinants of PNDM and TNDM (KCNJ11, ABCC8, INS, and defects of chromosome 6), while coverage of the less frequent causes will be left to a minimum.

Permanent Neonatal Diabetes Mellitus

K_{ATP} Channel Mutations as Cause of Human PNDM
The identification of K_{ATP} channels as key players in pancreatic β-cell physiology was a breakthrough in the understanding of the mechanism of glucose-stimulated insulin

secretion. K_{ATP} channels, through regulated changes in their activity, couple membrane excitability to glucose-stimulated insulin secretion, and thereby maintain blood glucose within a narrow physiologic range [26]. After a meal, glucose metabolism leads to an increase in the intracellular [ATP]:[ADP] ratio, which closes β-cell K_{ATP} channels, inducing membrane depolarization and opening voltage-dependent Ca^{2+} channels (Fig. 1a). Ca^{2+} influx increases intracellular $[Ca^{2+}]$, which triggers insulin vesicle fusion to the membrane and insulin secretion [26]. Conversely, a decrease in the metabolic signal keeps K_{ATP} channels open, suppressing the electrical trigger of insulin secretion. This electrical pathway is also modulated by K_{ATP}-independent mechanisms, e.g. nutrient metabolites and incretins, which affect secretion at various stages downstream of K_{ATP} channels [26, 27]. However, the ability of selective K_{ATP} channel inhibitors, sulfonylureas (SUs), to directly trigger insulin secretion underscores the critical role of K_{ATP}-dependent regulation [28–30].

Any mechanism that results in 'overactive' K_{ATP} channels should decrease membrane excitability, thereby impairing glucose sensing by the β-cell and reducing insulin secretion. Activating mutations in both the Kir6.2 (KCNJ11) [11] and the SUR1 (ABCC8) [12] genes that encode the pancreatic K_{ATP} channel subunits have now been identified as the commonest cause of human NDM [31, 32], both TNDM (see below) and PNDM. In approximately one-third of PNDM cases, K_{ATP} mutations are also associated with developmental delay (both motor and intellectual), epilepsy, and neonatal diabetes (DEND) syndrome, and extrapancreatic symptoms are likely the result of overactive K_{ATP} in muscle, peripheral nerves, and/or brain [11, 15, 33].

Molecular Mechanisms of PNDM Mutations
Nucleotide regulation of K_{ATP} channels [34, 35] (Fig. 1b) is unique among K channels. The channel is directly inhibited by ATP in the micromolar range. It is important to note that cytosolic ATP concentration is in the millimolar range (1–5 mM), and

Fig. 1. K_{ATP} channels and neonatal diabetes. **a** The physiologic and pathologic role of K_{ATP} in insulin secretion. In normal β-cells, metabolism is inhibited in low glucose, lowering the [ATP]/[ADP] ratio, promoting the opening of K_{ATP} channels, which hyperpolarizes the cell, inhibiting voltage-dependent Ca^{2+} channels and inhibiting insulin secretion. When glucose rises, metabolism is stimulated and the [ATP]/[ADP] ratio rises. This promotes K_{ATP} channel closure, depolarizing the cell, which opens Ca^{2+} channels, causing Ca^{2+} to rise, and triggers insulin secretion. Gain of function (GOF) in K_{ATP} results in maintained hyperpolarization in high glucose and failure of insulin secretion. **b** β-Cell K_{ATP} channels are octameric complexes of 4 pore-forming Kir6.2 subunits and 4 SUR1 subunits. Cytoplasmic ATP binding to Kir6.2 subunits stabilizes channel closure. MgATP binds to the two ATP-binding sites (ABS) formed at the NBF1-NBF2 interface on the SUR1 subunits. MgATP hydrolysis results in a conformational "activated" state that can open the channel. The "activated state" persists through ADP dissociation, and can be maintained by MgADP rebinding. Sulfonylurea or diazoxide, interacting with the SUR1 subunit, causes channel closure or opening, respectively. **c** Representation of SUR1 and Kir6.2, indicating approximate locations of mutations associated with permanent (PNDM) or transient neonatal diabetes (TNDM). *(For figure see next page.)*

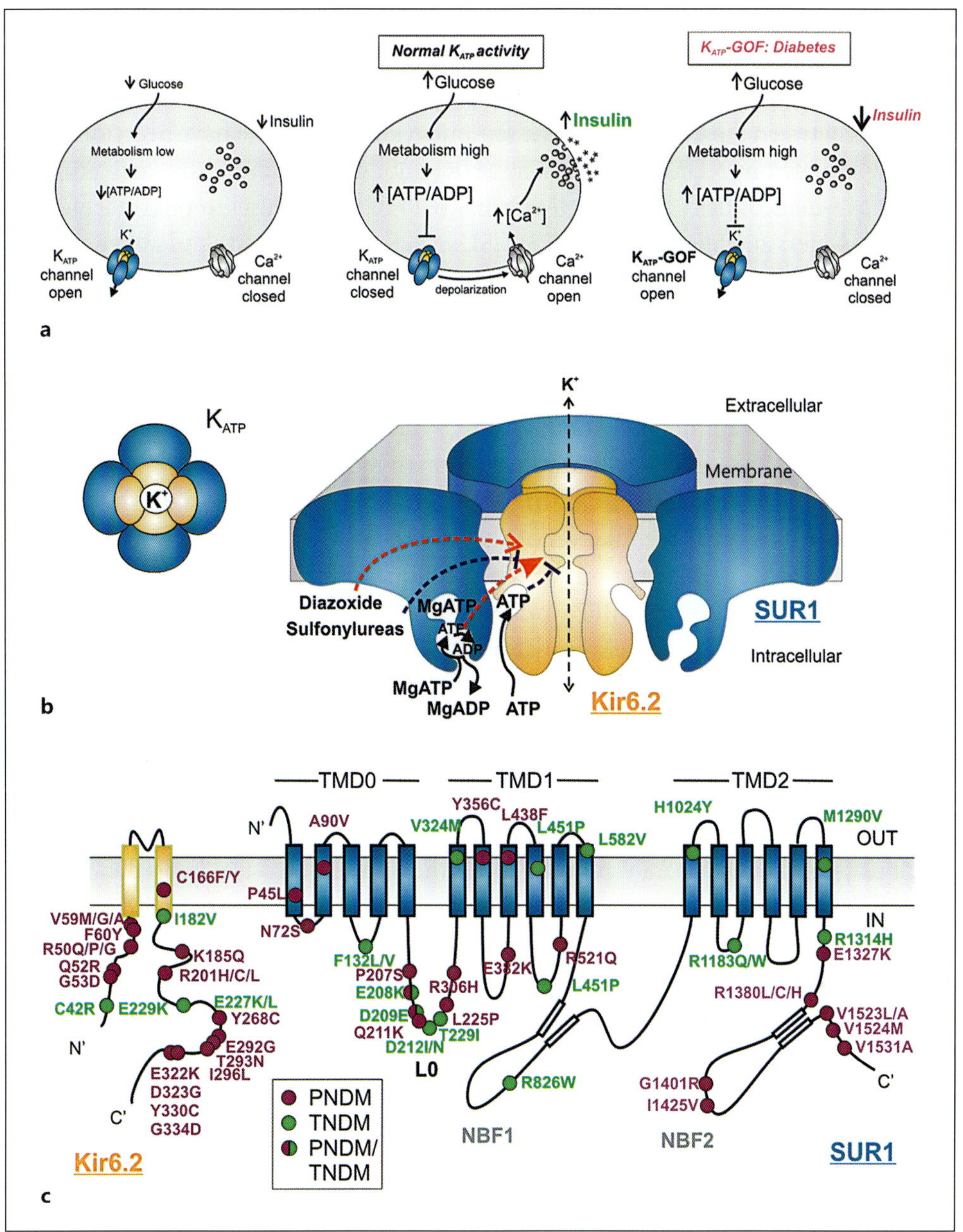

changes little with metabolism. Thus, [ATP] is probably always sufficient to almost fully inhibit channel activity. Channel activation arises from the activating effects of binding to the SUR subunit [36].

ATP-inhibition results from ATP binding to the Kir6.2 subunit [35] (Fig. 1b). Mutations causing NDM (Fig. 1c) all significantly decrease ATP sensitivity. Many mutations seem to affect ATP sensitivity allosterically by altering the intrinsic stability of the open state, but others directly affect the ATP-binding site. Residues R50, I182,

K185, R201, and G334, located at very different positions in the primary sequence, have all been identified as controlling ATP affinity (Fig. 1c). Satisfyingly, they are all predicted to be located at the inhibitory ATP-binding site [37] located at each of the interfaces between the 4 subunits in the tetramer (Fig. 1c), and all have been identified as being mutated in NDM patients. The SUR1 subunit determines the activating effects of Mg-nucleotides [36], as well as sensitivity of the channel to pharmacological channel openers and blockers [36, 38, 39]. SUs, such as tolbutamide and glibenclamide (glyburide), bind directly to the SUR1 subunit (Fig. 1b), leading to inhibition of K_{ATP} channel activity, membrane depolarization, and triggering of insulin secretion [35]. As with all other ABC proteins, SURs contain nucleotide-binding folds (NBFs) that typically dimerize to form two nucleotide-binding sites at the dimer interface. The first clue to the role of the SUR subunit in K_{ATP} channel gating was demonstrated by a mutation (G1479R) in NBF2 that caused human hyperinsulinism [36]. This mutation and other hyperinsulinism-causing NBF2 mutations selectively abolish MgADP- and diazoxide-mediated stimulation of channel activity, with no effect on ATP inhibition [35]. Mutation of the conserved lysine residues in the Walker A motifs of either NBF1 (mutation K719A) or NBF2 (mutation K1384M), predicted to reduce ATP hydrolytic activity, also block the stimulatory effect of MgADP [39] (Fig. 1c).

Multiple GOF mutations in Kir6.2 and SUR1 have now been found to underlie human NDM [32]. All show enhanced activity at any given [ATP]/[ADP] ratio [40], typically due to a decrease in the apparent affinity of the ATP-binding pocket or increased open state stability of the Kir6.2 subunit, or due to enhanced Mg-nucleotide activation of the SUR1 subunit. Several Kir6.2 residues (i.e., I182, R201, R50, K185), previously implicated as ATP binding and others (Y330 and F333) predicted to lie close to the phosphate tail of the ATP binding pocket [41] have been found to be mutated in patients with NDM (Fig. 1c). Other NDM mutations, located in both Kir6.2 and the TMD0 domain of the SUR1 subunit, alter channel gating (detected in the absence of ATP) and allosterically result in reduction of ATP sensitivity without changes in ATP-binding affinity (e.g., I296L, V59G, Q52R, C42R) (Fig. 1c). Q52 and V59 residues are located within the 'slide helix' of Kir6.2 (Fig. 1c), consistent with a role for this structure in linking ATP binding and gating.

Finally, in addition to a direct causal role in NDM, it should be noted that a common amino acid polymorphism (Glu23Lys, E23K) in the Kir6.2 subunit of the channel is one of the established risk factors for type 2 diabetes [42]. In this case, the polymorphism also causes a very weak loss of ATP sensitivity [43], leading to reduced insulin secretion, even in nondiabetic carriers, which seems to underlie the diabetes susceptibility.

Sulfonylurea Treatability in PNDM Patients
The realization that NDM results from mutations in the K_{ATP} channel has rapidly shifted therapy from insulin injections to oral SU drugs: by directly inhibiting the overactive K_{ATP} channels, these drugs can provide successful control of blood glucose levels, and

  Barbetti · Mammì · Liu · Grasso · Arvan · Remedi · Nichols

insulin requirements can be avoided (or reduced) in the majority of K_{ATP}-induced NDM [44–52]. Unlike exogenous insulin, which acts indiscriminately to lower blood glucose by promoting peripheral glucose uptake, SU drugs circumvent the metabolic signal in the β-cell and directly block K_{ATP} overactivity, thereby restoring endogenous insulin secretion, an effect which is then physiologically augmented in the presence of potentiating incretins. Approximately 92% of patients have successfully switched from insulin injections to oral SUs, blood glucose has been well controlled without insulin supplement, and HbA_{1C} levels fall, reducing the risk of diabetic complication [44, 53, 54]. Successful transfer has not proven to be possible in all cases: in general, transferability correlates negatively with the age of the patient and the severity of the disease [44, 55, 56]. It has been demonstrated that the younger the patient at the time of SU-transfer, the greater the chance for a successful complete transition from insulin to SU therapy [44, 57]. Importantly, however, in many cases the oral dosage of SUs at the beginning of therapy significantly exceeds by several fold the doses commonly used to treat type 2 diabetes [44, 53, 54], though it is usually tapered over time [58].

Although the success rate for transferability to SU is lower in patients with DEND symptoms, several patients have also demonstrated improved neurological features, motor tone and coordination [51, 59, 60], enhanced cognitive function [61, 62], and abolition of epileptic seizures [59] with SU treatment, suggesting that SUs also act on overactive K_{ATP} (Kir6.2 and SUR1) in central neurons to improve brain activity. Improvement of muscle weakness and ataxic gait was demonstrated in a patient with intermediate DEND treated with gliclazide (which only interacts with SUR1) [51], again suggesting that this effect is mainly through the improvement of the neuronal terminal activity.

Insights from Mouse Models of K_{ATP} NDM
Mouse models of KATP GOF-induced NDM, in which GOF mutations have been transgenically expressed in β-cells under either the insulin gene promoter or under a tamoxifen-inducible PDX1 promoter, show glucose intolerance shortly after birth (or after induction of the mutant gene), which progresses to severe diabetes within a few weeks, with unmeasurably high blood sugars, growth retardation, disruption of the pancreatic architecture, profound loss of β-cell mass, and dramatic reduction of total insulin content [63, 64]. These changes can be prevented by normalization of blood glucose levels, achieved by syngeneic islet transplantation or chronic SU therapy [63], indicating that they are secondary consequences of systemic hyperglycemia. Importantly, glibenclamide can prevent diabetes if administered at the onset of disease, but cannot reverse established chronic hyperglycemia, presumably because a profound loss of β-cells has already occurred [63]. Most strikingly, early aggressive acute SU treatment resulted in essentially permanent remission of diabetes in a subset of K_{ATP}-induced NDM mice [65], basically switching the disease from a permanent, progressively worsening form to a transient form, suggesting a potential mechanism for the differential TNDM and PNDM outcomes in humans [32, 44, 66] (see below). In this

case, the remission appears to be associated with enhanced insulin sensitivity [65], which may arise secondarily to the very low circulating insulin levels that are present following disease induction.

We would speculate that this sensitivity takes time to develop, resulting in a vulnerable window at the early stage of the disease, in which failed insulin secretion could result in dangerously high glucose levels that result in permanent damage to the islets, potentially β-cell death, or dedifferentiation [67], which results in even further lowering of insulin levels that cannot be compensated for by subsequent insulin hypersensitivity. Such a vulnerable window effect provides a further argument in support of early and aggressive control of blood glucose, potentially by early SU introduction, in all NDM patients.

Insulin Gene (INS) Mutations as a Cause of Diabetes and Its Permanent Neonatal Subtype

The human insulin (INS) gene was cloned in 1980 [68] and INS mutations giving rise to rare cases of familial hyperinsulinemia/familial hyper(pro)insulinemia were described over the subsequent 10 years [69]. The discovery of these genetic bases was linked to the (often serendipitous) finding of very high levels of immunoreactive serum insulin or (pro)insulin-like protein in patients presenting with mild alterations of glucose metabolism [69]. Using classic protein investigation tools, it was shown that the elevated insulin or (pro)insulin-like proteins were in fact mutant insulin gene products with amino acid changes in the insulin A- or B-chain or in the dibasic cleavage site between the A-chain and the C-peptide. These findings were then confirmed by genetic analyses that identified 3 heterozygous mutations leading to familial hyperinsulinemia [nomenclature of that time: Leu^{A3}Val, Phe^{B24}Ser, and Phe^{B25}Leu, now replaced by Leu92Val (L92V), Phe48Ser (F48S), and Phe49Leu (F49L) according to the position relative to the ATG encoding methionine 1 at the translation initiation site] and other mutations associated with familial hyper(pro)insulinemia [formerly His^{B10}Asp, Arg65His (R65H), ArgR65Leu (R65L), and Arg65Pro (R65P); currently His34Asp (H34D), R89H, R89L, and R89P] [69–71]. It turned out that all mutations inherited in the autosomal dominant mode greatly impair insulin receptor binding and, consequently, insulin biological activity [69]. As a consequence, mutant insulins/ (pro)insulins are secreted by β-cells, but fail to be cleared by receptor-mediated endocytosis, and accumulate in the plasma [69, 70]. Because patients with familial hyperinsulinemia or hyper(pro)insulinemia still secrete normal insulin encoded by the wild-type allele, they show normal glucose metabolism or mild diabetes [69]. Surprisingly, some of these patients may experience episodes of hypoglycemia, and this – with the concurrent presence of high levels of proinsulin-like material – can be mistaken for insulinoma [70].

More recently, novel heterozygous INS mutations have been discovered in patients with PNDM [13, 14]. Intriguingly, not only the patients' age at presentation was dramatically different from individuals with familial hyperinsulinemia/hyper(pro)-

insulinemia (usually identified in adolescence or later), but plasma C-peptide levels, an indicator of endogenous insulin secretion, was found to be either very low at diabetes onset [13, 14] or to rapidly decrease over time [14]. This clinical feature found in patients of 6 months of age or less was a clear indication of progressive and rapid β-cell failure. Interestingly, most, but not all, PNDM/INS mutations either disrupt 1 of the 3 invariant disulfide bonds of the insulin molecule, by substituting 1 of the 6 highly conserved cysteines with another amino acid, or introduce a new cysteine [13, 14]. A notable example is mutation INS/R89C (old nomenclature: R65C), which substitutes cysteine for the same arginine part of the cleavage site between the A-chain and C-peptide that is found mutated in familial hyperproinsulinemia. Not surprisingly, in silico modelling shows that insulin mutations associated with PNDM severely affect insulin tertiary structure [14]. Experiments performed on transfected HEK-293 cells reveal that mutant insulins causing PNDM are not found in the medium [14], i.e. are not secreted, in contrast to wild-type insulin or mutant insulins associated with familial hyper(pro)insulinemia. As a consequence, mutant insulins accumulate in the endoplasmic reticulum (ER), resulting in sustained ER-stress, and triggering a highly conserved signal transduction pathway called an "unfolded protein response" (UPR).

UPR uses 3 ER stress sensors/branches: IRE1α (inositol requiring enzyme 1α), PERK (pancreatic endoplasmic reticulum kinase), both ER-resident proteins, and ATF6 (activating transcription factor 6). In the presence of unfolded/misfolded proteins, IRE1α multimerizes and trans-autophosphorylates acquiring RNAse activity. Activated IRE1α excises a small intron from mRNA encoding a transcription factor, XBP-1 (X-box protein 1). After cytosolic splicing, XBP-1 translocates into the nucleus and induces transcription of hundreds of genes that increase the protein-folding capacity to counter ER stress. Experiments performed in HEK-293 cells show that although wild-type insulin or familial hyper(pro)insulinemia INS/R89L do not trigger UPR, PNDM-associated INS mutations like INS/R89C, INS/C95Y (old nomenclature: C^{A6}Y), INS/Y108X (old nomenclature: Y^{A19}X), and others strongly promote XBP-1 splicing [14], a sign that these mutant insulins are subjected to insurmountable terminal misfolding.

In a "professional" secretory cell such as the pancreatic β-cell, half of the amount of client proteins in the ER is insulin, which can be secreted at the striking rate of 10^6 molecules per minute. In such a cell, a high rate of production of an unfoldable insulin may trigger a UPR that fails to correct ER stress and rapidly becomes maladaptive, initiating downstream proapoptotic signals through each of its branches. Though the final effector of the apoptosis process of β-cells carrying proteotoxic mutations is not known, Colombo et al. [14] showed that in HEK-293 cells transfected with PNDM-associated insulin constructs, the percentage of cells expressing annexin V and/or positive to propidium iodide is significantly increased compared to cells transduced with wild-type insulin. Subsequent work has firmly established that several PNDM-associated INS proteotoxic mutations, but not familial hyperinsulinemia mutations, also impose dominant-negative inhibition on wild-type proinsulin transport [72–74]. Thus, two mechanisms of disease are probably at work in these patients: a secretory

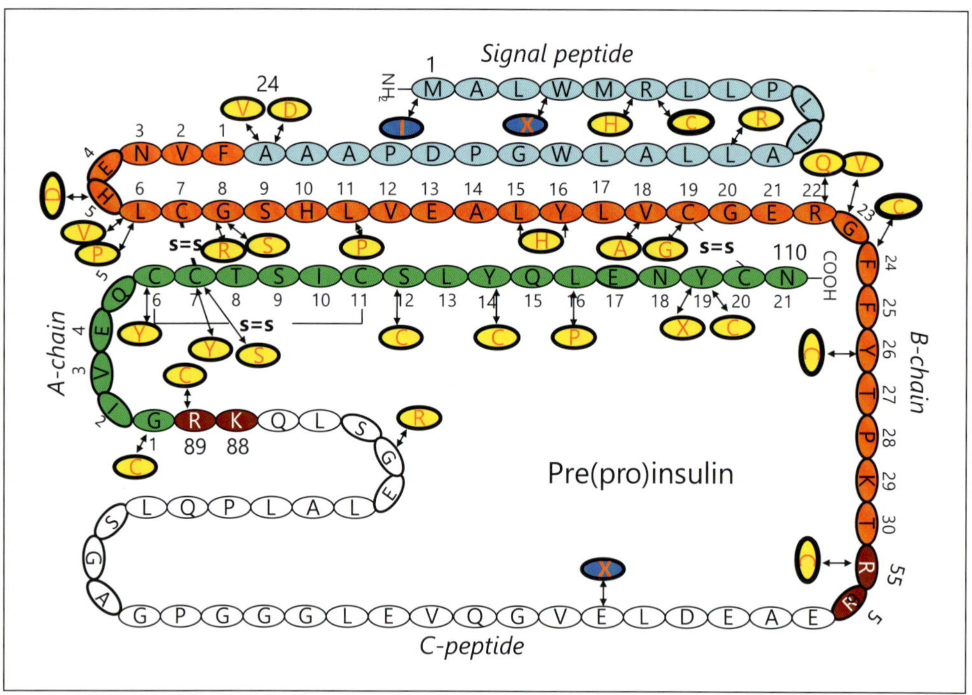

Fig. 2. Location of mutations in the coding region of the insulin gene associated with neonatal diabetes mellitus. The amino acid substitutions responsible of dominant form of diabetes (both neonatal or with onset in childhood or adulthood) are in yellow; recessive mutations leading to neonatal diabetes mellitus are in blue.

defect and progressive decrement of β-cell mass, which also leads to hyperglucagonemia [14]. Interestingly, even a noncoding, intronic mutation in intron 2 of the INS gene has been causally associated with PNDM by introducing an ectopic splice site that leads to synthesis of a longer INS mRNA that also results in disruption of normal disulfide bonds in the encoded mutant protein [75]. New insulin gene mutations with a proteotoxic effect causing autosomal-dominant PNDM or childhood-onset diabetes (i.e., INS/MODY, see chapter by Vaxillaire et al. [this vol., pp. 26–48) continue to be described and the total count has now reached 30 [76–82] (Fig. 2).

Loss-of-function recessive INS gene mutations may also cause neonatal diabetes via reduced insulin biosynthesis. Homozygous point mutations in the coding sequence of the gene, leading to substitution of the first methionine with isoleucine, or introduction of a premature stop codon in the signal peptide or in the C-peptide have been described [83–85]. In addition, a novel homozygous intronic mutation (c.187 + 241G>A) likely causing unstable insulin transcripts was discovered in a patient with undetectable levels of plasma insulin (but normal circulating amylin, which is co-secreted with C-peptide and usually absent in plasma of individuals with type 1 diabetes) and normal pancreas at ultrasound [86]. Homozygous or compound

Barbetti · Mammì · Liu · Grasso · Arvan · Remedi · Nichols

heterozygous partial deletions of the INS gene have also been reported [83, 87]. In addition, homozygous mutations located in the regulatory regions have been described leading to PNDM, but mainly to the transient form of the disease [83]. As expected, recessive mutations of the *INS* gene are more common in countries with high rates of consanguineous marriage [88].

Animal Models of Congenital Abnormalities of Expression of the Insulin Gene Product

Animal models have provided novel insights, but also introduce some complexities, in developing a mechanistic understanding of INS mutations in neonatal diabetes. Mice and rats in particular have two insulin genes including *Ins1* (mouse chromosome 19) and *Ins2* (mouse chromosome 7): Ins2 contains an exon that is lacking in Ins1, and the coding sequences of the two preproinsulins differ at certain positions in the signal peptide, C-peptide, and at residues 9 and 29 of the B-chain. As diploid species, all 4 rodent *Ins* alleles lead to a functional insulin gene product and normal expression of even one is sufficient to avoid immediate postnatal onset of DKA, both because of upregulated expression of the remaining allele in the absence of insulin synthesis from the other alleles and because of β-cell mass increases that occur much more readily in rodents [89]. Nevertheless, less-than-normal expression level of wild-type proinsulin protein is a definite susceptibility factor for onset of neonatal diabetes. For example, low (5%) expression of a tagged transgenic version of *Akita* proinsulin-C(A7)Y in wild-type mice produces little more than impaired glucose tolerance, whereas the same transgene expressed in *Ins2* knockout mice produces severe neonatal diabetes [90]. Authentic *Akita* mice are heterozygous for the proinsulin-C(A7)Y mutant expressed from the *Ins2* locus (a similar human mutation has also been reported), and these mice synthesize approximately one-third of all proinsulin as the misfolded mutant species (presumably one-half is synthesized in heterozygous humans) with all male *Akita* mice developing severe diabetes after weaning [91]. Moreover, a pig model in which the *Akita* proinsulin-C(A7)Y transgene is expressed at a high level (~80% of that of wild-type insulin mRNA) exhibits diabetes within the first week of life [92]. Similar to the *Akita* mouse, expression of the mutant proinsulin-C(A6)S in the *Munich* mouse also provokes neonatal diabetes [93]. All of these models lead to insulin deficiency with diminution of the storage pool of intraislet insulin leading to diabetes that can include insufficient circulating insulin as well as possible secondary de-repression of α-cell activity with increased circulating glucagon. However, a critical distinction that has emerged is that decreased production of proinsulin in the ER such as in *Ins* gene knockouts actually diminishes ER stress that is nontoxic to β-cells [94], whereas increased expression of misfolded proinsulin promotes its aggregation, with blockade of otherwise normal proinsulin bystander molecules, and increased ER stress that may be proteotoxic [95]. Ultimately, the resulting diabetes itself, via glucolipotoxicity, contributes to β-cell deterioration and β-cell death that yields an animal physiology similar to that seen in other forms of diabetes.

A major potential advantage of such animal models is as a first line for the study of potential therapies to ameliorate the disease. One approach involves increasing circulating leptin levels to suppress islet α-cell activity with improved glycemic control [96, 97]. A second idea is to alter ER molecular chaperones that promote the degradation of the misfolded proinsulin so as to rescue the wild-type bystander proinsulin molecules [97]. We expect that animal models will continue to be of value in proof-of-concept experiments that are critically needed to develop new therapies for INS/PNDM, and which may also eventually have broader applicability to other forms of diabetes.

PNDM and Defects of Other Genes Involved in Glucose Metabolism-Insulin Secretion Coupling in the Pancreatic β-Cell
Biallelic mutations of the GCK were the first example of PNDM in isolation (i.e., non-syndromic); the mechanism of the disease strongly supported the tenet of glucokinase as a glucose sensor of pancreatic β-cells [6]. A few patients with this genetic defect have been described in detail after the first report [24, 98–102]; remarkably, they all show severely reduced birth weight (1,500–1,700 g) and early detection of hyperglycemia, usually within the first week after birth [6, 98–100]. Though these patients may, in theory, respond to SU treatment, trials performed so far have been unsuccessful [99, 101]. More recently, mutations of the *SLC2A2* gene that are known to cause Fanconi-Bickel syndrome have been associated with 5 NDM cases, 4 of which showed transient hyperglycemia [103]. Interestingly, 4 out of those patients later developed features of the syndrome. This work supported the notion that GLUT2, the glucose transporter encoded by *SLC2A2* gene, likely teams up with glucokinase in the glucose-sensing machinery of the pancreatic β-cell.

PNDM Associated with Genetic Defects of Transcription Factors
After the pioneering work by Stoffers et al. [3], who identified a patient with biallelic mutations of PDX1 causing pancreatic agenesis, genetic defects in a host of transcription factors have been mainly associated with severe syndromic neonatal diabetes (Table 1). However, exceptions have been described: patients bearing "hypomorphic" mutations of *PDX1*, *GATA4*, *GATA6*, and *PTF1A* can present with isolated PNDM with or without pancreatic exocrine insufficiency, and even childhood-onset or adult-onset diabetes [104–108]. Most of these forms of PNDM are exceedingly rare, though GATA6 gene defects account for a sizeable number of cases [24]. For those interested in a detailed description of phenotypic features of each subtype, we refer to the original papers (Table 1).

Syndromic Form of Neonatal Diabetes Caused by PERK Deficiency (Wolcott-Rallison Syndrome)
After early reports of the association of biallelic mutations of *EIF2AK3* gene (encoding PERK) with Wolcott-Rallison syndrome [5, 109], several other reports have been published that suggest this condition is prevalent in consanguineous families [110,

                                Barbetti · Mammì · Liu · Grasso · Arvan · Remedi · Nichols

Table 1. Mechanisms of disease of PNDM/TNDM genes, excluding defects of chromosome 6

	Developmentally reduced number/absent β-cells	Reduced/absent β-cells due to autoimmune process	Apoptosis-related reduction of β-cells	Disruption of glucose-stimulated insulin secretion signaling	Reduced/absent insulin synthesis	Impaired insulin gene expression
Gene(s)						
Dominant	GATA6 [120], GATA4 [121]	STAT3 [128]	INS [13, 14]	KCNJ11 [15]; ABCC8 [16]		
Recessive	PTF1A [122], PDX1 [3], GLIS3 [123], NEUROG3 [124], NKX2.2 [125], MNX1 [125], RFX6[126], NEUROD1 [127]		EIF2AK3 [5]	GCK [17], SLC2A2 [18], EIF2AK3 [19]	INS [20]	PDX1, hypomorphic (?) NEUROD1 (?)
X-linked		FOXP3 [7, 8]				

111] and is a common cause of neonatal diabetes in the Middle-East, together with GCK [88, 111, 112]. One of the roles of PERK is to transiently repress protein synthesis via phosphorylation of eukaryotic initiation factor 2. Furthermore, the mechanism(s) of hyperglycemia of Wolcott-Rallison syndrome, which is characterized by the triad of PNDM, liver disease, and short stature, was initially linked to apoptosis of β-cells consequent to sustained ER stress and upregulation of CHOP [109, 110, 113]. More recently, however, it has been found that in tissue-specific PERK knockout mice, β-cell mass is reduced as a consequence of deficient β-cell proliferation, rather than increased apoptosis [114]. Moreover, acute pharmacological inhibition of PERK causes the blockade of glucose-stimulated Ca^{2+} uptake and inhibition of insulin secretion [115]. Which of these two mechanisms is more relevant in determining diabetes in Wolcott-Rallison syndrome is presently unknown.

PNDM and defects of the immune system are treated in detail in the chapter by Bacchetta et al. [this vol., pp. 78–90], but also listed in Table 1.

Transient Neonatal Diabetes Mellitus

6q24-Related Transient Neonatal Diabetes Mellitus

Transient neonatal diabetes mellitus 1 (TNDM1) (OMIM 601410), the first described form of TNDM, is an imprinting disorder related to human chromosomal region 6q24 (6q24 TNDM) and accounts for approximately 60–70% of TNDM. Genomic imprinting is a form of transcriptional regulation that results in the monoallelic expression of genes from the paternal or maternal allele, mediated by epigenetic modifications that do not involve changes in DNA sequence. The imprinted genes are often clustered together and share common *cis*-acting regulatory elements called imprinting control regions (ICRs). These ICRs are CpG-rich DNA sequences, differentially methylated regions (DMRs) at cytosines, in the paternal or maternal chromosome. Methylated alleles are typically not transcribed. Most DMRs are also marked by histone modifications because there is a link between these two epigenetic systems. In these clusters the presence of long noncoding RNAs is often demonstrated, some of which regulate the imprinting of the nearby genes. The monoallelic DNA methylation at ICRs is acquired during male and female gametogenesis by erasure (reset) of the old marks and establishment of new marks. Most methylation occurs in the oocyte postnatally, during oocyte growth, prior to ovulation, and more rarely ICRs are methylated in the male germline prenatally. After fertilization, the DMRs are maintained despite the extensive demethylation that occurs in the preimplantation embryo, through fetal development and postnatal life. *cis*-acting sequences and *trans*-acting factors play a role in DMR protection, but underlying mechanisms are not fully understood.

The Chromosomal Region 6q24
The human imprinted 6q24 chromosomal region is a relatively small imprinted locus with 2 CTCF/cohesin regions separated by more than 70 kb that interact physically and restrict imprinting to only those genes contained within this chromatin loop [116]: PLAGL1 (OMIM 603044) (pleomorphic adenoma gene-like 1) also known as ZAC (zinc finger protein, which regulates apoptosis and cell cycle arrest), and HYMAI (OMIM 606546) (hydatidiform mole associated and imprinted transcript). The microimprinted domain is regulated by a DMR that is methylated in oocytes but not in sperm, located within the promoter (P1) of PLAGL1, in the first exon of the gene. The promoter P1 is also shared with the HYMAI gene. Imprinting monoallelic expression of PLAGL1 and HYMAI has been observed in human placenta and in most fetal tissues, but in adults has only been reported in skin fibroblasts. PLAGL1 has a second nonimprinted promoter (P2), 55 kb upstream from the P1, which promotes biallelic expression in some tissues as peripheral blood leucocytes. PLAGL1 is a zinc finger transcription factor that regulates apoptosis and cell cycle. Downstream targets of the gene are not fully characterized, but PLAGL1 plays an important role in a co-regulated imprinted gene network involved in fetal growth. Maternal intakes of alcohol and vitamin B$_2$ have also been positively correlated with PLAGL1 DMR methylation, highlighting the role of the maternal environment in regulation of DNA methylation at the 6q24 region. Loss of PLAGL1 expression is frequently observed in many human tumors, consistent with its role as a tumor-suppressor gene. HYMAI is a noncoding gene, transcribed but not translated (long noncoding RNA), and is located in the first intron of human PLAGL1. Its functions are unknown, but unlike other known imprinted long ncRNAs with a repressive role, HYMAI may act to keep the unmethylated paternal PLAGL1 allele in a transcriptionally permissive state.

Etiology of TNDM1
TNDM1 is not associated with mutations in PLAGL1 or HYMAI genes, but rather with their overexpression via 3 genetic mechanisms that result in the doubling of the normal gene dosage [117, 118]:

		Barbetti·Mammì·Liu·Grasso·Arvan·Remedi·Nichols

Partial or Complete Paternal Uniparental Disomy of Chromosome 6 (UPD6pat) (41% of Cases). Uniparental disomy (UPD) is defined as the presence in a diploid genome of both homologous chromosomes of a pair from one parent (maternal or paternal UDP) and no copy from the second parent. UPD is also classified as heterodisomic when the two chromosomes are both chromosomes of a single parent or as isodisomic when the two chromosomes are two identical homologs of a single parent. In the partial UDP, only a region of the chromosome is inherited uniparentally. Fetal trisomy rescue with loss of the extra chromosome or fetal monosomy rescue with the duplication of the single chromosome has been proposed as a potentially more frequent pathogenic mechanism leading to complete UPD. UPD can also occur by other rare mechanisms, including gamete complementation in which a gamete, by chance, is disomic for the same nullisomic chromosome of the second gamete. Mitotic recombination can also be causative of partial UDP. In TNDM1 patients with paternal UDP6, two chromosomal regions 6q24 are inherited from the father and none from the mother, and this is in general a de novo event. Complete iUDP6pat is more frequent (>90%), but hUDP6pat and partial UDP6pat have been reported.

Paternal Duplication of 6q24 (29–33%). In these subtypes of TNDM1, there is an unbalanced paternal microduplication of the chromosomal region 6q24 that may be inherited (with a pathogenic result only if inherited from the father) or de novo. Occasionally it arises as part of a more complex chromosomal rearrangement in a parent, which in such cases may be visible via cytogenetics analysis.

Hypomethylation of the Maternal 6q24 Region (26–30%). In TNDM1 patients with hypomethylation of the maternal 6q24 region, the methylated maternal allele loses its methylation, resulting in biallelic expression of PLAGL1 and HYMAI genes (relaxing of imprinting). This group is clinically heterogeneous and can be subdivided into two subgroups based on the epimutation type: isolated maternal hypomethylation (40%), with maternal hypomethylation only at locus 6q24, and hypomethylation at multiple imprinted loci (HIL) (60%), with a mosaic pattern of hypomethylation affecting other maternally methylated loci, caused in about 50% of the cases by recessive mutations in ZFP57 gene (ZFP57-HIL) (OMIM 612192)

Pathogenesis of TNDM1

In line with mouse models, human overexpression of PLAGL1 might cause TNDM1 by reducing the absolute number of islet β-cells during fetal development, followed by a postnatal increase prior to diabetes remission. This increase might become insufficient during metabolic stress, such as intercurrent illness or pregnancy, and physiologic decrease of insulin sensitivity, as occurs in adolescence. It is has also been proposed that 6q24 region overexpression causes a specific defect of insulin secretion through downregulation of PACAP receptor 1 or RASGRF1 genes.

Clinical Findings in TNDM1

In the natural history of the disease, three distinct phases are normally apparent: phase1 (neonatal diabetes), phase 2 (apparent remission), and phase 3 (relapse of diabetes). There are no obvious differences in the severity, duration, or relapse rate of diabetes between the three TNDM1 groups [118], although nondiabetes manifestations, such as congenital malformations and others functional defects, may vary between the three causative genetic mechanisms.

Phase 1 (neonatal diabetes). Three cardinal features are observed in TNDM1 neonates: (1) low birth weight with severe intrauterine growth retardation by the third trimester of pregnancy; (2) hyperglycemia usually during the first week of life and lasting on average 3 months, but in some cases as long as 18 months; and (3) dehydration with absence of ketoacidosis. Intrauterine growth retardation and low birth weight are caused by low levels of insulin, a prenatal growth factor, in utero. In a series of 163 confirmed cases of TNDM1 [118], the mean birth weight was 2,001 g and the 30.1% of the patients were born at <37 weeks of gestation. Hyperglycemia was detected at a median age of 4 days and the median for remission was 3 months. The age of presentation with diabetes was positively correlated with gestational age and there was earlier remission in patients with higher birth weight. Compared to TNDM associated with *ABCC8* or *KCNJ11* mutations (also referred as to TNDM2 and TNDM3) (see below), TNDM1 patients have lower birth weight, earlier diagnosis and remission, and lower frequency of diabetic ketoacidosis at onset. Macroglossia and umbilical hernia, also present in Beckwith-Wiedemann syndrome, another human imprinting disorder, are the most frequently observed congenital abnormalities (44 and 21%, respectively). Less frequently reported congenital abnormalities include dysmorphic facial appearance (18%), renal tract abnormalities (9%), cardiac anomalies (9%), short finger abnormalities (8%), and hypothyroidism (4%). In TNDM1 patients with 6q24 microduplication, congenital abnormalities occurred significantly less frequently, while in TNDM1 patients with isolated maternal hypomethylation at 6q24, the macroglossia was the only reported anomaly. Conversely, TNDM1 patients with hypomethylation at imprinted loci (HIL) typically have a more complex but highly variable phenotype. In these patients, macroglossia, umbilical hernia, congenital heart disease, ear lobe abnormalities, hemihypertrophy of extremities, pectus carinatum, brain malformations, and developmental delay have all been described. These findings may be explained by additional imprinted loci other than 6q24 involved in HIL.

Phase 2 (apparent remission). On resolution of neonatal diabetes there is often significant catch-up growth and some infants become overweight in the first year. During this period some TNDM1 infants might develop hyperinsulinemic hypoglycemia of varying severity and intermittent episodes of hyperglycemia may occur in childhood, particularly during intercurrent illnesses.

Phase 3 (relapse of diabetes). About 50–60% of TNDM1 patients in remission may subsequently develop diabetes in late childhood, adolescence, or early adulthood, and TNDM1 women are at risk for relapse or development of gestational diabetes during pregnancy. The earliest age of relapse reported is 4 years and the average age of relapse is 14 years. Relapse clinically resembles early-onset type 2 diabetes and is characterized by a loss of the first-phase insulin secretion. There is usually response to oral SUs and, if at all needed, required insulin doses are lower than in patients with typical type 1 diabetes.

Penetrance

Reduced penetrance of TNDM1 has been reported and the clinical presentation of an imprinted 6q24 aberration may not invariably include a neonatal presentation. Gestational diabetes or adult type 2 diabetes, without any history of NDM, has been described in individuals with 6q24 paternal duplication, suggesting that other genetic or epigenetic factors may influence the clinical expression alterations of chromosome 6q24. In addition, TNDM1 ZFP57-HIL shows inter- and intrafamilial clinical variability with features ranging from severe neurological disability and early infant death to a normal phenotype [119].

Treatment of TNDM1

Rehydration and intravenous insulin are usually required at the onset of diabetes. Subcutaneous injection of insulin is introduced as soon as possible. Both continuous insulin pump therapy and treatment with subcutaneous insulin glargine have been reported. Despite the severity of the initial presentation, the majority of patients do not require any treatment by a median age of 12 weeks. In the relapse phase, successful targeting of the GLP1 pathway with a dipeptidyl peptidase-4 (DPP4) GLP1 inhibitor has been described.

Genetic Counseling

The genetic risk for developing TNDM1 in relatives of a proband differs depending on the underlying molecular mechanism. Generally, this risk is low in TNDM1-UPD6, higher in TNDM1 with paternal duplication, and low or unpredictable in TNDM1 with isolated maternal hypomethylation. For those interested in this very specialized area, we suggest reading Temple et al. [117].

K_{ATP} Channel and TNDM

Mutations in KCNJ11 (Kir6.2) (TNDM3, OMIM 610582) and ABCC8 (SUR1) (TNDM2, OMIM 610374) have now clearly been associated with TNDM. Of note, mutations in Kir6.2 have been found mostly in association with very early forms of diabetes, usually before 6 months of age, whereas the phenotypic variability of SUR1 mutations is broader [49, 50]. Indeed, mutations in SUR1 can be linked to ketoacidosis in a newborn, as well as to bona fide type 2 diabetes in a young adult [49].

The reason for postnatal resolution in these patients remains unknown. TNDM patients with KCNJ11 mutations differ from subjects with 6q24 imprinting defects, as previously described: the birth weight is typically higher, the mean age of diagnosis is later (mean: 5.2 vs. 1.0 weeks), and the time to remission is longer (mean: 76 vs. 16 weeks). This suggests that Kir6.2-TNDM subjects have a less severe β-cell defect in utero and early life, but compensatory mechanisms take longer to achieve euglycemia than in 6q24-TNDM. This would fit with the idea of a relatively constant but mild β-cell defect associated with K_{ATP} mutations. Importantly, several mutations (e.g., G53S, G53R, or I182V) have been associated with both TNDM and PNDM. Although the apparently different clinical presentations could represent undiagnosed remission in the latter, it is likely that there is modification of the phenotype by other genetic or environmental factors. Patients with the common PNDM KCNJ11/R201H mutation have varying levels of C-peptide, ranging from undetectable to the normal range [54]. Variability in response is also evident with the KCNJ11/V59M mutation [15]: while the majority of patients show a severe DEND phenotype, others exhibit none of the syndromic features. In one striking example [57], three family members with KCNJ11/R201H demonstrated remarkably different responses to SUs: in one child and in the mother, first treated at 6 years of age and as an adult, respectively, adequate glucose control required an extremely high dose and still occasional insulin, but in a second affected child, treated with glibenclamide from birth, the SU dose was extremely low and no insulin was required to maintain normoglycemia, such that the patient was essentially in remittance.

TNDM and Mutations in Regulatory Regions of the INS Gene
Homozygous as well as compound heterozygous mutations in regulatory regions of the INS gene (c.-332C>G, c.-331C>G, c.-331C>A, c.-218A>C) have been found in very few patients (about 2%) with TNDM [83]; these individuals enter remission at a median age of 12 weeks. Mutations are located in cyclic-AMP response elements, which are highly conserved through species. Functional studies in the MIN-6 cell line showed that INS gene promoter constructs bearing these mutations have severely reduced transcriptional activity [83]. The reason(s) why these defects may lead to transient neonatal diabetes (and the permanent subtype) is currently unknown.

Conclusions

NDM represents a tiny fraction of diabetes, probably accounting for less than 1% of cases referred to the pediatric diabetes clinic [82]. Nevertheless, the identification of NDM genes has shed light on various biological aspects of the pancreatic β-cell, and has led to the "therapeutic miracle" of weaning from insulin most of patients carrying mutations in the K_{ATP} genes, adding new meaning to precision medicine. New insights into the mechanism(s) of pancreatic β-cell failure (e.g., ER stress-induced apoptosis, decreased β-cell mass) provided by the studies presented in this chapter may pave the way for new drugs and new forms of therapy that specifically tackle these genetic defects.

References

1 Engleson G, Zetterqvist P: Congenital diabetes mellitus and neonatal pseudodiabetes mellitus. Arch Dis Child 1957;32:193–196.

2 Temple IK, James RS, Crolal JA, Sitch FL, Jacobs PA, Howel WM, Betts P, Baum JD, Shield JP: An imprinted gene(s) for diabetes? Nat Genet 1995;9:110–112.

3 Stoffers DA, Zinkin NT, Stanojevic V, Clarke WL, Habener JF: Pancreatic agenesis attributable to a single nucleotide deletion in the human IPF1 gene coding sequence. Nat Genet 1997;15:106–110.

4 Von Muhlendahl KE, Herkenhoff H: Long-term course of neonatal diabetes. N Engl J Med 1995;333:704–708.

5 Delepine M, Nicolino M, Barrett T, Golamaully M, Lathrop GM, Julier C: EIF2AK3, encoding translation initiation factor 2-alpha kinase 3, is mutated in patients with Wolcott-Rallison syndrome. Nat Genet 2000;25:406–409.

6 Njolstad PR, Sovik O, Cuesta-Munoz A, Bjorkhaug L, Massa O, Barbetti F, Undlien D, Shiota C, Magnuson MA, Molven A, Matschinsky FM, Bell GI: Neonatal diabetes mellitus due to complete glucokinase deficiency. N Engl J Med 2001;344:1588–1592.

7 Wildin RS, Ramsdell F, Peake J, Faravelli F, Casanova J-L, Buist N, Levy-Lahada E, Mazzella M, Goulet O, Perroni L, Dagna Bricarelli F, Byrne G, McEuen M, Proll S, Appleby M, Brunkow ME: X-linked neonatal diabetes mellitus, enteropathy and endocrinopathy syndrome is the human equivalent of mouse scurfy. Nat Genet 2001;27:18–20.

8 Bennet CL, Christie J, Ramsdell F, Brunkow ME, Ferguson PJ, Whitesekk L, Kelly TE, Saulbury FT, Chance PF, Ochs HD: The immune dysregulation, polyendocrinopathy, enteropathy, X-linked syndrome (IPEX) is caused by mutations of *FOXP3*. Nat Genet 2001;27:20–21.

9 Koster JC, Marshall BA, Ensor N, Corbett JA, Nichols CG: Targeted overactivity of beta cell K(ATP) channels induces profound neonatal diabetes. Cell 2000;100:645–654.

10 Iafusco D, Stazi MA, Cotichini R, Cotellessa M, Martinucci ME, Mazzella M, Cherubini V, Barbetti F, Martinetti M, Cerutti F, Prisco F; Early Onset Diabetes Study Group of the Italian Society of Paediatric Endocrinology and Diabetology: Permanent diabetes mellitus in the first year of life. Diabetologia 2002;45:798–804.

11 Gloyn AL, Pearson ER, Antcliff JF, Proks P, Bruining GJ, Slingerland AS, Howard N, Srinivasan S, Silva JMCL, Molnes J, Edghill EL, Frayling TM, Temple IK, Mackay D, Shiled JPH, Sumnik Z, van Rhijn A, Wales JKH, Clark P, Gorman S, Aisenberg J, Ellard S, Njolstad PR, Ashcroft FM, Hattersley AT: Activating mutations in the ATP-sensitive potassium channel subunit Kir6.2 gene are associated with permanent neonatal diabetes. N Engl J Med 2004;350:1838–1849.

12 Babenko AP, Polak M, Cave H, Busiah K, Czernichow P, Scharfmann R, Bryan J, Aguilar-Bryan L, Vaxillaire M, Froguel P: Activating mutations in the ABCC8 gene in neonatal diabetes mellitus. N Engl J Med 2006;355:456–466.

13 Støy J, Edghill EL, Flanagan SE, Ye H, Paz VP, Pluzhnikov A, Below JE, Hayes MG, Cox NJ, Lipkind GM, Lipton RB, Greeley SA, Patch AM, Ellard S, Steiner DF, Hattersley AT, Philipson LH, Bell GI; Neonatal Diabetes International Collaborative Group: Insulin gene mutations as a cause of permanent neonatal diabetes. Insulin gene mutations as a cause of permanent neonatal diabetes. Proc Natl Acad Sci USA 2007;104:15040–15044.

14 Colombo C, Porzio O, Liu M, Massa O, Vasta M, Salardi S, Beccaria L, Monciotti C, Toni S, Pedersen O, Hansen T, Federici L, Pesavento R, Cadario F, Federici G, Ghirri P, Arvan P, Iafusco D, Barbetti F; Early Onset Diabetes Study Group of the Italian Society of Pediatric Endocrinology and Diabetes (SIEDP): Seven mutations in the human insulin gene linked to permanent neonatal/infancy-onset diabetes mellitus. J Clin Invest 2008;118:2148–2156.

15 Massa O, Iafusco D, D'Amato E, Gloyn AL, Hattersley AT, Pasquino B, Tonini G, Dammacco F, Zanette G, Meschi F, Porzio O, Bottazzo GF, Crinò A, Lorini R, Cerutti F, Vanelli M, Barbetti F; Early Onset Diabetes Study Group of the Italian Society of Pediatric Endocrinology and Diabetology: KCNJ11 activating mutations in Italian patients with permanent neonatal diabetes. Hum Mutat 2005;25:22–27.

16 Russo L, Iafusco D, Brescianini S, Nocerino V, Bizzarri C, Toni S, Cerutti F, Monciotti C, Pesavento R, Iughetti L, Bernardini L, Bonfanti R, Gargantini L, Vanelli M, Aguilar-Bryan L, Stazi A, Grasso V, Colombo C, Barbetti F; ISPED Early Diabetes Study Group: Permanent diabetes during the first year of life: multiple gene screening in 54 patients. Diabetologia 2011;54:1693–1701.

17 Edghill EL, Dix RJ, Flanagan SE, Bingley PJ, Hattersley AT, Ellard S, Gillespie KM: HLA genotyping supports a nonautoimmune etiology in patients diagnosed with diabetes under the age of six months. Diabetes 2006;55:1895–1898.

18 Stanik J, Gasperikova D, Paskova M, Barak L, Javorkova J, Jamncova E, Ciljakova M, Hlava P, Michalek J, Flanagan SE, Pearson E, Hattersley AT, Ellard S, Klimes I: Prevalence of permanent neonatal diabetes in Slovakia and successful replacement of insulin with sulfonylurea therapy in KCNJ11 and ABCC8 mutation carriers. J Clin Enodcrinol Metab 2007;92:1276–1282.

19 Iafusco D, Massa O, Pasquino B, Colombo C, Iughetti L, Bizzarri C, Mammì C, Lo Presti D, Suprani T, Schiaffini R, Nichols CG, Russo L, Grasso V, Meschi F, Bonfanti R, Brescianini S, Barbetti F; Early Diabetes Study Group of ISPED: Minimal incidence of neonatal/infancy onset diabetes in Italy is 1:90,000 live births. Acta Diabetol 2012;49:405–408.

20 Shield JPH, Gardner RJ, Wadsworth EJK, Whiteford ML, James RS, Robinson DO, Baum JD, Temple IK: Aetiopathology and genetic basis of neonatal diabetes. Arch Dis Child 1997;76:F39–F42.

21 Demirbilek H, Arya VB, Ozbek MN, Hoghton JAL, Baran RT, Akar M, Tekes S, Tuzun H, Mackay DJ, Flanagan SE, Hattersley AY, Ellard S, Hussein S: Clinical characteristics and molecular genetic analysis of 22 patients with neonatal diabetes from the South-Eastern region of Turkey: predominance of non-K_{ATP} channel mutations. Eur J Endocrinol 2015;172:697–705.

22 Habeb AM, Al-Magamsi MSF, Eid IM, Ali MI, Hattersley AT, Hussain K, Ellard S: Incidence, genetics, and clinical phenotype of permanent neonatal diabetes mellitus in northwest Saudi Arabia. Pediatr Diabetes 2012;13:499–505.

23 Flanagan SE, De Franco E, Lango Allen H, Zerah M, Abdul-Rasoul MM, Edge JA, Stewart H, Alamiri E, Hussain K, Wallis S, de Vries L, Rubio-Cabezas O, Houghton JAL, Edghill EL, Patch A-M, Ellard S, Hattersley AT: Analysis of transcription factors key for mouse pancreatic development establishes NKX2–2 and MNX1 mutations as causes of neonatal diabetes in man. Cell Metab 2014;19:146–154.

24 De Franco E, Flanagan SE, Houghton JA, Lango Allen H, Mackay DJ, Temple IK, Ellard S, Hattersley AT: The effect of early, comprehensive genomic testing on clinical care of neonatal diabetes: an international cohort study. Lancet 2015;386:957–963.

25 Vaxillaire M, Froguel P: Monogenic diabetes: implementation of translational genomic research towards precision medicine. J Diabetes 2016;8:782–795.

26 Kurata HT, Marton LJ, Nichols CG: The polyamine binding site in inward rectifier K^+ channels. J Gen Physiol 2006;127:467–480.

27 Aizawa T, Komatsu M, Asanuma M, Sato Y, Sharp GW: Glucose action "beyond ionic events" in the pancreatic beta cell. Trends Pharmacol Sci 1998;19:496–499.

28 Henquin JC: Triggering and amplifying pathways of regulation of insulin secretion by glucose. Diabetes 2000;49:1751–1760.

29 Trube G, Rorsman P, Ohno-Shosaku T: Opposite effects of tolbutamide and diazoxide on the ATP-dependent K+ channel in mouse pancreatic beta-cells. Pflugers Arch 1986;407:493–499.

30 Simonson DC, Ferrannini E, Bevilacqua S, Smith D, Barrett E, Carlson R, DeFronzo RA: Mechanism of improvement in glucose metabolism after chronic glyburide therapy. Diabetes 1984;33:838–845.

31 Hattersley AT, Ashcroft FM: Activating mutations in Kir6.2 and neonatal diabetes: new clinical syndromes, new scientific insights, and new therapy. Diabetes 2005;54:2503–2513.

32 Flanagan SE, Clauin S, Bellanné-Chantelot C, de Lonlay P, Harries LW, Gloyn AL, Ellard S: Update of mutations in the genes encoding the pancreatic beta-cell K(ATP) channel subunits Kir6.2 (KCNJ11) and sulfonylurea receptor 1 (ABCC8) in diabetes mellitus and hyperinsulinism. Hum Mutat 2009;30:170–180.

33 Vaxillaire M, Populaire C, Busiah K, Cavé H, Gloyn AL, Hattersley AT, Czernichow P, Froguel P, Polak M: Kir6.2 mutations are a common cause of permanent neonatal diabetes in a large cohort of French patients. Diabetes 2004;53:2719–2722.

34 Ashcroft SJ, Ashcroft FM: Properties and functions of ATP-sensitive K-channels. Cell Signal 1990;2:197–214.

35 Nichols CG: KATP channels as molecular sensors of cellular metabolism. Nature 2006;440:470–476.

36 Nichols CG, Shyng SL, Nestorowicz A, Glaser B, Clement JP 4th, Gonzalez G, Aguilar-Bryan L, Permutt MA, Bryan J: Adenosine diphosphate as an intracellular regulator of insulin secretion. Science 1996;272:1785–1787.

37 Enkvetchakul D, Nichols CG: Gating mechanism of KATP channels: function fits form. J Gen Physiol 2003;122:471–480.

38 Aguilar-Bryan L, et al: Cloning of the beta cell high-affinity sulfonylurea receptor: a regulator of insulin secretion. Science 1995;268:423–426.

39 Gribble FM, Tucker SJ, Ashcroft FM: The essential role of the Walker A motifs of SUR1 in K-ATP channel activation by Mg-ADP and diazoxide. EMBO J 1997;16:1145–1152.

40 Remedi MS, Koster JC: K(ATP) channelopathies in the pancreas. Pflugers Arch 2010;460:307–320.

41 Haider S, Antcliff JF, Proks P, Sansom MS, Ashcroft FM: Focus on Kir6.2: a key component of the ATP-sensitive potassium channel. J Mol Cell Cardiol 2005;38:927–936.

42 Florez JC: Newly identified loci highlight beta cell dysfunction as a key cause of type 2 diabetes: where are the insulin resistance genes? Diabetologia 2008;51:1100–1110.

43 Schwanstecher C, Meyer U, Schwanstecher M: K(IR)6.2 polymorphism predisposes to type 2 diabetes by inducing overactivity of pancreatic beta-cell ATP-sensitive K(+) channels. Diabetes 2002;51:875–879.

44 Pearson ER, Flechtner I, Njølstad PR, Malecki MT, Flanagan SE, Larkin B, Ashcroft FM, Klimes I, Codner E, Iotova V, Slingerland AS, Shield J, Robert JJ, Holst JJ, Clark PM, Ellard S, Søvik O, Polak M, Hattersley AT; Neonatal Diabetes International Collaborative Group: Switching from insulin to oral sulfonylureas in patients with diabetes due to Kir6.2 mutations. N Engl J Med 2006;355:467–477.

45 Tonini G, Bizzarri C, Bonfanti R, Vanelli M, Cerutti F, Faleschini E, Meschi F, Prisco F, Ciacco E, Cappa M, Torelli C, Cauvin V, Tumini S, Iafusco D, Barbetti F; Early Onset Diabetes Study Group of the Italian Society of Paediatric Endocrinology and Diabetology: Sulfonylurea treatment outweighs insulin therapy in short-term metabolic control of patients with permanent neonatal diabetes mellitus due to activating mutations of the *KCNJ11* gene. Diabetologia 2006;49:2210–2213.

46 Gloyn AL, Siddiqui J, Ellard S: Mutations in the genes encoding the pancreatic beta-cell KATP channel subunits Kir6.2 (KCNJ11) and SUR1 (ABCC8) in diabetes mellitus and hyperinsulinism. Hum Mutat 2006;27:220–231.

47 Sperling MA: ATP-sensitive potassium channels – neonatal diabetes mellitus and beyond. New Engl J Med 2006;355:456–466.

48 Masia R, De Leon DD, MacMullen C, McKnight H, Stanley CA, Nichols CG: A mutation in the TMD0-L0 region of sulfonylurea receptor-1 (L225P) causes permanent neonatal diabetes mellitus (PNDM). Diabetes 2007;56:1357–1362.

49 Patch AM, Flanagan SE, Boustred C, Hattersley AT, Ellard S: Mutations in the ABCC8 gene encoding the SUR1 subunit of the KATP channel cause transient neonatal diabetes, permanent neonatal diabetes or permanent diabetes diagnosed outside the neonatal period. Diabetes Obes Metab 2007;9(suppl 2):28–39.

50 Vaxillaire M, Dechaume A, Busiah K, Cavé H, Pereira S, Scharfmann R, de Nanclares GP, Castano L, Froguel P, Polak M; SUR1-Neonatal Diabetes Study Group: New ABCC8 mutations in relapsing neonatal diabetes and clinical features. Diabetes 2007;56:1737–1741.

51 Koster JC, Cadario F, Kurata HT, Peruzzi C, Colombo C, Nichols CG, Barbetti F: The G53D mutation in Kir6.2 (KCNJ11) is associated with neonatal diabetes and motor dysfunction in adulthood that is improved with sulfonylurea therapy. J Clin Endocrinol Metab 2008;93:1054–1061.

52 Ashcroft FM: New uses for old drugs: neonatal diabetes and sulphonylureas. Cell Metab 2010;11:179–181.

53 Sagen JV, Raeder H, Hathout E, Shehadeh N, Gudmundsson K, Baevre H, Abuelo D, Phornphutkul C, Molnes J, Bell GI, Gloyn AL, Hattersley AT, Molven A, Søvik O, Njølstad PR: Permanent neonatal diabetes due to mutations in KCNJ11 encoding Kir6.2: patient characteristics and initial response to sulfonylurea therapy. Diabetes 2004;53:2713–2718.

54 Zung A, Glaser B, Nimri R, Zadik Z: Glibenclamide treatment in permanent neonatal diabetes mellitus due to an activating mutation in Kir6.2. J Clin Endocrinol Metab 2004;89:5504–5507.

55 Hattersley AT, Pearson ER: Minireview: pharmacogenetics and beyond: the interaction of therapeutic response, beta-cell physiology, and genetics in diabetes. Endocrinology 2006;147:2657–2663.

56 Flechtner I, Vaxillaire M, Cavé H, Scharfmann R, Froguel P, Polak M: Diabetes in very young children and mutations in the insulin-secreting cell potassium channel genes: therapeutic consequences. Endocr Dev 2007;12:86–98.

57 Wambach JA, Marshall BA, Koster JC, White NH, Nichols CG: Successful sulfonylurea treatment of an insulin-naive neonate with diabetes mellitus due to a KCNJ11 mutation. Pediatr Diabetes 2010;11:286–288.

58 Iafusco D, Bizzarri C, Cadario F, Pesavento R, Tonini G, Tumini S, Cauvin V, Colombo C, Bonfanti R, Barbetti F: No beta cell desensitisation after a median of 68 months on glibenclamide therapy in patients with *KCNJ11*-associated permanent neonatal diabetes. Diabetologia 2011;54:2736–2738.

59 Shimomura K, Hörster F, de Wet H, Flanagan SE, Ellard S, Hattersley AT, Wolf NI, Ashcroft F, Ebinger F: A novel mutation causing DEND syndrome: a treatable channelopathy of pancreas and brain. Neurology 2007;69:1342–1349.

60 Slingerland AS, Nuboer R, Hadders-Algra M, Hattersley AT, Bruining GJ: Improved motor development and good long-term glycaemic control with sulfonylurea treatment in a patient with the syndrome of intermediate developmental delay, early-onset generalised epilepsy and neonatal diabetes associated with the V59M mutation in the KCNJ11 gene. Diabetologia 2006;49:2559–2563.

61 Mlynarski W, Tarasov AI, Gach A, Girard CA, Pietrzak I, Zubcevic L, Kusmierek J, Klupa T, Malecki MT, Ashcroft FM: Sulfonylurea improves CNS function in a case of intermediate DEND syndrome caused by a mutation in KCNJ11. Nat Clin Pract Neurol 2007;3:640–645.

62 Slingerland AS, Hurkx W, Noordam K, Flanagan SE, Jukema JW, Meiners LC, Bruining GJ, Hattersley AT, Hadders-Algra M: Sulphonylurea therapy improves cognition in a patient with the V59M KCNJ11 mutation. Diabet Med 2008;25:277–281.

63 Remedi MS, Kurata HT, Scott A, Wunderlich FT, Rother E, Kleinridders A, Tong A, Brüning JC, Koster JC, Nichols CG: Secondary consequences of beta cell inexcitability: identification and prevention in a murine model of K(ATP)-induced neonatal diabetes mellitus. Cell Metab 2009;9:140–151.

64 Girard CA, Wunderlich FT, Shimomura K, Collins S, Kaizik S, Proks P, Abdulkader F, Clark A, Ball V, Zubcevic L, Bentley L, Clark R, Church C, Hugill A, Galvanovskis J, Cox R, Rorsman P, Brüning JC, Ashcroft FM: Expression of an activating mutation in the gene encoding the KATP channel subunit Kir6.2 in mouse pancreatic beta cells recapitulates neonatal diabetes. J Clin Invest 2009;119:80–90.

65 Remedi MS, Agapova SE, Vyas AK, Hruz PW, Nichols CG: Acute sulfonylurea therapy at disease onset can cause permanent remission of KATP-induced diabetes. Diabetes 2011;60:2515–2522.

66 Gloyn AL, Reimann F, Girard C, Edghill EL, Proks P, Pearson ER, Temple IK, Mackay DJ, Shield JP, Freedenberg D, Noyes K, Ellard S, Ashcroft FM, Gribble FM, Hattersley AT: Relapsing diabetes can result from moderately activating mutations in KCNJ11. Hum Mol Genet 2005;14:925–934.

67 Wang Z, York NW, Nichols CG, Remedi MS: Pancreatic beta cell dedifferentiation in diabetes and re-differentiation following insulin therapy. Cell Metab 2014;19:872–882.

68 Bell GI, Pictet RL, Rutter WJ, Cordell B, Tischer E, Goodman HM: Sequence of the human insulin gene. Nature 1980;284:26–32.

69 Steiner DF, Tager HS, Chan SJ, Nanjo K, Sanke T, Rubenstein AH: Lessons learned from molecular biology of insulin-gene mutations. Diabetes Care 1990; 13:600–609.

70 Barbetti F, Raben N, Kadowaki T, Cama A, Accili D, Merenich JH, Gabbay KH, Taylor SI, Roth J: Two unrelated patients with familial hyperproinsulinemia due to a mutation substituting histidine for arginine at position 65 in the proinsulin molecule: identification of the mutation by direct sequencing of genomic DNA amplified by polymerase chain reaction. J Clin Endocrinol Metab 1990;71:164–169.

71 Warren-Perry MG, Manley SE, Ostrega D, Polonsky K, Musset S, Brown P, Turner RC: A novel point mutation in the insulin gene giving rise to hyperproinsulinemia. J Clin Endocrinol Metab 1997;82:1629–1631.

72 Liu M, Haataja L, Wright J, Wickramasinghe NP, Quing-Xin H, Phillps NF, Barbetti F, Weiss MA, Arvan P: Mutant INS-gene induced diabetes of youth: proinsulin cysteine residues impose dominant-negative inhibition on wild-type proinsulin transport. PLoS One 2010;5:e13333.

73 Liu M, Lara-Lemus R, Shan SO, Wright J, Hataaja L, Barbetti F, Guo H, Larkin D, Arvan P: Impaired cleavage of preproinsulin signal peptide linked to autosomal dominant diabetes. Diabetes 2012;61:828–837.

74 Liu M, Sun J, Cui J, Chen W, Guo H, Barbetti F, Arvan P: INS-gene mutations: from genetics and beta cell biology to clinical disease. Mol Aspect Med 2015; 42:3–18.

75 Garin I, Perez de Nanclares G, Gastaldo E, Harries LW, Rubio-Cabezas O, Castano L: Permanent neonatal diabetes caused by creation of an ectopic splice site within the INS gene. PLoS One 2012;7:e290205.

76 Edghill EL, Flanagan SE, Patch A-M, Bousterd C, Parrish A, Shields B, Shepherd MH, Hussain K, Kapoor RR, Malecki M, MacDonald MJ, Stoy J, Steiner DF, Philipson PH, Bell GI, Hattersely AT, Ellard S: Insulin mutations screening in 1,044 patients with diabetes. Diabetes 2008;57:1034–1042.

77 Stoy J, Steiner DF, Park S-Y, Honggang Y, Philipson LH, Bell GI: Clinical and molecular genetics of neonatal diabetes due to mutations in the insulin gene. Rev Endocr Metab Disord 2010;11:205–215.

78 Hussain S, Ali JM, Jalaludin MY, Harun F: Permanent neonatal diabetes due to a novel insulin signal peptide mutation. Pediatr Diabetes 2013;14:299–303.

79 Dimova R, Tankova T, Guergueltcheva V, Tournev I, Kostantinova M: A family with permanent neonatal diabetes due to a novel mutation in insulin gene. Diabetes Res Clin Pract 2015;108:e28–e30.

80 Ortolani F, Piccinno E, Grasso V, Papadia F, Panzeca R, Cortese C, Felappi B, Tummolo A, Vendemiale M, Barbetti F: Diabetes associated with dominant insulin gene mutations: outcome of 24-month, sensor-augmented insulin pump treatment. Acta Diabetol 2016;53:599–601.

81 Piccini B, Artuso R, Lenzi L, Guasti M, Braccesi G, Barni F, Casalini E, Giglio S, Toni S: Clinical and molecular characterization of a novel insulin mutation identified in patients with a MODY phenotype. Eur J Med Genet 2016;59:590–595.

82 Delvecchio M, Mozzillo E, Salzano G, Iafusco D, Frontino G, Patera PI, Rabbone I, Cherubini V, Grasso V, Tinto N, Giglio S, Contreas G, Di Paola R, Salina A, Cauvin V, Tumini S, d'Annunzio G, Iughetti L, Mantovani V, Maltoni G, Toni S, Marigliano M, Barbetti F; Diabetes Study Group of the Italian Society of Pediatric Endocrinology and Diabetes (ISPED): Monogenic diabetes accounts for 6.3% of cases referred to 15 Italian pediatric diabetes centers during 2007–2012. J Clin Endocrinol Metab; accepted for publication.

83 Garin I, Edghill EL, Akerman I, Rubio-Cabezas O, Rica I, Locke JM, Maestro MA, Alshaikh A, Bundak R, del Castillo G, Deeb A, Deiss D, Fernandez JM, Godbole K, Hussain K, O'Connell M, Klupa T, Kolouskova S, Mohsin F, Perlman K, Sumnik Z, Rial JM, Ugarte E, Vasanthi T; Neonatal Diabetes International Group, Johnstone K, Flanagan SE, Martínez R, Castaño C, Patch AM, Fernández-Rebollo E, Raile K, Morgan N, Harries LW, Castaño L, Ellard S, Ferrer J, Perez de Nanclares G, Hattersley AT: Recessive mutations in the insulin gene result in neonatal diabetes through reduced insulin biosynthesis. Proc Natl Acad Sci USA 2010;107:3105–3110.

84 Rachmiel M, Rubio-Cabezas O, Ellard S, Hattersley AT, Perlman K: Early-onset, severe insulin lipoatrophy in a patient with permanent neonatal diabetes mellitus secondary to a recessive mutation in the INS gene. Pediatr Diabetes 2012;13:e26–e29.

85 Di Benedetto M, Richard O, Pelissier P, Darteyre S, Cavé H, Stephan J-L: Permanent neonatal diabetes and recessive mutation of the INS gene: a familial history. Arch Pediatr 2013;20:199–202.

86 Carmody D, Park S-Y, Ye H, Perrone ME, Aranburu GA, Highland HM, Hanis CL, Philipson LH, Bell GI, Greeley SAW: Continued lessons from the INS gene: an intronic mutation causing diabetes through a novel mechanism. J Med Genet 2015;52:612–616.

87 Raile K, O'Connel M, Galler A, Werther G, Kuhnen P, Krude H, Blankstein O: Diabetes caused by insulin gene (INS) deletion: clinical characteristics of homozygous and heterozygous individuals. Eur J Endocrinol 2011;165:255–260.

88 Deeb A, Habeb A, Kaplan W, Attia S, Hadi S, Osman A, Al-Jubeh J, Flanagan S, DeFranco E, Ellard S: Genetic characteristics, clinical spectrum, and incidence of neonatal diabetes in the emirate of Abu Dhabi, United Arab Emirates. Am J Med Genet A 2016;170:602–609.

89 Leroux L, Desbois P, Lamotte L, Duvillié B, Cordonnier N, Jackerott M, Jami J, Bucchini D, Joshi RL: Compensatory responses in mice carrying a null mutation for Ins1 or Ins2. Diabetes 2001;50(suppl 1):S150–S153.

90 Hodish I, Absood A, Liu L, Liu M, Haataja L, Larkin D, Al-Khafaji A, Zaki A, Arvan P: In vivo misfolding of proinsulin below the threshold of frank diabetes. Diabetes 2011;60:2092–2101.

91 Liu M, Haataja L, Wright J, Wickramasinghe NP, Hua QX, Phillips NF, Barbetti F, Weiss MA, Arvan P: Mutant INS-gene induced diabetes of youth: proinsulin cysteine residues impose dominant-negative inhibition on wild-type proinsulin transport. PLoS One 2010;5:e13333.

92 Renner S, Braun-Reichhart C, Blutke A, Herbach N, Emrich D, Streckel E, Wünsch A, Kessler B, Kurome M, Bähr A, Klymiuk N, Krebs S, Puk O, Nagashima H, Graw J, Blum H, Wanke R, Wolf E: Permanent neonatal diabetes in INS(C94Y) transgenic pigs. Diabetes 2013;62:1505–1511.

93 Herbach N, Rathkolb B, Kemter E, Pichl L, Klaften M, de Angelis MH, Halban PA, Wolf E, Aigner B, Wanke R: Dominant-negative effects of a novel mutated Ins2 allele causes early-onset diabetes and severe beta-cell loss in Munich Ins2C95S mutant mice. Diabetes 2007;56:1268–1276.

94 Szabat M, Page MM, Panzhinskiy E, Skovsø S, Mojibian M, Fernandez-Tajes J, Bruin JE, Bround MJ, Lee JT, Xu EE, Taghizadeh F, O'Dwyer S, van de Bunt M, Moon KM, Sinha S, Han J, Fan Y, Lynn FC, Trucco M, Borchers CH, Foster LJ, Nislow C, Kieffer TJ, Johnson JD: Reduced insulin production relieves endoplasmic reticulum stress and induces β cell proliferation. Cell Metab 2016;23:179–193.

95 Liu M, Hodish I, Rhodes CJ, Arvan P: Proinsulin maturation, misfolding, and proteotoxicity. Proc Natl Acad Sci USA 2007;104:15841–15846.

96 Naito M, Fujikura J, Ebihara K, Miyanaga F, Yokoi H, Kusakabe T, Yamamoto Y, Son C, Mukoyama M, Hosoda K, Nakao K: Therapeutic impact of leptin on diabetes, diabetic complications, and longevity in insulin-deficient diabetic mice. Diabetes 2011;60:2265–2273.

97 Cunningham CN, He K, Arunagiri A, Paton AW, Paton JC, Arvan P, Tsai B: Chaperone-driven degradation of a misfolded proinsulin mutant in parallel with restoration of wild type insulin secretion. Diabetes 2016; pii: db161338, Epub ahead of print.

98 Njolstad P, Sagen JV, Biorkhaug L, Odili S, Shehadeh N, Bakry D, Umit Sarici S, Alpai F, Molnes J, Molven A, Sovik O, Matschinsky FM: Permanent neonatal diabetes caused by glucokinase deficiency. Diabetes 2003;52:2854–2860.

99 Turkkahraman D, Bircan I, Tribble ND, Ackurin S, Ellard S, Gloyn A: Permanent neonatal diabetes mellitus caused by a novel homozygous (T168A) glucokinase mutation: initial response to oral sulphonylurea therapy. J Pediatr 2008;153:122–126.

100 Bennet K, James C, Mutair A, Al-Shaik H, Sinani A, Hussain K: Four novel cases of permanent neonatal diabetes caused by homozygous mutations in the glucokinase gene. Pediatr Diabet 2011;12:192–196.

101 Oriola J, Moreno F, Gutierrez-Nogues A, Luon S, Garcia-Herrero C-M, Vincent O, Navas M-A: Lack of glibenclamide response in a case of permanent neonatal diabetes caused by incomplete inactivation of glucokinase. JIMD Rep 2015;20:21–26.

102 Esquiaveto-Aun AM, De Mello MO, Paulino MF, Minicucci WJ, Guerra-Junior G, De Lemos-Marini SH: A new compound heterozygous for inactivating mutations in the glucokinase gene as cause of permanent neonatal diabetes mellitus (PNDM) in double-first cousins. Diabetol Metab Syndr 2015;7: 101.

103 Sansbury FH, Flanagan SE, Houghton JAL, Shuixian Shen FL, Al-Senani AMS, Habeb AM, Abdullah M, Kariminejad A, Ellard S, Hattersley AT: *SLC2A2* mutations can cause neonatal diabetes, suggesting GLUT2 may have a role in human insulin secretion. Diabetologia 2012;55:2381–2385.

104 Nicolino M, Claiborn KC, Senée V, Boland A, Stoffers DA, Julier C: A novel hypomorphic PDX1 mutation responsible for permanent neonatal diabetes with subclinical exocrine deficiency. Diabetes 2010; 59:733–740.

105 De Franco E, Shaw-Smith C, Flanagan SE, Edhill EL, Wolf J, Otte V, Ebinger F, Varthakavi P, Vasanthi P, Edvardsson S, Hattersley AT, Ellard S: Biallelic PDX1 (insulin promoter factor 1) mutations causing neonatal diabetes without exocrine pancreas insufficiency. Diabet Med 2013;30:e197–e200.

106 De Franco E, Shaw-Smith C, Flanagan SE, Shepherd MH; International NDM Consortium, Hattersley AT, Ellard S: GATA6 mutations cause a broad phenotypic spectrum of diabetes from pancreatic agenesis to adult-onset diabetes without exocrine pancreatic insufficiency. Diabetes 2013; 62:993–997.

107 Shaw-Smith C, De Franco E, Lango Allen H, Battle A, Flanagan SE, Borowiec M, Taplin CE, van Alfen-van der Velden J, Cruz-Rojo J, Perez de Nanclares G, Miedzybrodzka Z, Deja G, Wlodarska I, Mlynarski W, Ferrer J, Hattersley AT, Ellard S: GATA4 mutations are a cause of neonatal and childhood-onset diabetes. Diabetes 2014;63:2888–2894.

108 Houghton JA, Swift GH, Shaw-Smith C, Flanagan SE, de Franco E, Caswell R, Hussain K, Mohamed S, Abdulrasoul M, Hattersley AT, MacDonald RJ, Ellard S: Isolated pancreatic aplasia due to a hypomorphic PTF1A mutation. Diabetes 2016;65:2810–2815.

109 Biason-Lauber A, Lang-Muritano M, Vaccaro T, Schoenle EJ: Loss of kinase activity in a patient with Wolcott-Rallison syndrome caused by a novel mutation in the EIF2AK3 gene. Diabetes 2002;51: 2301–2305.

110 Senee V, Vattem KM, Delepine M, Rainbow LA, Haton C, Lecoq A, Shaw NJ, Robert J-J, Rooman R, Diatloff-Zito C, Michaud JL, Bin-Abbas B, Taha D, Zabel B, Franceschini P, Topaglu AK, Lathrop GM, Barrett TG, Nicolino M, Wek RC, Julier C: Wolcott-Rallison syndorme. Clinical, genetic and functional study of EIF2AJK3 mutations and suggestion of genetic heterogeneity. Diabetes 2004;53:1876–1883.

111 Rubio-Cabezas O, Patch A-M, Minton JAL, Flanagan SE, Edghill EL, Hussain K, Balafrej A, Deeb A, Buchanan CR, Jefferson IG, Mutair A; Neonatal Diabetes International Collaborative Group, Hattersley AT, Ellard S: Wolcott-Rallison syndrome is the most common genetic cause of permanent neonatal diabetes in consanguineous families. J Clin Endocrinol Metab 2009;94:4162–4170.

112 Habeb AM, Flanagan SE, Deeb A, Al-Alwan I, Alawneh H, Balafrej AAL, Mutair A, Hattersley AT, Hussain K, Ellard S: Permanent neonatal diabetes: different aetiology in Arabs compared to Europeans. Arch Dis Child 2012;97:721–723.

113 Harding HP, Novoa I, Zhang Y, Zeng H, Wek R, Schapira M, Ron D: Regulated translation initiation controls stress-induced gene expression in mammalian cells. Mol Cell 2000;6:1099–1108.

114 Cavener DR, Gupta S, McGrath BC: PERK in beta cell biology and insulin biogenesis. Trends Endocrinol Metab 2010;21:714–721.

115 Wang R, McGrath BC, Kopp RF, Roe MW, Tang X, Chen G, Cavener DR: Insulin secretion and Ca^{2+} dynamics in β-cells are regulated by PERK (EIF2AK3) in concert with calcineurin. J Biol Chem 2013;288:33824–33836.

116 Iglesias-Platas I, Court F, Camprubi C, Sparago A, Guillaumet-Adkins A, Martin-Trujillo A, Riccio A, Moore E, Monk D: Imprinting at the PLAGL1 domain is contained within a 70-kb CTCF/cohesin-mediated non-allelic chromatin loop. Nucleic Acids Res 2013;41:2171–2179.

117 Temple IK, Docherty LE, Mackay DJG: Diabetes Mellitus, 6q24-Related Transient Neonatal; in Pagon RA, Adam MP, Ardinger HH, Wallace SE, Amemiya A, Bean LJH, Bird TD, Ledbetter N, Mefford HC, Smith RJH, Stephens K (eds): GeneReviews®. Seattle, University of Washington, 2015.

118 Docherty LE, Kabwama S, Lehmann A, Hawke E, Harrison L, Flanagan SE, Ellard S, Hattersley AT, Shield JPH, Ennis S, Mackay DJ, Temple IK: 6q24 transient neonatal diabetes mellitus (6q24 TNDM) – clinical presentation and genotype phenotype correlation in an international cohort of cases. Diabetologia 2013;56:758–762.

119 Mackay DJG, Callaway JLA, Marks SM, White HE, Acerini CL, Boonen SE, Dayanikli P, Firth HV, Goodship JA, Haemers AP, Hahnemann JMD, Kordonouri O, Masoud AF, Oestergaard E, Storr J, Ellard S, Hattersley AT, Robinson DO, Temple IK: Hypomethylation of multiple imprinted loci in patients with transient neonatal diabetes is associated with mutations in ZFP57. Nat Genet 2008;40:949–951.

120 Lango Allen H, et al: GATA6 haploinsufficiency causes pancreatic agenesis in humans. Nat Genet 2012;44:20–22.

121 D'Amato E, et al: Genetic investigation in an Italian child with an unusual combination of atrial septal defect, attributable to a new familial GATA4 gene mutation, and neonatal diabetes due to pancreatic agenesis. Diabetic Med 2010;27:1195–1200.

122 Sellick GS, et al: Mutations in PTF1A cause pancreatic and cerebellar agenesis. Nat Genet 2004;36: 1301–1305.

123 Senee V, et al: Mutations in GLIS3 are responsible for a rare syndrome with neonatal diabetes mellitus and congenital hypothyroidism. Nat Genet 2006; 38:682-687.

124 Rubio-Cabezas O, et al: Permanent neonatal diabetes and enteric anendocrinosis associated with biallelic mutations in NEUROG3. Diabetes 2011;60: 1349–1353.

125 Flanagan SE, et al: Analysis of transcription factors key for mouse pancreatic development establishes NKX2-2 and MNX1 mutations as cause of neonatal diabetes in man. Cell Metab 2014;19:146–154.

126 Smith FB, et al: Rfx6 directs islet formation and insulin production in mice and humans. Nature 2010;463:775–780.

127 Rubio-Cabezas O, et al: Homozygous mutations in NEUROD1 are responsible for a novel syndrome of permanent neonatal diabetes and neurological abnormalities. Diabetes 2010;59:2326–2331.

128 Flanagan SE, et al: Activating germline mutations in STAT3 cause early-onset multi-organ autoimmune disease. Nat Genet 2014;46:812–814.

Fabrizio Barbetti, MD, PhD
Department of Experimental Medicine and Surgery
University of Rome Tor Vergata
Via Montpellier 1
IT–00133 Rome (Italy)
E-Mail Fabrizio.Barbetti@uniroma2.it

Colin G. Nichols, PhD, FRS
Department of Cell Biology and Physiology
Washington University School of Medicine
Campus Box 8228
660 South Euclid Avenue
Saint Louis, MO 63110 (USA)
E-Mail cnichols@wustl.edu

Barbetti F, Ghizzoni L, Guaraldi F (eds): Diabetes Associated with Single Gene Defects and Chromosomal Abnormalities. Front Diabetes. Basel, Karger, 2017, vol 25, pp 26–48 (DOI: 10.1159/000454695)

Maturity-Onset Diabetes of the Young: From Genetics to Translational Biology and Personalized Medicine

Martine Vaxillaire[a–c] · Philippe Froguel[a–d]

[a]CNRS-UMR 8199, Integrative Genomics and Modelling of Metabolic Diseases, Lille Pasteur Institute, [b]Lille University, and [c]European Genomic Institute for Diabetes (EGID), Lille, France; [d]Department of Genomics of Common Diseases, School of Public Health, Hammersmith Hospital, Imperial College Faculty of Medicine, London, UK

Abstract

Monogenic diabetes is defined as diabetes resulting from a rare causal deleterious mutation of a single gene that usually impairs pancreatic β-cell function. There is a large spectrum of clinical presentations of monogenic diabetes, depending on the affected gene and the nature of the mutation. Maturity-onset diabetes of the young (MODY) is the most frequent, representing 1–2% of all diabetes cases. MODY is dominantly inherited with early-onset nonautoimmune diabetes. At least 14 MODY genes have been identified so far, including key genes involved in developmental and/or functional processes of the pancreatic β-cell physiology. These discoveries remarkably modified patients' care, improving their quality of life and long-term evolution, and offer proof-of-concepts of successful genomic diabetes medicine. Further, recent advances in genome editing and pluripotent stem-cell reprogramming technologies are providing new opportunities and challenges for in vitro human cell-based diabetes modelling and for novel drugs and cell-based diabetes therapy discovery. This review chapter focuses on the lessons learned from MODY gene identification to clinical translational research and implementation of personalized genomic medicine, as well as on future directions to further elucidate and better understand the pathophysiological mechanisms underlying early-onset monogenic diabetes. © 2017 S. Karger AG, Basel

This review chapter focuses on the lessons learned from MODY gene identification to clinical translational research and implementation of personalized genomic medicine, as well as on future directions to further elucidate and better understand the pathophysiological mechanisms underlying early-onset monogenic diabetes.

Etiopathogenic Characteristics of Maturity-Onset Diabetes of the Young

Maturity-onset diabetes of the young (MODY) was initially reported in the early 1970s by Fajans and Tattersall, and recognized as a mild or even asymptomatic form of diabetes in young people with a strong familial clustering and in absence of insulin dependence [1, 2]. Subsequently, the familial pattern of MODY was suggested to have an autosomal dominant mode of inheritance, and the following clinical criteria for diagnosing MODY patient were proposed: (1) nonautoimmune early-onset diabetes, usually diagnosed in early childhood, adolescence or young adulthood (typically before 25 years of age, although some patients aged >40 years at diagnosis have been reported); (2) vertical transmission of early-onset diabetes in at least 3 generations within a family; (3) no insulin dependence (not requiring exogenous insulin even after 3 years of diagnosis); and (4) absence of autoimmune biomarkers (particularly the lack of islet autoantibodies) [2, 3]. Based on these criteria, the prevalence of MODY is estimated at 1–2% of all diabetic cases in Europe, although it might be largely underestimated in clinical settings, perhaps because the phenotypes overlap with classical forms of diabetes (either type 1 or type 2 diabetes) [4, 5]. Numerous studies have indicated that only a small proportion of MODY are correctly diagnosed: the prevalence of MODY in the UK population has been reported to be approximately 10 cases/100,000 [5], whereas estimations from population-based childhood diabetes registries were between 2.5–5 cases/100,000 in several European countries and 2.1 cases/100,000 in American children from the SEARCH for Diabetes in Youth Study [6, 7]. A high frequency (27%) of clinically suspected MODY was also reported among patients with type 2 diabetes younger than 25 years of age in South India [8].

MODY is mainly due to primary defects in pancreatic β-cell function [3, 9]. However, residual insulin secretion may still be maintained for many years after diagnosis; therefore, exogenous insulin is generally not required at the time of diagnosis or even later, depending on the disease-causing genetic defect. Interestingly, MODY is rarely associated with obesity, which is not required for its development.

Overview of the MODY Genetic Subtypes

Researchers began to unravel the molecular genetic basis of MODY in the 1990s with the identification of *GCK* (encoding glucokinase) and *HNF1A* (encoding hepatocyte nuclear factor-1α [HNF1-α]) as MODY2 and -3 genes, respectively [10, 11]. These familial linkage studies performed in large French MODY families led to the definition of MODY1–5 due to either decreased glucose phosphorylation or impaired activity of pancreatic β-cell expressed transcription factors [3]. Since these proof-of-concept discoveries, an expanding amount of genetic data has revealed a marked genetic heterogeneity of the disease with 14 MODY genes reported so far, which harbor heterozygous mutations or partial/whole gene deletions that are involved in the MODY phenotype (Table 1) [12, 13].

Table 1. Main characteristics of the MODY genetic subtypes

Gene name and locus	Protein/Function	Phenotypes/syndromes	OMIM	Association with T2D (low-frequency or common variants)
HNF4A 20q12	HNF-4α Transcription factor	MODY1, in adolescence or early adulthood (and neonatal hyper-insulinism)	125850 600281	+
GCK 7p13	Glucokinase Glycolytic enzyme	MODY2, mild hyperglycemia (onset in early childhood, and life-long) (frequent)	138079 125851	+
HNF1A 12q24.2	HNF-1α Transcription factor	MODY3, in adolescence or early adulthood [frequent]	600496 142410	+
PDX1 13q12.1	IPF1 Transcription factor	MODY4, in early adulthood (similar to HNF1A but rare)	606392 600733	+
HNF1B 17q21	HNF-1β Transcription factor	MODY5, in early adulthood, RCAD	137920 189907	+
NEUROD1 2q31.3	NeuroD1 or β2 Transcription factor	MODY6, in early adulthood (similar to HNF1A but rare)	606394 601724	
KLF11 2p25	Krüppel-like factor 11 Transcription factor	MODY7, in childhood and early-adulthood	603301 610508	
CEL 9q34	Carboxyl-ester Lipase enzyme	MODY8, in early-adulthood Pancreatic exocrine insufficiency, pancreatic atrophy and lipomatosis	114840 609812	
PAX4 7q32	Paired box gene 4 Transcription factor	MODY9, in early-adulthood	167413 612225	+
INS 11p15.5	Preproinsulin, insulin Hypoglycemic hormone, effect on anabolism	MODY10, in childhood and early-adulthood	613370 176730	
BLK 8p23	B lymphocyte kinase Nonreceptor tyrosine kinase	MODY11, in early-adulthood	191305 613375	+
ABCC8 11p15.1	SUR1 (sulfonylurea receptor) K_{ATP} channel regulatory subunit	MODY12, in childhood and early-adulthood	600509	+
KCNJ11 11p15.1	Kir6.2 K_{ATP} channel pore-forming subunit	MODY13, in childhood and early-adulthood	600937	+
WFS1 4p16	Wolfram syndrome 1 Wolframin	MODY14, in early-adulthood	606201 222100	+

The OMIM (Online Mendelian Inheritance in Man) numbers depict the phenotype and/or gene MIM numbers. A detailed overview and recent update on T2D-associated genetic variants are given in [79]. K_{ATP}, ATP-sensitive potassium channel; RCAD, renal cysts and diabetes.

	MODY	NDM/MDI	Syndromic NDM/MDI
Nucleus, regulation of gene transcription and transcriptional networks			
	HNF1A, HNF4A, KLF11, PAX4, PCBD1/DCoH	*MNX1* *PLAGL1/ZAC (6q24)* *ZFP57*	*GATA4, GATA6, GLIS3, HNF1B, NEUROD1, NEUROG3, NKX2.2, PAX6, PTF1A, RFX6*
	HNF1B, NEUROD1, PDX1		
Glucose uptake and phosphorylation, cellular metabolism and insulin secretion			
	BLK	*SLC2A2*	*SLC19A2*
	GCK		
Endoplasmic reticulum, insulin production and secretion			
	WFS1		*CISD2, EIF2AK3, IER3IP1, WFS1*
	INS		
K+(ATP-sensitive) channel, insulin secretion			
	ABCC8, KCNJ11		
Exocrine pancreas, lipase enzymatic activity			
	CEL		

Fig. 1. Key genes involved in the different subtypes of monogenic diabetes (MODY, NDM, and MDI) and their role in the pancreatic β-cell function. Several of these genes are known to contribute to a continuum of early-onset diabetes phenotypes from NDM to MODY, depending on the severity of functional defects and the nature of the mutation (as reviewed in [12]. * Biallelic *PCBD1/DCoH* mutations were recently identified as causing early-onset antibody-negative diabetes in consanguineous families [72]. MODY, maturity-onset diabetes of the young; NDM, neonatal diabetes mellitus; MDI, monogenic diabetes of infancy.

Most of the MODY genes encode pancreatic β-cell-expressed proteins that have a crucial role in the fetal development of the pancreas and β-cells, in the maturation and maintenance of β-cell function, or in regulating glucose sensing of the pancreatic β-cell and cell signaling to insulin secretion (Figure 1) [12]. The molecular defects underlying these early-onset diabetes phenotypes result from impaired insulin production with regard to in vivo hyperglycemia levels and/or abnormal regulation of insulin secretion. However, there are marked clinical differences within and among the different genetic subtypes, as well as extrapancreatic features that may be seen in specific cases (as described below and in Table 1).

Mild Fasting Hyperglycemia Due to Glucokinase Gene Mutations (GCK-MODY, MODY2)

Over 600 different heterozygous inactivating *GCK* mutations (missense, nonsense, frameshift, splice site, and exon deletion) distributed throughout the gene have been reported to be responsible for MODY in more than 1,500 families worldwide [14], representing one of the most common forms of MODY in European countries (accounting for 30–60% of all subtypes depending on geographic origin). Glucokinase is mainly expressed in pancreatic β-cells and hepatocytes, where it catalyzes the first rate-limiting step of glucose metabolism (i.e., production of glucose-6-P) [15]. Glucokinase acts as the pancreatic glucose sensor and plays a major role in regulating glucose-stimulated insulin secretion through glucose uptake and glycolytic flux in the cell [15]. Loss-of-function *GCK* mutations result in both an increased threshold of pancreatic glucose-stimulated insulin secretion and impaired hepatic glycogen synthesis, which lead to moderate nonprogressive fasting hyperglycemia (5.5–8.0 mmol/L) from birth and impaired glucose tolerance at the oral glucose tolerance test. Indeed, very few affected individuals will have overt diabetes, and nearly half of the mutation carriers may remain asymptomatic for many years. Pharmacological treatment for MODY2 patients is not usually required [16]. Conversely, homozygous loss-of-function mutations cause permanent neonatal diabetes requiring lifelong insulin treatment, whereas heterozygous activating *GCK* mutations may cause persistent hyperinsulinemic hypoglycemia of infancy.

A broad range of in vitro defects for more than 70 *GCK*-MODY mutations, particularly altered kinetic properties and protein instability depending on the mutation severity, has been shown to contribute to enzyme dysfunction [17]. In vivo, there is compensation of the mutated allele by the wild-type allele, which is posttranslationally upregulated by glucose [18]. Nevertheless, variability in the clinical phenotypes of MODY2 patients has been described, and patients carrying severe inactivating *GCK* mutations may have high postchallenge glucose values, possibly resulting from a marked liver component of the disease [19]. Importantly, a recent study assessed the prevalence and severity of vascular complications among patients with *GCK* mutations and chronic mild hyperglycemia, and showed that they had a low prevalence of microvascular and macrovascular complications despite their lifelong hyperglycemia (median duration of 48.6 years in 99 *GCK* mutation carriers) [20]. Corroborating with the mild clinical symptoms in MODY2, metabolomic analyses revealed that *GCK*-MODY patients present a normal (or supernormal) metabolic profile, most of which were similar to that of healthy individuals, with lower levels of free fatty acids and triglycerides, which likely contribute to the nonprogressive nature of MODY2 [21].

Another important effect of *GCK*-MODY mutations is that they give rise to a reduced birth weight by affecting insulin-mediated fetal growth in mutation carriers, whereas maternal *GCK* mutations will indirectly increase the birth weight by increasing fetal insulin secretion as a consequence of maternal hyperglycemia during fetal life [22].

Familial Early-Onset Diabetes Due to Mutations in Transcription Factor Genes
Heterozygous mutations or partial/whole deletions of several genes coding for transcription factors involved in fetal pancreas development and/or pancreatic β-cell maturation and function have been described as being involved in MODY: HNF-1α *(HNF1A)*, HNF-1β *(HNF1B)*, HNF-4α *(HNF4A)*, PDX1 (also known as IPF1), NEUROD1, KLF11, and Pax-4 (Table 1) [12].

HNF4A-MODY (MODY1) and HNF1A-MODY (MODY3)
Inactivating mutations of the 2 related transcription factors, HNF-4α and HNF-1α, are responsible for the MODY1 and MODY3 forms [23], respectively, with *HNF1A*-MODY3 being the most common MODY subtype reported in Northern Europe (accounting for >30% of MODY cases), whereas *HNF4A*-MODY1 accounts for approximately 10% of MODY cases without *HNF1A* mutations [5, 24, 25]. More than 400 different *HNF1A* mutations located in the promoter and coding regions have been described in more than 1,200 families of various ethnic origins; the most common mutation was p.P291fsinsC, which was reported in more than 60 families [23]. *HNF4A* mutations are a rarer cause of MODY, with about 105 mutations reported in more than 170 families to date [23].

Mutations in *HNF1A* and *HNF4A* lead to a progressive insulin secretory defect resulting in a severe form of diabetes as early as adolescence and young adulthood, which requires hypoglycemic drugs or even insulin therapy at young ages owing to a severe deterioration in glucose tolerance. *HNF1A* mutations in the dimerization and DNA-binding domains of HNF-1α have been associated with an earlier age of diabetes diagnosis compared to mutation in the transactivation domain. The shared phenotype of MODY1 and MODY3 is consistent with the interdependence of HNF-1α and HNF-4α, forming part of a wide regulatory network not only in pancreatic β-cells, but also in the liver and the kidney [3]. HNF-1α and HNF-4α can bind and activate each other's promoter, and also regulate the expression of common targets, such as *SLC2A2* coding for the GLUT2 transporter. Thus, the mutation effects may extend beyond pancreatic β-cells with impaired GLUT2 activity in the kidney and altered proximal renal tubular reabsorption of glucose, which in turns leads to renal glycosuria [26]. Due to the progressive nature and early age at diagnosis of *HNF1A*-MODY3 and *HNF4A*-MODY1, patients are at risk of long-term microvascular and macrovascular complications, similarly to patients with type 1 and type 2 diabetes, which are strongly influenced by the degree of glycemic control [2]. *HNF1A*-MODY3 patients may be predisposed to liver adenomatosis, likely through somatic inactivation of the remaining wild-type allele, although reports of such cases are quite rare [27].

HNF1A and *HNF4A* mutations may also lead to a dual phenotype of macrosomia, neonatal hypoglycemia and increased birth weight by determining hyperinsulinism in utero that may persist several months after birth before evolving to decreased insulin secretion and diabetes later in life [28]. The mechanisms behind the dysregulation causing hyperinsulinism and then MODY are still unknown, highlighting the interdependence of these transcription factors.

Renal Cysts and Diabetes Syndrome (HNF1B-MODY, MODY5)

Germline heterozygous mutations in *HNF1B* (also termed *TCF2*) give rise to a wide clinical spectrum with either isolated renal developmental disease, isolated diabetes, or both as a multisystem disorder called renal cysts and diabetes syndrome (RCAD) [29]. The transcription factor HNF-1β plays a major role in embryonic endodermal development, namely of the kidney, pancreas, liver, genital tract, and gut. The severity of the renal disease is extremely variable, including hypoplastic glomerulocystic kidney disease, cystic renal dysplasia, horseshoe kidney, or atypical familial juvenile hyperuricemic nephropathy, while in some patients the renal abnormalities are mild or absent [30]. Most of the patients with *HNF1B* mutations have pancreatic hypoplasia (particularly of the pancreas tail) and reduced exocrine function, and calcifications in the pancreas head have been reported in some patients [31]. Additional clinical features besides renal disease and diabetes include abnormal liver and biliary function, urogenital tract malformations, hyperuricemia, and gout [29].

HNF1B mutations associated with RCAD consist of point/splice site mutations, small deletions/insertions, and large/whole gene deletion (106 different *HNF1B* mutations have been reported in >230 families) [32]. De novo mutations were reported in approximately 50% of cases where a family history is absent (but with a distinct phenotype of RCAD), and are thought to arise from nonallelic homologous recombination between segmental duplications flanking the region that encompasses *HNF1B*. There is no evidence to suggest a genotype-phenotype correlation (between large deletions, large genomic rearrangements, and point mutations) that is consistent with haploinsufficiency as the disease mechanism [29].

Although *HNF1B* mutations were initially associated with diabetes (MODY5), renal abnormalities are very frequent in the mutation carriers, particularly in pediatric cases before the development of diabetes [30, 32]. More recent studies have reported that neurodevelopmental features, such as autism spectrum disorders, can be part of the phenotype in subjects with a chr17q12 deletion encompassing the *HNF1B* locus [33]. The 1.4-Mb deleted region on chr17q12, which was found in several patients referred for clinical genetic testing for autism spectrum disorders, developmental delay, or cognitive impairments, contains 15 genes (including *HNF1B*); therefore, the genetic mechanism giving rise to the neurodevelopmental phenotypes remains to be clearly described [33].

Other Transcription Factor Genes Involved in MODY

Heterozygous missense or frameshift mutations in *PDX1* (MODY4), *NEUROD1* (MODY6), *KLF11* (MODY7), and *PAX4* (MODY9) have been reported in only a few families, each subtype representing a rare cause of MODY (Table 1) [12].

PDX1, NEUROD1, and PAX4 have an important role in the early development of the endocrine pancreas, and/or in the maturation and maintenance of pancreatic β-cells, as well as in transcriptional regulation of insulin, GLUT2, glucokinase, ghrelin, and glucagon genes in mature pancreatic endocrine cells. Very rare homozygous *NEUROD1* mutations are associated with neonatal diabetes, cerebellar hypoplasia, learning difficulties, and visual and hearing impairment, highlighting the critical role of NEUROD1 in the development of both the endocrine pancreas and central nervous system [3, 9].

KLF11 is a transcriptional factor of the Krüppel-like factor family, which regulates the transcription of genes important in the pancreatic β-cell function such as *PDX1/IPF1* and insulin [34]. Heterozygous missense *KLF11* mutations have been found to cosegregate with early-onset diabetes in a few families with a clinical pattern similar to MODY, but *KLF11* deficiency has not been confirmed to cause MODY in other cohorts [12].

Other Genetic Defects Impairing Pancreatic β-Cell Function and Insulin Secretion
INS-MODY (MODY10)
Heterozygous mutations in the *INS* gene were first described in patients with mild diabetes and hyperinsulinemia, resembling type 2 diabetes, and in several cohorts of neonatal diabetes mellitus (NDM) patients (as de novo or inherited mutations) [35]. The dominance of these mutations is explained by the misfolding of mutant proinsulin, leading to intracellular accumulation of abnormal proteins and dysfunctional β-cell ER stress responses, and the retention of wild-type insulin molecules in the ER, thus strongly decreasing insulin production in the pancreatic β-cells leading to severe diabetes [35, 36]. However, some family members carrying a NDM-associated mutation have mild diabetes at 30 years of age or older. It turns out that the phenotypic spectrum is quite broad, with patients fulfilling classical MODY criteria: they are non-obese, generally diagnosed before age 25, have a family history of diabetes consistent with autosomal dominant inheritance, and the diabetes is nonketotic. The extent of β-cell failure can be progressive, as some patients had declining C-peptide levels over time [36, 35]. Therefore, the *INS*-MODY10 subtype is characterized by a marked clinical heterogeneity regarding age at onset and severity of diabetes, and thus the therapeutic options range from diet only (in individuals who are particularly protected from a severe evolution) to oral hypoglycemic agents or insulin (in more severely affected cases) [37].

BLK-MODY (MODY11)
BLK (B lymphocyte kinase) encodes a nonreceptor tyrosine kinase of the SRC family of proto-oncogenes, which is expressed in pancreatic islet β-cells and may act as an enhancer of insulin secretion. Five rare mutations at the *BLK* locus, including only 1 missense variant (p.A71T), were reported to segregate with diabetes in 3 MODY families [38]. The p.A71T mutation was shown to blunt insulin secretion in vitro.

However, *BLK* has not been confirmed in other cohorts to cause MODY, but instead the p.A71T mutation was reported to be a low-frequency coding variant in Europeans, which could influence type 2 diabetes risk in a context of obesity [39].

ABCC8-MODY (MODY12) and *KCNJ11*-MODY (MODY13)

Heterozygous gain-of-function mutations in *KCNJ11* and *ABCC8*, which encode the 2 subunits (Kir6.2 and SUR1, respectively) of the pancreatic β-cell expressed ATP-sensitive potassium (K_{ATP}) channel, have been shown to cause a wide spectrum of phenotypes, ranging from permanent or transient forms of NDM (often involving de novo mutations responsible for severe hyperglycemia in neonates or in the first 6 months of life) to later onset forms of dominantly inherited diabetes developing in the 3rd or 4th decades of life and resembling MODY in a few families [40, 41]. Gain-of-function mutations of *KCNJ11* and *ABCC8* impair K_{ATP} channel closure by reducing the ATP-binding affinity on Kir6.2 or altering channel gating via the interaction of Mg^2-ADP with SUR1, which leads to persistent channel overactivity, β-cell membrane hyperpolarization, and consequently to a severe reduction of insulin secretion. In case of mutations that severely affect channel function, diabetes may be associated with speech and developmental delay, epilepsy, and muscular hypotonia, known as DEND or iDEND syndrome (reviewed in [12]). This is a good example of how different mutations affecting a same gene may cause a wide spectrum of clinical phenotypes ranging from NDM to inherited late-onset diabetes with a lower penetrance appearing in childhood or adulthood.

WFS1-MODY (MODY14)

Genetic variations in *WFS1* (Wolfram syndrome 1 gene) lead to a spectrum of clinical phenotypes, including Wolfram syndrome (WS, also called DIDMOAD for "diabetes insipidus, diabetes mellitus, optic atrophy, and deafness"), which is a rare and progressive autosomal recessive neurodegenerative disorder, and a milder form of sensorineural hearing impairment, which is inherited as an autosomal dominant condition caused by heterozygous missense *WFS1* mutations [42], as well as to susceptibility to type 1 and type 2 diabetes [43]. *WFS1* encodes a multispan transmembrane protein (named wolframin) localized to the endoplasmic reticulum and expressed in pancreatic β-cells that participates in insulin production, processing, and secretion as well as the regulation of endoplasmic reticulum calcium levels [42]. More recently, an exome sequencing study of a 3-generation Finnish family reported a novel heterozygous missense *WFS1* mutation (p.W314R) associated with dominantly inherited nonsyndromic early-onset diabetes [44]. Functionally, the *WFS1*-W314R mutation appeared to alter the ability of WFS1 to protect against endoplasmic reticulum stress, which probably damages β-cell function over time, leading to insufficient insulin production and diabetes via a dominant-negative mechanism [44]. The heterozygous mutation carriers in the family had none of the other syndromic features of WS, but high penetrance of diabetes with relative insulin insufficiency, and most of them are treated with insulin [44].

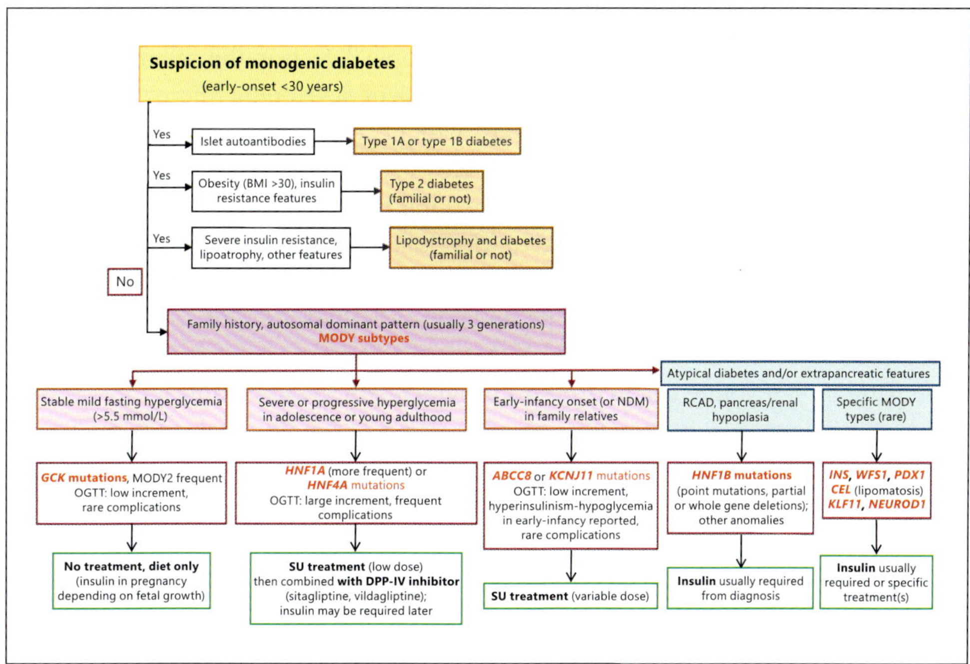

Fig. 2. Diagnostic criteria and clinical features for differentiating the main genetic subtypes of MODY, and impact of the genetic defect on the recommended therapeutic options. Gene symbol names are described in Table 1. NDM, neonatal diabetes mellitus; OGTT, oral glucose tolerance test; RCAD, renal cysts and diabetes; SU, sulfonylurea.

Diabetes Secondary to Exocrine Pancreas Deficiency (CEL-MODY, MODY8)

Mutations in *CEL*, encoding the carboxyl-ester lipase enzyme, cause a rare subtype of pancreatic lipomatosis with exocrine and endocrine pancreatic insufficiency and subsequent progressive diabetes (mean age at onset of 35 years) [45]. Extensive pancreatic imaging studies have revealed very characteristic alterations in pancreatic texture and a reduction of pancreatic size (around 50% of pancreas volume) in *CEL* mutation carriers compared with healthy controls [31]. Protein misfolding with intracellular and extracellular aggregation may exert a cytotoxic effect and lead to disease progression involving the islets of Langerhans, which will lead to endocrine dysfunction and diabetes mellitus.

Evidence for Personalized Pharmacogenomic Medicine in MODY

Clinical investigation studies carried out in patients with the more common MODY subtypes have shed light on their respective clinical and metabolic features according to genetic and molecular defects, which have also shown marked differences and specificities in drug therapy response (Fig. 2).

The fasting hyperglycemia associated with *GCK* mutations is most often mild and stable over the patient's lifetime, despite the multiple defects in the pancreas and the liver. As HbA_{1c} levels are mildly increased, the risk of developing microvascular diabetic complications is very low in MODY2 patients compared to the other MODY subtypes and late-onset type 2 diabetes [2]. However, the development of insulin resistance with age may have an impact on the long-term deterioration of glucose tolerance in MODY2 patients, compared to what is seen in the general population [46]. The majority of MODY2 patients do not require the use of pharmacotherapy, as they are usually well responsive to diet alone, and low-carbohydrate diets are recommended for good glycemic control in GCK-MODY [47]. It is thus important to recognize these patients at a young age in order to provide them the best clinical care, as they may be misdiagnosed with type 1 or type 2 diabetes. A longitudinal study of 20 subjects who had been treated with insulin or oral hypoglycemic agents showed no change in HbA_{1c} when treatment was discontinued after the diagnosis of GCK-MODY. Therefore, the consensus is that antidiabetic drugs can be stopped in most MODY2 patients. The only exception is during pregnancy when fetal macrosomia is suspected and insulin treatment is generally recommended in order to control fetal growth.

In contrast, the diabetic phenotype of *HNF1A*-MODY3 and *HNF4A*-MODY1 patients is more severe at diagnosis and quickly progressive with a deterioration throughout life, especially when superimposed environmental factors are present [2]. Typically, *HNF1A* or *HNF4A* mutation carriers are normoglycemic in childhood, but have progressively impaired insulin secretion, with diabetes usually diagnosed in the second to fifth decades. Tight glycemic control and management of cardiovascular risk factors are essential for long-term care of these MODY patients. The effectiveness of oral sulfonylurea (SU) treatment is a feature of both MODY1 and MODY3 patients, and consensus guidelines for diabetes management of *HNF1A*- and *HNF4A*-MODY recommend low-dose SU as the first-line treatment. According to animal and cellular models of HNF-1α and HNF-4α deficiency, the pancreatic β-cell defect is upstream of the pancreatic K_{ATP} channel, where SU molecules directly bind the SUR1 channel regulatory subunit and lead to channel closure, thereby stimulating insulin release from pancreatic β-cells. Subsequently, this effect can result in symptomatic hypoglycemia in some hyperresponsive patients. The hypersensitivity to SU means that patients who have been misdiagnosed as type 1 diabetes and treated with long-term insulin from diagnosis can be switched safely and successfully from insulin to oral SU with improved glycemic control in most cases [48]. Good control may be maintained for many years, although SU treatment may become insufficient in many MODY3 patients, thus often requiring combined therapy with insulin. Interestingly, the new class of dipeptidyl peptidase-IV inhibitors, which act by prolonging the activity of circulating incretins, was also reported to be an effective adjuvant therapy in *HNF1A*-MODY patients who no longer responded to SU monotherapy, as they were found to improve β-cell function in those patients as documented by increased insulin secretion during intravenous glucose tolerance tests performed in fasting conditions [49]. In contrast, MODY5 patients with *HNF1B* mutations are not sensitive to SU treatment, and early insulin therapy is generally required from diabetes diagnosis to prevent long-term complications.

Although rare, etiological diagnosis of adult-onset K_{ATP} channel-associated diabetes has significant clinical and therapeutic implications, as good metabolic control may be achieved for many years with oral SU treatment alone [12]. For example, a study that evaluated the metabolic features of adult-onset diabetes associated with *ABCC8* mutations showed impaired insulin secretion capacity that was restored after a 4-week SU trial in 2 patients [40].

Furthermore, it has been hypothesized that MODY patients with different genetic etiologies of diabetes could have distinct metabolic profiles, which may uncover novel biomarkers that might be useful to prioritize or select subgroups of patients for molecular genetic testing, early diagnosis, and therapy monitoring. A good example of such genotype-biochemical phenotype relationships was the observation that lower serum levels of high-sensitivity C-reactive protein, which is under transcriptional control by HNF1A, can significantly discriminate *HNF1A*-MODY patients from other subtypes of diabetes [50]. A large European study has demonstrated that low concentrations of high-sensitivity C-reactive protein (<0.25–0.75 mg/L, depending on the assay used) is a clinically valid biomarker for diagnosis of *HNF1A*-MODY with high sensitivity (78%) and specificity (80%) [51]. Besides being a useful tool as a diagnostic discriminator, high-sensitivity C-reactive protein may also become a reliable tool to assist in the interpretation of novel mutations of uncertain pathogenic significance. The urinary C-peptide-to-creatinine ratio is a stable measure of endogenous insulin secretion, which may also be used as a noninvasive biomarker for differential diagnosis between type 1 diabetes and *HNF1A/4A*-MODY (AUC: 0.98 with a cutoff urinary C-peptide-to-creatinine ratio ≥0.2 nmol/mmol for MODY) [52].

More recent studies have attempted to stratify nontargeted metabolomic profiling data from MODY patients of different genetic subgroups compared to type 2 diabetes and normoglycemic controls, which allows for examining changes of whole-body metabolism in the development and progression of different types of diabetes. Interestingly, unbiased metabolite profiling from serum samples of patients with *HNF4A*-MODY1, *GCK*-MODY2, *HNF1A*-MODY3, and type 2 diabetes, and from samples of healthy individuals has revealed that *GCK*-MODY patients present normal or supernormal metabolic control characterized by lower free fatty acid and triglyceride levels (a 52% decrease in free fatty acids compared with healthy controls was reported), which is usually a sign of high insulin sensitivity, despite chronic high fasting glucose levels [21]. In contrast, the other forms of diabetes differed markedly from healthy controls in their metabolite profiles [21]. These findings provide evidence that *GCK*-MODY is a metabolically normal condition, which may explain the lack of microvascular complications and the nonprogressive nature of MODY2. However, another metabolomic profiling study did not identify any single urine metabolite contributing significantly to the separation of *GCK*-MODY and *HNF1A*-MODY subgroups, compared to type 2 diabetes and normoglycemic controls, despite the distinct molecular pathways affected according to genetic basis [53]. Alternative 'omics' approaches such as proteomics or lipidomics might be more powerful in identifying robust biomarkers for monogenic diabetes subtype discrimination.

Other circulating biomarkers such microRNAs (miRNAs) have emerged as potent regulators of gene expression, and they may have an important role in pancreas development and β-cell differentiation, as well as in insulin production, secretion, and action [54]. To date, one representative study investigated changes in miRNA expression in INS-1 insulinoma cells inducibly expressing the *HNF1A*-Pro291fsinsC hot-spot mutation and in serum from 31 cases with *HNF1A*-MODY [55]. Two miRNAs, miR-103 and miR-224, were significantly upregulated upon suppression of endogenous HNF-1α function in the INS-1 cell line, and both miRNAs were found strongly elevated in the serum of *HNF1A*-MODY patients when compared with family controls (mean levels 47- and 293-fold higher, respectively) [55]. Furthermore, miR-103 may distinguish *HNF1A*-MODY patients from HbA_{1c}-matched type 2 diabetes subjects. Such findings with validated and replicated data may lead to new potential biomarkers and novel targets for therapeutic intervention.

Clinical Relevance of a Molecular Diagnosis for MODY

A differential genetic diagnosis of MODY will provide a molecular confirmation of a clinical diagnosis of MODY, which will have important clinical implications in some patients, particularly for choosing the best therapeutic option related to the genetic defect. Indeed, making the molecular diagnosis of a specific genetic subtype will guide the most appropriate clinical management and pharmacological treatment (notably for *GCK*-MODY, *HNF1A/HNF4A*-MODY, and *ABCC8/KCNJ11*-MODY, as described in the above sections); this will also help to anticipate the long-term clinical course of the disease and high or low risk of complications. Furthermore, genetic counseling in the family may trigger molecular testing in other family members, which may be important in children with incidental hyperglycemia or in undiagnosed patients. It could also eventually lead to reclassifying diabetes in patients misdiagnosed with type 1 or type 2 diabetes with beneficial effects upon therapeutic adaptation.

Best practice consensus guidelines for MODY genetic testing have been proposed to assist physicians in their decision to test for a MODY diagnosis, and also to improve the rate of a positive molecular diagnosis [56, 57]. These recommendations are mainly based on the previously established clinical criteria for the MODY definition, which are a family history of diabetes in 1 parent and first-degree relatives (although isolated

MODY cases with de novo mutations may exist, recognizable with less strict clinical criteria of early-onset diabetes despite a negative family history of diabetes), lack of islet autoantibodies, age at diagnosis usually before 25 years, low or no insulin requirements 2 years after diagnosis, and absence of obesity, as discussed in the report by the European Molecular Genetics Quality Network (EMGQN) MODY Group [13, 56]. Mainly based on these full criteria, a MODY calculator has been validated and proposed to assess the probability that a particular patient has MODY with a probability score, taking into account age at diagnosis, BMI, HbA$_{1c}$ level, treatment with insulin or oral hypoglycemic agents, and whether a parent has or does not have diabetes [58]. An English version is available online at http://www.diabetesgenes.org/content/mody-probability-calculator, and a French version is available at http://files-good.ibl.fr/childhood-obesity-fr/. A second prediction model including additional clinical parameters of insulin resistance was also proposed to help better differentiate early-onset type 2 diabetes to *HNF1A*-MODY [24], which particularly contrasts with type 2 diabetes in adolescents in whom obesity and features of insulin resistance are almost always associated with diabetes.

Notwithstanding, the question of a lack of family history of diabetes is a recurring one in genetic testing practices, i.e., whether to test patients with a clinical suspicion of MODY apart from a familial inheritance. Interestingly, a recent study showed that de novo mutations in the most prevalent MODY genes (*GCK, HNF1A,* and *HNF4A*) may be more frequent than previously thought by systematically investigating a target group of 150 patients without a family history of diabetes who fulfilled the remaining diagnostic criteria for MODY (representing 16.3% of the referrals for MODY testing in 2 national monogenic diabetes registries): 11 cases with de novo mutations (6 *GCK,* 4 *HNF1A,* and 1 *HNF4A*) were identified, i.e., 7.3% of the probands tested [59]. A report from the Young Diabetes in Oxford (YDX) study showed that less than 50% of probands who identified with a mutation fulfilled all the diagnostic criteria for MODY [60]. These 2 studies clearly support that MODY diagnosis genetic testing should be extended beyond current guidelines to include patients with measurable C-peptide ≥3 years from diagnosis and age of diabetes diagnosis under 30 years despite a negative family history of diabetes.

Otherwise, a 7-item clinical flowchart (called 7-iF) has been proposed to specifically identify candidate patients for *GCK*-MODY2 genetic testing on the basis of 7 simple binary questions (again largely based on the EMGQN guidelines) [61]. This flowchart was retrospectively and prospectively validated in several Italian cohorts from the ISPED registry and diabetic outpatient clinics in Italy, resulting in 80% of MODY2 patients being identified [61]. This approach can be useful to select patients in clinical settings for a *GCK*-MODY2 genetic testing with a strong impact on reducing health care costs by avoiding unnecessary pharmacological treatment and follow-up care in those patients.

The questions of genetic testing costs and health care benefits, both for patients' care and educational perspectives, are also being discussed to explore the next steps towards best practices [62]. To this end, a recent study used a simulation model for diabetes complications to evaluate the cost-effectiveness of a genetic testing policy for mutations in *GCK-*, *HNF1A-*, and *HNF4A*-MODY in a hypothetical base case cohort with a MODY prevalence of 2% [63]. With a conservative interpretation of cost-effectiveness and based on incremental cost-effectiveness ratio thresholds in the US, the model sensitivity analyses showed that small increases in MODY prevalence in the base case cohort (from 2 to 6%) made the genetic screening policy cost-effective [63]. Moreover, as genetic testing costs are markedly decreasing with the recent progresses and ongoing developments made in high-throughput sequencing technologies, it seems important to offer broader screening for all the currently known MODY subtypes in selected young-onset type 2 diabetes patients, besides strict clinical criteria of MODY. We can expect this will actually allow us to move towards the new era of personalized genetic medicine.

Next-Generation Sequencing as a Diagnostic Tool for MODY and Future Research Perspectives

Over the past 15 years, the practice of molecular genetic diagnosis for monogenic diabetes in most of the specialized centers has relied on the selection and Sanger sequencing of a few potentially candidate genes selected on the basis of knowledge and availability of phenotype information in the patients (e.g., presence of a renal disease in *HNF1B*-MODY, macrosomia, and/or neonatal hypoglycemia in *HNF4A*-MODY), but this greatly limited the likelihood of making a genetic diagnosis in a substantial number of the clinically relevant tested patients. As MODY is a genetically heterogeneous group of disorders, the ability to move to next-generation sequencing (NGS) approaches to evaluate a defined set of candidate genes simultaneously has proven to be a reliable, accurate, rapid, and cost-effective means, compared to whole-exome or whole-genome sequencing, for increasing the rate of molecular diagnosis in several cohorts of MODY patients [64–67].

However, among the different NGS platforms dedicated to targeted gene panel sequencing, a perfect sequencing coverage of the targets was not fully obtained by all the existing enrichment methods, which are based either on DNA sonication (Custom Agilent SureSelect exon capture or Raindance microdroplet-based PCR enrichment) [64, 65] or enzymatic DNA fragmentation (Nextera Custom Rapid Capture or Halo-Plex Custom Kit) [66]. It is of high importance for routine diagnosis that these targeted sequencing methods provide high sensitivity and reliability data for an accurate genetic diagnosis in each of the tested patients. To this end, the study by Bonnefond et al. [64] reported that the microdroplet-based PCR enrichment RainDance technology coupled with Illumina sequencing has great performance and advantages to accurately detect all the causal mutations previously identified in 40 patients with monogenic diabetes or obesity (except 1 complex indel variant) from a custom panel of 43 genes, and notably with most of the targeted coding regions perfectly sequenced in all participants. This NGS method was found to be highly sensitive, very fast, and cost-effective for mutation screening based on a targeted multigene panel analysis [64].

The question of which NGS technique yields the highest diagnosis rate is frequently discussed and is still open [68]. From our NGS experience and based on comparative analysis data, the RainDance enrichment method and SureSelect exon capture provide the best results in terms of high quality of sequencing and sensitivity of variant detection (with RainDance's best advantage) [A. Bonnefond, personal communication].

These targeted NGS methods may serve as a prescreening tool before using more sophisticated and expensive methods aiming at a broader or almost complete genome sequencing with the potential of discovering new disease-causing genes. Given the extensive genetic and clinical heterogeneity of MODY, the alternative approach is to carry out whole-exome sequencing in place of testing specific genes, which may allow a first evaluation of a large predefined set of genes implicated in glucose metabolism [67]. Improvements in sequence coverage for disease-associated genes are still needed and are currently being performed in order to propose a "medical exome" that could be used as a fully optimized diagnostic tool [69]. Furthermore, the hypothesis-free whole-exome sequencing approach will provide a significantly larger number of variants of unknown clinical significance, as well as variants of incidental findings, which requires development of integrated and sophisticated analysis pipelines (including filtering out the vast majority of known variants from various public databases, and a comprehensive functional annotation of all novel potentially deleterious mutations). For diagnosis purposes, the increased number of genes tested will result in a higher detection rate of MODY mutations, and may also lead to identify cases of possible digenic MODY presentation, as this was evidenced in 2 recent reports by the coinheritance of 2 pathogenic *HNF1A* and *GCK* variants in 2 MODY families [70, 71].

Yet, numerous MODY patients still have undefined genetic defects (at least 20–30% according to the published cohorts), which actually hampers the establishment of a pathogenesis-oriented treatment and our understanding of diabetes pathophysiology in those patients. A recent study that used whole-genome sequencing with linkage analysis to study a consanguineous family with early-onset antibody-negative diabetes reported interesting novel findings with the identification of a novel deletion in *PCBD1* (encoding pterin-4-α-carbinolamine dehydratase, also known as dimerization cofactor of HNF-1α); subsequently, 3 additional biallelic *PCBD1* mutations were found in 3 patients with mild neonatal hyperphenylalaninemia who had developed *HNF1A*-MODY-like diabetes from independent families [72]. Furthermore, a morpholino-mediated knockdown in *Xenopus* revealed that Pcbd1 activity is required for proper establishment of early pancreatic fate within the endoderm [72]. Importantly, patients with *PCBD1* deficiency could be detected through a newborn screening for phenylketonuria, and they can be treated with oral antidiabetic drugs (SU or glinide) instead of insulin.

The availability of NGS approaches will help unravel the full spectrum of early-onset diabetes genes, ranging from truly monogenic to digenic or possibly more complex inherited traits, depending on the phenotypes associated with diabetes [70, 71]. Notably, with whole-genome sequencing on the horizon and rapid progress in understanding regulatory DNA sequences, it is conceivable that noncoding mutations will be identified in subsets of patients. Altogether, we can expect the new developments in genomic analyses will allow us to go further into our comprehension of disease mechanisms and will lead to optimized mechanistic-based therapeutic approaches for specific (genetic) subtypes of diabetes. Functional analyses in vitro and in vivo should help define such specific gene-related therapies.

Perspectives on Monogenic Diabetes Modelling: The New Era of Induced Pluripotent Stem Cell Biology

One of the promising approaches to better understand the molecular mechanisms underlying different forms of diabetes is to use pluripotent stem cells (PSCs), including embryonic stem cells and induced PCSs (iPSCs), which have great potential to differentiate into all cell types and to reestablish the disease phenotype in vitro (review in [73]).

Several iPSC lines have recently been generated from patients with different types of diabetes, including several MODY subtypes, and some of these cell lines were able to differentiate into insulin-secreting β-cells [74–78]. These biotechnological advances are important for diabetes physiopathology issues as the molecular mechanisms underlying MODY in humans are still incompletely understood.

The proof-of-concept of such an approach was provided by Hua et al. [75] with human iPSCs derived from MODY2 patients who carry GCK mutations. These cells have been differentiated into mature β-cells with similar efficiency as control counterparts, and they recapitulated well the clinical phenotype of the patients. Another study has successfully generated human iPSC lines from patients with different types of MODY including HNF4A-MODY1, GCK-MODY2, HNF1A-MODY3, HNF1B-MODY5, and CEL-MODY8 [74]. This study used a polycistronic lentiviral vector for reprogramming, which gave a higher efficiency than the frequently used retroviruses, and the derived MODY human iPSCs showed no karyotypic defects, although the authors did not perform pancreatic differentiation of those cells [74]. The generation of these cells and other MODY patient-specific iPSCs is important to investigate the role played by the MODY genes in pancreatic development and islet-cell dysfunction in diabetes. However, the extent to which these cells are representative of functionally mature adult β-cells remains unclear. Pagliuca et al. [76] reported a novel in vitro differentiation approach leading to the generation of functional human pancreatic β-cells, and a gene expression analysis showed that these cells are more similar to adult rather than fetal β-cells. In short, they obtained stem cell-derived glucose-responsive and monohormonal insulin-producing cells with features of mature adult β-cells [76]. These new approaches used for generating patient-specific human iPSC lines will enable the direct comparison of mutated and corrected cells sharing the same genetic background, which is particularly important in cases of patients with an established single-gene defect [73].

Interestingly, the study by Shang et al. [77] took a cell biology approach after successfully generating in vitro iPSC-derived β-cells from skin cells of WS patients to validate the role of *WFS1* in insulin production, insulin secretion, and protection against ER stress in β-cells. The "WS-iPSC-derived β-cells" were found to have increased ER stress levels and decreased insulin content, and upon exposure to experimental ER stress, they showed impaired insulin processing and defective insulin secretion in response to glucose and other secretagogues [77]. Moreover, this study also showed that a chemical protein folding and trafficking chaperone (4-phenylbutyric acid) can restore normal insulin synthesis and the ability to upregulate insulin secretion in these WS-iPSC-derived β-cells [77], which suggests 4-phenylbutyric acid and potentially other chemical chaperones might protect β-cells from death arising from ER stress. Otherwise, such β-cell models could be used to test the efficacy of other candidate drugs that may be effective in preventing or delaying β-cell dysfunction and ultimately to develop novel treatments for other forms of diabetes.

The pathogenic mechanisms and/or the functional hierarchy of defective molecular processes that are responsible for the clinical outcome of diabetic patients are not fully understood in several MODY subtypes, mainly due to the poor accessibility of affected tissues, including pancreatic β-cells. Thus, the generation of patient-specific iPSCs towards glucose-responsive insulin-secreting cells represents a pivotal key step to address some of the important issues of diabetes cellular models and of human cell-based diabetes therapy in the near future of precision and regenerative medicine.

Conclusion and Future Perspectives

Over the past 25 years, the scientific community has been strongly committed to investigating the genetic determinants of MODY and its pathophysiology, mainly related to pancreatic β-cell defects, through various powerful human genome-based and cell biology-based approaches. This research has delivered outstanding achievements and insightful information which have greatly broadened our knowledge of both normal and pathologic β-cell biology and of the many faces of its functional regulation at the basis of dynamically and temporally controlled insulin secretion in humans. Most of these discoveries have proven to be crucial for a better understanding of many components involved in the pathophysiology of monogenic diabetes, particularly of the MODY subtypes.

Currently used NGS approaches are key to deciphering the large spectrum of known genetic defects underlying pancreatic islet β-cell dysfunction in diabetic conditions. In addition, they can inform us about novel genetic etiologies of familial or atypical early-onset diabetes. Then, a crucial issue will be to make timely and accurate translations of the new findings into pathophysiological events and underlying defective cellular targets. Above all, this will provide new insights to guide improved diagnosis, prevention, and therapeutic policies.

In the near future, we can expect the rapidly expanding fields of integrative genomic research and translational biology on both monogenic and polygenic forms of diabetes will open new ways towards a broader knowledge of human diabetes and foster transdisciplinary research for improved mechanistic-based treatments and a cure of some specific types of diabetes.

References

1 Tattersall RB, Fajans SS: A difference between the inheritance of classical juvenile-onset and maturity-onset type diabetes of young people. Diabetes 1975; 24:44–53.

2 Fajans SS, Bell GI: MODY: history, genetics, pathophysiology, and clinical decision making. Diabetes Care 2011;34:1878–1884.

3 Vaxillaire M, Froguel P: Monogenic diabetes in the young, pharmacogenetics and relevance to multifactorial forms of type 2 diabetes. Endocr Rev 2008;29: 254–264.

4 Ledermann HM: Maturity-onset diabetes of the young (MODY) at least ten times more common in Europe than previously assumed? Diabetologia 1995;38:1482.

5 Shields BM, Hicks S, Shepherd MH, Colclough K, Hattersley AT, Ellard S: Maturity-onset diabetes of the young (MODY): how many cases are we missing? Diabetologia 2010;53:2504–2508.

6 Irgens HU, Molnes J, Johansson BB, Ringdal M, Skrivarhaug T, Undlien DE, Søvik O, Joner G, Molven A, Njølstad PR: Prevalence of monogenic diabetes in the population-based Norwegian Childhood Diabetes Registry. Diabetologia 2013;56:1512–1519.

7 Pihoker C, Gilliam LK, Ellard S, Dabelea D, Davis C, Dolan LM, Greenbaum CJ, Imperatore G, Lawrence JM, Marcovina SM, Mayer-Davis E, Rodriguez BL, Steck AK, Williams DE, Hattersley AT: Prevalence, characteristics and clinical diagnosis of maturity onset diabetes of the young due to mutations in HNF1A, HNF4A, and glucokinase: results from the SEARCH for Diabetes in Youth. J Clin Endocrinol Metab 2013;98:4055–4062.

8 Sahu RP, Aggarwal A, Zaidi G, Shah A, Modi K, Kongara S, Aggarwal S, Talwar S, Chu S, Bhatia V, Bhatia E: Etiology of early-onset type 2 diabetes in Indians: islet autoimmunity and mutations in hepatocyte nuclear factor 1alpha and mitochondrial gene. J Clin Endocrinol Metab 2007;92:2462–2467.

9 Murphy R, Ellard S, Hattersley AT: Clinical implications of a molecular genetic classification of monogenic beta-cell diabetes. Nat Clin Pract Endocrinol Metab 2008;4:200–213.

10 Froguel P, Vaxillaire M, Sun F, Velho G, Zouali H, Butel MO, Lesage S, Vionnet N, Clément K, Fougerousse F: Close linkage of glucokinase locus on chromosome 7p to early-onset non-insulin-dependent diabetes mellitus. Nature 1992;356:162–164.

11 Vaxillaire M, Boccio V, Philippi A, Vigouroux C, Terwilliger J, Passa P, Beckmann JS, Velho G, Lathrop GM, Froguel P: A gene for maturity onset diabetes of the young (MODY) maps to chromosome 12q. Nat Genet 1995;9:418–423.

12 Vaxillaire M, Bonnefond A, Froguel P: The lessons of early-onset monogenic diabetes for the understanding of diabetes pathogenesis. Best Pract Res Clin Endocrinol Metab 2012;26:171–187.

13 Colclough K, Saint-Martin C, Timsit J, Ellard S, Bellanné-Chantelot C: Clinical utility gene card for: maturity-onset diabetes of the young. Eur J Hum Genet 2014;22:e1–e7.

14 Osbak KK, Colclough K, Saint-Martin C, Beer NL, Bellanné-Chantelot C, Ellard S, Gloyn AL: Update on mutations in glucokinase (GCK), which cause maturity-onset diabetes of the young, permanent neonatal diabetes, and hyperinsulinemic hypoglycemia. Hum Mutat 2009;30:1512–1526.

15 Matschinsky FM: Regulation of pancreatic beta-cell glucokinase: from basics to therapeutics. Diabetes 2002;51(suppl 3):S394–S404.

16 Stride A, Shields B, Gill-Carey O, Chakera AJ, Colclough K, Ellard S, Hattersley AT: Cross-sectional and longitudinal studies suggest pharmacological treatment used in patients with glucokinase mutations does not alter glycaemia. Diabetologia 2014;57:54–56.

17 García-Herrero CM, Galán M, Vincent O, Flández B, Gargallo M, Delgado-Alvarez E, Blázquez E, Navas MA: Functional analysis of human glucokinase gene mutations causing MODY2: exploring the regulatory mechanisms of glucokinase activity. Diabetologia 2007;50:325–333.

18 Sagen JV, Odili S, Bjørkhaug L, Zelent D, Buettger C, Kwagh J, Stanley C, Dahl-Jørgensen K, de Beaufort C, Bell GI, Han Y, Grimsby J, Taub R, Molven A, Søvik O, Njølstad PR, Matschinsky FM: From clinicogenetic studies of maturity-onset diabetes of the young to unraveling complex mechanisms of glucokinase regulation. Diabetes 2006;55:1713–1722.

19 Cuesta-Muñoz AL, Tuomi T, Cobo-Vuilleumier N, Koskela H, Odili S, Stride A, Buettger C, Otonkoski T, Froguel P, Grimsby J, Garcia-Gimeno M, Matschinsky FM: Clinical heterogeneity in monogenic diabetes caused by mutations in the glucokinase gene (GCK-MODY). Diabetes Care 2010;33:290–292.

20 Steele AM, Shields BM, Wensley KJ, Colclough K, Ellard S, Hattersley AT: Prevalence of vascular complications among patients with glucokinase mutations and prolonged, mild hyperglycemia. JAMA 2014;311:279–286.

21 Spégel P, Ekholm E, Tuomi T, Groop L, Mulder H, Filipsson K: Metabolite profiling reveals normal metabolic control in carriers of mutations in the glucokinase gene (MODY2). Diabetes 2013;62:653–661.

22 Velho G, Hattersley AT, Froguel P: Maternal diabetes alters birth weight in glucokinase-deficient (MODY2) kindred but has no influence on adult weight, height, insulin secretion or insulin sensitivity. Diabetologia 2000;43:1060–1063.

23 Colclough K, Bellanne-Chantelot C, Saint-Martin C, Flanagan SE, Ellard S: Mutations in the genes encoding the transcription factors hepatocyte nuclear factor 1 alpha and 4 alpha in maturity-onset diabetes of the young and hyperinsulinemic hypoglycemia. Hum Mutat 2013;34:669–685.

24 Bellanné-Chantelot C, Lévy DJ, Carette C, Saint-Martin C, Riveline J-P, Larger E, Valéro R, Gautier J-F, Reznik Y, Sola A, Hartemann A, Laboureau-Soares S, Laloi-Michelin M, Lecomte P, Chaillous L, Dubois-Laforgue D, Timsit J; French Monogenic Diabetes Study Group: Clinical characteristics and diagnostic criteria of maturity-onset diabetes of the young (MODY) due to molecular anomalies of the HNF1A gene. J Clin Endocrinol Metab 2011;96:E1346–E1351.

25 Kyithar MP, Bacon S, Pannu KK, Rizvi SR, Colclough K, Ellard S, Byrne MM: Identification of HNF1A-MODY and HNF4A-MODY in Irish families: phenotypic characteristics and therapeutic implications. Diabetes Metab 2011;37:512–519.

26 Pontoglio M, Prié D, Cheret C, Doyen A, Leroy C, Froguel P, Velho G, Yaniv M, Friedlander G: HNF1alpha controls renal glucose reabsorption in mouse and man. EMBO Rep 2000;1:359–365.

27 Reznik Y, Dao T, Coutant R, Chiche L, Jeannot E, Clauin S, Rousselot P, Fabre M, Oberti F, Fatome A, Zucman-Rossi J, Bellanne-Chantelot C: Hepatocyte nuclear factor-1 alpha gene inactivation: cosegregation between liver adenomatosis and diabetes phenotypes in two maturity-onset diabetes of the young (MODY)3 families. J Clin Endocrinol Metab 2004; 89:1476–1480.

28 Stanescu DE, Hughes N, Kaplan B, Stanley CA, De León DD: Novel presentations of congenital hyperinsulinism due to mutations in the MODY genes: HNF1A and HNF4A. J Clin Endocrinol Metab 2012; 97:E2026–E2030.

29 Bellanné-Chantelot C, Chauveau D, Gautier J-F, Dubois-Laforgue D, Clauin S, Beaufils S, Wilhelm J-M, Boitard C, Noël L-H, Velho G, Timsit J: Clinical spectrum associated with hepatocyte nuclear factor-1beta mutations. Ann Intern Med 2004;140:510–517.

30 Bingham C, Hattersley AT: Renal cysts and diabetes syndrome resulting from mutations in hepatocyte nuclear factor-1beta. Nephrol Dial Transplant 2004; 19:2703–2708.

31 Haldorsen IS, Ræder H, Vesterhus M, Molven A, Njølstad PR: The role of pancreatic imaging in monogenic diabetes mellitus. Nat Rev Endocrinol 2012;8:148–159.

32 Alvelos MI, Rodrigues M, Lobo L, Medeira A, Sousa AB, Simão C, Lemos MC: A novel mutation of the HNF1B gene associated with hypoplastic glomerulocystic kidney disease and neonatal renal failure: a case report and mutation update. Medicine (Baltimore) 2015;94:e469.

33 Clissold RL, Hamilton AJ, Hattersley AT, Ellard S, Bingham C: HNF1B-associated renal and extra-renal disease – an expanding clinical spectrum. Nat Rev Nephrol 2014;11:102–112.

34 Bonnefond A, Lomberk G, Buttar N, Busiah K, Vaillant E, Lobbens S, Yengo L, Dechaume A, Mignot B, Simon A, Scharfmann R, Neve B, Tanyolaç S, Hodoglugil U, Pattou F, Cavé H, Iovanna J, Stein R, Polak M, Vaxillaire M, Froguel P, Urrutia R: Disruption of a novel Kruppel-like transcription factor p300-regulated pathway for insulin biosynthesis revealed by studies of the c.-331 INS mutation found in neonatal diabetes mellitus. J Biol Chem 2011;286:28414–28424.

35 Støy J, Steiner DF, Park S-Y, Ye H, Philipson LH, Bell GI: Clinical and molecular genetics of neonatal diabetes due to mutations in the insulin gene. Rev Endocr Metab Disord 2010;11:205–215.

36 Colombo C, Porzio O, Liu M, Massa O, Vasta M, Salardi S, Beccaria L, Monciotti C, Toni S, Pedersen O, Hansen T, Federici L, Pesavento R, Cadario F, Federici G, Ghirri P, Arvan P, Iafusco D, Barbetti F; Early Onset Diabetes Study Group of the Italian Society of Pediatric Endocrinology and Diabetes (SIEDP): Seven mutations in the human insulin gene linked to permanent neonatal/infancy-onset diabetes mellitus. J Clin Invest 2008;118:2148–2156.

37 Meur G, Simon A, Harun N, Virally M, Dechaume A, Bonnefond A, Fetita S, Tarasov AI, Guillausseau P-J, Boesgaard TW, Pedersen O, Hansen T, Polak M, Gautier J-F, Froguel P, Rutter GA, Vaxillaire M: Insulin gene mutations resulting in early-onset diabetes: marked differences in clinical presentation, metabolic status, and pathogenic effect through endoplasmic reticulum retention. Diabetes 2010;59:653–661.

38 Borowiec M, Liew CW, Thompson R, Boonyasrisawat W, Hu J, Mlynarski WM, El Khattabi I, Kim S-H, Marselli L, Rich SS, Krolewski AS, Bonner-Weir S, Sharma A, Sale M, Mychaleckyj JC, Kulkarni RN, Doria A: Mutations at the BLK locus linked to maturity onset diabetes of the young and beta-cell dysfunction. Proc Natl Acad Sci U S A 2009;106:14460–14465.

39 Bonnefond A, Yengo L, Philippe J, Dechaume A, Ezzidi I, Vaillant E, Gjesing AP, Andersson EA, Czernichow S, Hercberg S, Hadjadj S, Charpentier G, Lantieri O, Balkau B, Marre M, Pedersen O, Hansen T, Froguel P, Vaxillaire M: Reassessment of the putative role of BLK-p.A71T loss-of-function mutation in MODY and type 2 diabetes. Diabetologia 2013;56:492–496.

40 Riveline J-P, Rousseau E, Reznik Y, Fetita S, Philippe J, Dechaume A, Hartemann A, Polak M, Petit C, Charpentier G, Gautier J-F, Froguel P, Vaxillaire M: Clinical and metabolic features of adult-onset diabetes caused by ABCC8 mutations. Diabetes Care 2012;35:248–251.

41 Bonnefond A, Philippe J, Durand E, Dechaume A, Huyvaert M, Montagne L, Marre M, Balkau B, Fajardy I, Vambergue A, Vatin V, Delplanque J, Le Guilcher D, De Graeve F, Lecoeur C, Sand O, Vaxillaire M, Froguel P: Whole-exome sequencing and high throughput genotyping identified KCNJ11 as the thirteenth MODY gene. PloS One 2012;7:e37423.

42 Rigoli L, Lombardo F, Di Bella C: Wolfram syndrome and WFS1 gene. Clin Genet 2011;79:103–117.

43 Zalloua PA, Azar ST, Delépine M, Makhoul NJ, Blanc H, Sanyoura M, Lavergne A, Stankov K, Lemainque A, Baz P, Julier C: WFS1 mutations are frequent monogenic causes of juvenile-onset diabetes mellitus in Lebanon. Hum Mol Genet 2008;17:4012–4021.

44 Bonnycastle LL, Chines PS, Hara T, Huyghe JR, Swift AJ, Heikinheimo P, Mahadevan J, Peltonen S, Huopio H, Nuutila P, Narisu N, Goldfeder RL, Stitzel ML, Lu S, Boehnke M, Urano F, Collins FS, Laakso M: Autosomal dominant diabetes arising from a Wolfram syndrome 1 mutation. Diabetes 2013;62:3943–3950.

45 Raeder H, Johansson S, Holm PI, Haldorsen IS, Mas E, Sbarra V, Nermoen I, Eide SA, Grevle L, Bjørkhaug L, Sagen JV, Aksnes L, Søvik O, Lombardo D, Molven A, Njølstad PR: Mutations in the CEL VNTR cause a syndrome of diabetes and pancreatic exocrine dysfunction. Nat Genet 2006;38:54–62.

46 Martin D, Bellanné-Chantelot C, Deschamps I, Froguel P, Robert J-J, Velho G: Long-term follow-up of oral glucose tolerance test-derived glucose tolerance and insulin secretion and insulin sensitivity indexes in subjects with glucokinase mutations (MODY2). Diabetes Care 2008;31:1321–1323.

47 Klupa T, Solecka I, Nowak N, Szopa M, Kiec-Wilk B, Skupien J, Trybul I, Matejko B, Mlynarski W, Malecki MT: The influence of dietary carbohydrate content on glycaemia in patients with glucokinase maturity-onset diabetes of the young. J Int Med Res 2011;39:2296–2301.

48 Shepherd M, Pearson ER, Houghton J, Salt G, Ellard S, Hattersley AT: No deterioration in glycemic control in HNF-1alpha maturity-onset diabetes of the young following transfer from long-term insulin to sulphonylureas. Diabetes Care 2003;26:3191–3192.

49 Katra B, Klupa T, Skupien J, Szopa M, Nowak N, Borowiec M, Kozek E, Malecki MT: Dipeptidyl peptidase-IV inhibitors are efficient adjunct therapy in HNF1A maturity-onset diabetes of the young patients – report of two cases. Diabetes Technol Ther 2010;12:313–316.

50 McDonald TJ, Shields BM, Lawry J, Owen KR, Gloyn AL, Ellard S, Hattersley AT: High-sensitivity CRP discriminates HNF1A-MODY from other subtypes of diabetes. Diabetes Care 2011;34:1860–1862.

51 Thanabalasingham G, Shah N, Vaxillaire M, Hansen T, Tuomi T, Gašperíková D, Szopa M, Tjora E, James TJ, Kokko P, Loiseleur F, Andersson E, Gaget S, Isomaa B, Nowak N, Raeder H, Stanik J, Njolstad PR, Malecki MT, Klimes I, Groop L, Pedersen O, Froguel P, McCarthy MI, Gloyn AL, Owen KR: A large multicentre European study validates high-sensitivity C-reactive protein (hsCRP) as a clinical biomarker for the diagnosis of diabetes subtypes. Diabetologia 2011;54:2801–2810.

Vaxillaire · Froguel

52 Besser RE, Shepherd MH, McDonald TJ, Shields BM, Knight BA, Ellard S, Hattersley AT: Urinary C-peptide creatinine ratio is a practical outpatient tool for identifying hepatocyte nuclear factor 1-{alpha}/hepatocyte nuclear factor 4-{alpha} maturity-onset diabetes of the young from long-duration type 1 diabetes. Diabetes Care 2011;34:286–291.

53 Gloyn AL, Faber JH, Malmodin D, Thanabalasingham G, Lam F, Ueland PM, McCarthy MI, Owen KR, Baunsgaard D: Metabolic profiling in maturity-onset diabetes of the young (MODY) and young onset type 2 diabetes fails to detect robust urinary biomarkers. PloS One 2012;7:e40962.

54 Guay C, Regazzi R: Role of islet microRNAs in diabetes: which model for which question? Diabetologia 2015;58:456–463.

55 Bonner C, Nyhan KC, Bacon S, Kyithar MP, Schmid J, Concannon CG, Bray IM, Stallings RL, Prehn JHM, Byrne MM: Identification of circulating microRNAs in HNF1A-MODY carriers. Diabetologia 2013;56:1743–1751.

56 Ellard S, Bellanné-Chantelot C, Hattersley AT: Best practice guidelines for the molecular genetic diagnosis of maturity-onset diabetes of the young. Diabetologia 2008;51:546–553.

57 Rubio-Cabezas O, Hattersley AT, Njølstad PR, Mlynarski W, Ellard S, White N, Chi DV, Craig ME: The diagnosis and management of monogenic diabetes in children and adolescents. Pediatr Diabetes 2014;15(suppl 20):47–64.

58 Shields BM, McDonald TJ, Ellard S, Campbell MJ, Hyde C, Hattersley AT: The development and validation of a clinical prediction model to determine the probability of MODY in patients with young-onset diabetes. Diabetologia 2012;55:1265–1272.

59 Stanik J, Dusatkova P, Cinek O, Valentinova L, Huckova M, Skopkova M, Dusatkova L, Stanikova D, Pura M, Klimes I, Lebl J, Gasperikova D, Pruhova S: De novo mutations of GCK, HNF1A and HNF4A may be more frequent in MODY than previously assumed. Diabetologia 2014;57:480–484.

60 Thanabalasingham G, Pal A, Selwood MP, Dudley C, Fisher K, Bingley PJ, Ellard S, Farmer AJ, McCarthy MI, Owen KR: Systematic assessment of etiology in adults with a clinical diagnosis of young-onset type 2 diabetes is a successful strategy for identifying maturity-onset diabetes of the young. Diabetes Care 2012; 35:1206–1212.

61 Pinelli M, Acquaviva F, Barbetti F, Caredda E, Cocozza S, Delvecchio M, Mozzillo E, Pirozzi D, Prisco F, Rabbone I, Sacchetti L, Tinto N, Toni S, Zucchini S, Iafusco D; Italian Study Group on Diabetes of the Italian Society of Pediatric Endocrinology and Diabetology: Identification of candidate children for maturity-onset diabetes of the young type 2 (MODY2) gene testing: a seven-item clinical flowchart (7-iF). PloS One 2013;8:e79933.

62 Van der Zwaag AM, Weinreich SS, Bosma AR, Rigter T, Losekoot M, Henneman L, Cornel MC: Current and best practices of genetic testing for maturity onset diabetes of the young: views of professional experts. Public Health Genomics 2015;18:52–59.

63 Naylor RN, John PM, Winn AN, Carmody D, Greeley SAW, Philipson LH, Bell GI, Huang ES: Cost-effectiveness of MODY genetic testing: translating genomic advances into practical health applications. Diabetes Care 2014;37:202–209.

64 Bonnefond A, Philippe J, Durand E, Muller J, Saeed S, Arslan M, Martínez R, De Graeve F, Dhennin V, Rabearivelo I, Polak M, Cavé H, Castaño L, Vaxillaire M, Mandel J-L, Sand O, Froguel P: Highly sensitive diagnosis of 43 monogenic forms of diabetes or obesity through one-step PCR-based enrichment in combination with next-generation sequencing. Diabetes Care 2014;37:460–467.

65 Ellard S, Lango Allen H, De Franco E, Flanagan SE, Hysenaj G, Colclough K, Houghton JA, Shepherd M, Hattersley AT, Weedon MN, Caswell R: Improved genetic testing for monogenic diabetes using targeted next-generation sequencing. Diabetologia 2013; 56:1958–1963.

66 Alkorta-Aranburu G, Carmody D, Cheng YW, Nelakuditi V, Ma L, Dickens JT, Das S, Greeley SA, del Gaudio D: Phenotypic heterogeneity in monogenic diabetes: the clinical and diagnostic utility of a gene panel-based next-generation sequencing approach. Mol Genet Metab 2014;113:315–320.

67 Dusatkova P, Fang M, Pruhova S, Gjesing AP, Cinek O, Hansen T, Pedersen OB, Xu X, Lebl J: Lessons from whole-exome sequencing in MODYX families. Diabetes Res Clin Pract 2014;104:e72–e74.

68 Sun Y, Ruivenkamp CAL, Hoffer MJV, Vrijenhoek T, Kriek M, van Asperen CJ, den Dunnen JT, Santen GWE: Next Generation Diagnostics: Gene Panel, Exome or Whole Genome? Hum Mutat 2015;36: 648–655.

69 Yang Y, Muzny DM, Xia F, Niu Z, Person R, Ding Y, et al: Molecular findings among patients referred for clinical whole-exome sequencing. JAMA 2014;312: 1870–1879.

70 López-Garrido MP, Herranz-Antolín S, Alija-Merillas MJ, Giralt P, Escribano J: Co-inheritance of HNF1a and GCK mutations in a family with maturity-onset diabetes of the young (MODY): implications for genetic testing. Clin Endocrinol (Oxf) 2013;79: 342–347.

71 Bennett JT, Vasta V, Zhang M, Narayanan J, Gerrits P, Hahn SH: Molecular genetic testing of patients with monogenic diabetes and hyperinsulinism. Mol Genet Metab 2015;114:451–458.

72 Simaite D, Kofent J, Gong M, Rüschendorf F, Jia S, Arn P, Bentler K, Ellaway C, Kühnen P, Hoffmann GF, Blau N, Spagnoli FM, Hübner N, Raile K: Recessive mutations in PCBD1 cause a new type of early-onset. Diabetes 2014;63:3557–3564.

73 Abdelalim EM, Bonnefond A, Bennaceur-Griscelli A, Froguel P: Pluripotent stem cells as a potential tool for disease modelling and cell therapy in diabetes. Stem Cell Rev 2014;10:327–337.

74 Teo AKK, Windmueller R, Johansson BB, Dirice E, Njolstad PR, Tjora E, Raeder H, Kulkarni RN: Derivation of human induced pluripotent stem cells from patients with maturity onset diabetes of the young. J Biol Chem 2013;288:5353–5356.

75 Hua H, Shang L, Martinez H, Freeby M, Gallagher MP, Ludwig T, Deng L, Greenberg E, Leduc C, Chung WK, Goland R, Leibel RL, Egli D: iPSC-derived β cells model diabetes due to glucokinase deficiency. J Clin Invest 2013;123:3146–3153.

76 Pagliuca FW, Millman JR, Gürtler M, Segel M, Van Dervort A, Ryu JH, Peterson QP, Greiner D, Melton DA: Generation of functional human pancreatic β cells in vitro. Cell 2014;159:428–439.

77 Shang L, Hua H, Foo K, Martinez H, Watanabe K, Zimmer M, Kahler DJ, Freeby M, Chung W, LeDuc C, Goland R, Leibel RL, Egli D: β-Cell dysfunction due to increased ER stress in a stem cell model of Wolfram syndrome. Diabetes 2014;63:923–933.

78 Yabe SG, Iwasaki N, Yasuda K, Hamazaki TS, Konno M, Fukuda S, Takeda F, Kasuga M, Okochi H: Establishment of maturity onset diabetes of the young (MODY)-iPS cells from Japanese patient. J Diabetes Investig 2015;6:543–547.

79 Bonnefond A, Froguel P: Rare and Common genetic events in type 2 diabetes: what should biologists know? Cell Metab 2015;21:357–368.

Martine Vaxillaire, PharmD, PhD
CNRS-UMR 8199, Integrative Genomics and Modelling of Metabolic Diseases
European Genomic Institute for Diabetes (EGID)
Faculty of Medicine – Pole Recherche (1st Floor)
1 place de Verdun
FR–59045 Lille (France)
E-Mail martine.vaxillaire@cnrs.fr

Philippe Froguel, MD, PhD
Department of Genomics of Common Diseases
School of Public Health, Hammersmith Hospital
Imperial College Faculty of Medicine
Room E303, Burlington-Danes Building
Du Cane Road, London W12 0NN (UK)
E-Mail p.froguel@imperial.ac.uk

Barbetti F, Ghizzoni L, Guaraldi F (eds): Diabetes Associated with Single Gene Defects and Chromosomal Abnormalities. Front Diabetes. Basel, Karger, 2017, vol 25, pp 49–54 (DOI: 10.1159/000454700)

Thiamine-Responsive Megaloblastic Anemia Syndrome

Adriana Franzese · Valentina Fattorusso · Enza Mozzillo

Section of Pediatrics, Department of Translational Sciences, Federico II University of Naples, Naples, Italy

Abstract

Thiamine-responsive megaloblastic anemia (TRMA) syndrome (OMIM No. 249270) is an autosomal recessive disorder and an example of a rare form of monogenic diabetes coexisting with anemia and deafness. The disease is caused by mutations in the SLC19A2 gene encoding the high-affinity thiamine transporter 1 (h-THTR1), which is the major route of delivery thiamine in a variety of cells lines: pancreatic β-cells, cochlear cells, hemopoietic tissues, and retinal pigment epithelial cells. Deficiency of the transport mechanism leads to an inadequate intracellular concentration of thiamine and cell apoptosis. Treatment with pharmacological doses of thiamine ameliorates megaloblastic anemia and diabetes mellitus, while sensorineural hearing loss is irreversible and may not be prevented even if therapy is started in infancy. Optic atrophy and retinal dystrophy have been seen in patients, but no studies are present in the literature showing the efficacy of treatment, started in infancy, with thiamine on maculopathy.   © 2017 S. Karger AG, Basel

Thiamine-responsive megaloblastic anemia (TRMA) syndrome (OMIM No. 249270) is a rare autosomal recessive inherited disorder of thiamine metabolism due to loss-of-function mutations in the thiamine transport *SLC19A2* gene, which resides on chromosome 1q23.2-23 and encodes the high-affinity thiamine transporter 1 (h-THTR1) [1]; it is also called Rogers' syndrome [2]. It is a rare condition and only around 80 cases have been described (Orphanet 2014), with only a few in Europe [3–6]. This syndrome is clinically defined by the occurrence of megaloblastic anemia, diabetes, and sensorineural deafness. In addition to the classic triad of symptoms, a number of other, more rare, organ defects including congenital heart malformations [7, 8], trilineage myelodysplasia, optic atrophy and retinal degeneration [9, 10], and situs viscerum inversus; aminoaciduria; polycystic ovary syndrome; and stroke have been reported [11–14]. *SLC19A2* is widely expressed in human tissues; indeed h-THTR1, which it encodes, is the major route of thiamine delivery in a variety of cells lines, such as pancreatic β-cells, cochlear cells, hemopoietic tissues, and retinal pigment epithelial ARPE-19 cells [15–17], with the highest expression in skeletal muscle [18]. Deficiency of h-THTR1 results in a defective transport mechanism of the thiamine, which leads to an inadequate intracellular concentration of thiamine and apoptosis [19]. Thiamine is a water-soluble vitamin found in high concentrations in all tissues including skeletal muscle, heart, liver, kidney, and the brain. It plays a role in several major metabolic processes, such as carbohydrate metabolism and biosynthesis of cell constituents, including neurotransmitters. Furthermore, it is involved in the production of reducing equivalents in oxidant stress defenses and in the synthesis of pentoses considered as nucleic acid precursors [20]. Normal thiamine homeostasis involves 4 steps: (1) uptake of thiamine from the gut, (2) transport to tissues and into cells, (3) conversion of thiamine into the cofactor form thiamine pyrophosphate by thiamine pyrophosphokinase, and (4) binding of thiamine pyrophosphate to apoenzymes [21–23]. Two uptake pathways exist for thiamine intracellular absorption. Firstly, at concentrations lower than 1 μmol/l, thiamine is transported mainly by an active carrier-mediated system that involves the intracellular phosphorylation of the vitamin [21]. Secondly, at higher concentrations, simple passive diffusion prevails [24]. In fact, TRMA can be clinically improved through administration of pharmacological doses.

Anemia

Anemia in TRMA syndrome is usually an early finding in infancy or early childhood [25]. The classic hematological profile in this syndrome is macrocytic anemia with ringed sideroblasts, but a number of different types of anemia have been reported in TRMA, such as sideroblastic and aplastic anemia, thrombocytopenia, and neutropenia [11]. Anemia is responsive within a few weeks of starting high-dose thiamine treatment, but erythrocytes remain macrocytic [24, 26]. Very different doses have been administered to the patients reported by the literature, ranging from 25 to 250 mg/day [27, 28]. During puberty the supplementation might become ineffective and blood transfusions could be necessary [29].

Diabetes

In TRMA, another component is nonautoimmune diabetes mellitus, the onset of which is usually early, i.e., in childhood, in TRMA patients [27]. Recent studies indicate that TRMA syndrome should be considered when additional features like parental consanguinity are present, in case of neonatal diabetes [30]. Thiamine is required by pancreatic β-cells for glucose transport across the cell membrane and its physiological utilization, as well as for insulin secretion. In addition, thiamine administration improves glucose tolerance in patients with TRMA. Diabetes mellitus in TRMA is most likely secondary to impairment of β-cell function and secondary to β-cell apoptosis because of intracellular thiamine deficiency. β-Cells are able to produce and secrete insulin after stimulation with glucagon, but they are probably affected by an impaired response after glucose stimulation in TRMA patients [3]. Early institution of appropriate integration of thiamine improves diabetes in TRMA and may result in prolonged periods of noninsulin treatment [3, 4], but during puberty the supplementation could become ineffective and the insulin requirement might increase [4, 29].

Deafness

Another cardinal finding of TRMA syndrome is sensorineural deafness because h-THTR1 is expressed in the inner hair cells within the cochlea [31], and the loss of *SLC19A2* results in selective inner hair cell loss and an auditory neuropathy phenotype [32], a consequence of metabolic abnormalities in the auditory pathways. Hearing loss is progressive and mild hearing loss may not be noticed by parents in the early months of life. Most of the TRMA cases reported to date have been diagnosed after infancy when hearing loss was already present at the time of diagnosis. Sensorineural deafness is irreversible in all patients, although some investigators have reported that thiamine therapy prevented further progression of deafness [33], but did not prevent deafness onset when treatment was started at 20 months of age [34].

Ocular Pathology

Some reports have shown the involvement of h-THTR1 in the uptake process of thiamine in a cellular model of human retinal pigment epithelium. The retinal pigment epithelium is part of the blood-retinal barrier and plays an important role in the delivery of nutrients to the highly differentiated and metabolically active retina. Mutations of h-THTR1 lead to impaired cell surface expression and to an impairment in the nutrient transport function of these cells that may adversely affect the retina [15]. The ophthalmic features of TRMA patients include cone rod dystrophy, optic atrophy, and retinitis pigmentosa [35, 36]. It has been argued that optic atrophy or retinal dystrophy could be extreme consequences seen in older patients who had a delayed diagnosis [36]. A recent case report showed that retinal maculopathy progressed in a 13-year-old girl after 5 years of follow-up despite a special thiamine diet, but in this case thiamine treatment was not started in infancy [37]. To date, there are no studies on the efficacy of thiamine treatment, started in infancy, in preventing ocular pathology in the literature.

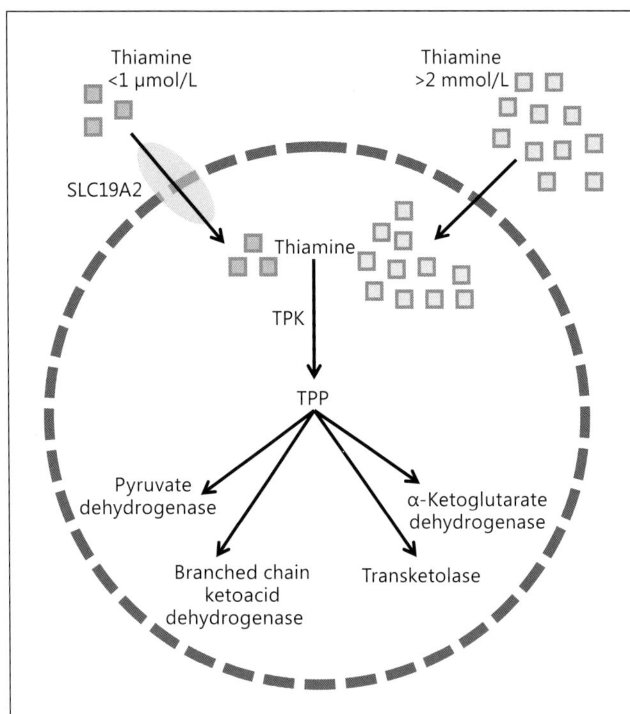

Fig. 1. The metabolic pathways of thiamine in mammalian cells. Thiamine enters in the cells either through nonsaturable low-affinity uptake or by SLC19A2. In the cells, thiamine is converted to thiamine diphosphate (TPP) by the thiamine pyrophosphokinase enzyme (TPK). TPP is a cofactor for 4 enzymes.

Discussion

Thiamine is essential for all tissues, and thiamine uptake into the cells follows a biphasic curve: nonlinear at low concentrations and linear at high concentrations. Under physiological circumstances (low thiamine concentrations), SLC19A2, the saturable high-affinity low-capacity carrier, transports thiamine, while at high concentrations (>2 mmol/L), thiamine diffuses passively over the cell membrane via a low affinity/high-capacity mechanism. In the cell, thiamine is converted to thiamine diphosphate by the enzyme thiamine pyrophosphokinase (Fig. 1). Diagnosis of TRMA should be suspected in patients with syndromic diabetes including hearing loss and anemia, even if the latter is only very mild. Deafness, a cardinal component of the syndrome, may not be present at the onset of disease in infancy. If TRMA is diagnosed or suspected, investigations of cardiac function and an ophthalmologic examination should be carried out because of the variable additional symptoms. Early institution of appropriate thiamine supplementation does not appear to prevent hearing loss in these patients, but early diagnosis is essential because substitutive therapy with adequate doses of thiamine after diagnosis can prevent or significantly delay anemia and diabetes. Data about thiamine treatment efficacy to prevent ocular maculopathy (cone rod dystrophy, optic atrophy, and/or retinitis pigmentosa) are not present in the literature.

References

1 Neufeld EJ, Fleming JC, Tartaglini E, Steinkamp MP: Thiamine-responsive megaloblastic anemia syndrome: a disorder of high-affinity thiamine transport. Blood Cells Mol Dis 2001;27:135–138.

2 Rogers LE, Porter FS, Sidbury JB Jr: Thiamine-responsive megaloblastic anemia. J Pediatr 1969;74:494–504.

3 Mozzillo E, Melis D, Falco M, Fattorusso V, Taurisano R, Flanagan SE, Ellard S, Franzese A: Thiamine responsive megaloblastic anemia: a novel SLC19A2 compound heterozygous mutation in two siblings. Pediatr Diabetes 2013;14:384–387.

4 Valerio G, Franzese A, Poggi V, Tenore A: Long-term follow-up of diabetes in two patients with thiamine-responsive megaloblastic anemia syndrome. Diabetes Care 1998;21:38–41.

5 Pichler H, Zeitlhofer P, Dworzak MN, Diakos C, Haas OA, Kager L: Thiamine-responsive megaloblastic anemia (TRMA) in an Austrian boy with compound heterozygous SLC19A2 mutations. Eur J Pediatr 2012;171:1711–1715.

6 Mikstiene V, Songailiene J, Byckova J, Rutkauskiene G, Jasinskiene E, Verkauskiene R, Lesinskas E, Utkus A: Thiamine responsive megaloblastic anemia syndrome: a novel homozygous SLC19A2 gene mutation identified. Am J Med Genet A 2015;167:1605–1609.

7 Gritli S, Omar S, Tartaglini E, Guannouni S, Fleming JC, Steinkamp MP, Berul CI, Hafsia R, Jilani SB, Belhani A, Hamdi M, Neufeld EJ: A novel mutation in the SLC19A2 gene in a Tunisian family with thiamine-responsive megaloblastic anaemia, diabetes and deafness syndrome. Br J Haematol 2001;113:508–513.

8 Lorber A, Gazit AZ, Khoury A, Schwartz Y, Mandel H: Cardiac manifestations in thiamine-responsive megaloblastic anemia syndrome. Pediatr Cardiol 2003;24:476–481.

9 Meire FM, Van Genderen MM, Lemmens K, Ens-Dokkum MH: Thiamine-responsive megaloblastic anemia syndrome (TRMA) with cone-rod dystrophy. Ophthalmic Genet 2000;21:243–250.

10 Rindi G, Casirola D, Poggi V, De Vizia B, Patrini C, Laforenza U: Thiamine transport by erythrocytes and ghosts in thiamine-responsive megaloblastic anaemia. J Inherit Metab Dis 1992;15:231–242.

11 Oishi K, Diaz GA: Thiamine-responsive megaloblastic anemia syndrome; in Pagon RA, Adam MP, Ardinger HH, Wallace SE, Amemiya A, Bean LJH, Bird TD, Fong CT, Mefford HC, Smith RJH, Stephens K (eds): GeneReviews® (Internet). Oct 24, 2003 (updated November 20, 2014), Seattle, University of Washington.

12 Gritli S, Omar S, Tartaglini E, Guannouni S, Fleming JC, Steinkamp MP, Berul CI, Hafsia R, Jilani SB, Belhani A, Hamdi M, Neufeld EJ: A novel mutation in the SLC19A2 gene in a Tunisian family with thiamine-responsive megaloblastic anaemia, diabetes and deafness syndrome. Br J Haematol 2001;113:508–513.

13 Viana MB, Carvalho RI: Thiamine-responsive megaloblastic anemia, sensorineural deafness, and diabetes mellitus: a new syndrome? J Pediatr 1978;93:235–238.

14 Setoodeh A, Haghighi A, Saleh-Gohari N, Ellard S, Haghighi A: Identification of a SLC19A2 nonsense mutation in Persian families with thiamine-responsive megaloblastic anemia. Gene 2013;519:295–297.

15 Subramanian VS, Mohammed ZM, Molina A, Marchant JS, Vaziri ND, Said HM: Vitamin B_1 (thiamine) uptake by human retinal pigment epithelial (ARPE-19) cells: mechanism and regulation. J Physiol 2007;582:73–85.

16 Ashokkumar B, Vaziri ND, Said HM: Thiamin uptake by the human-derived renal epithelial (HEK-293) cells: cellular and molecular mechanisms. Am J Physiol Renal Physiol 2006;291:F796–F805.

17 Mee L, Nabokina SM, Sekar VT, Subramanian VS, Maedler K, Said HM: Pancreatic beta cells and islets take up thiamin by a regulated carrier-mediated process: studies using mice and human pancreatic preparations. Am J Physiol Gastrointest Liver Physiol 2009;297:G197–G206.

18 Dutta B, Huang W, Molero M, Kekuda R, Leibach FH, Devoe LD, Ganapathy V, Prasad PD: Cloning of the human thiamine transporter, a member of the folate transporter family. J Biol Chem 1999;274:31925–31929.

19 Alzahrani A, Baitei E, Zou M, Shi Y: Thiamine transporter mutation: an example of monogenic diabetes mellitus. Eur J Endocrinol 2006;155:787–792.

20 Singleton CK, Martin PR: Molecular mechanisms of thiamine utilization. Curr Mol Med 2001;1:197–207.

21 Rindi G, Ferrari G: Thiamine transport by human intestine in vitro. Experientia 1977;33:211–213.

22 Hoyumpa AM Jr, Strickland R, Sheehan JJ, Yarborough G, Nichols S: Dual system of intestinal thiamine transport in humans. J Lab Clin Med 1982;99:701–708.

23 Laforenza U, Patrini C, Alvisi C, Faelli A, Licandro A, Rindi G: Thiamine uptake in human intestinal biopsy specimens, including observations from a patient with acute thiamine deficiency. Am J Clin Nutr 1997;66:320–326.

24 Kurtoglu S, Hatipoglu N, Keskin M, Kendirci M, Akcakus M: Thiamine withdrawal can lead to diabetic ketoacidosis in thiamine responsive megaloblastic anemia: report of two siblings. J Pediatr Endocrinol Metab 2008;21:393–397.

25 Zmysłowska A, Młynarski W: Megaloblastic anaemia in infancy or early childhood and diabetes as leading symptoms of the TRMA syndrome. Pediatr Endocrinol Diabetes Metab 2012;18:37–39.

26 Zhao R, Goldman ID: Folate and thiamine transporters mediated by facilitative carriers (SLC19A1-3 and SLC46A1) and folate receptors. Mol Aspects Med 2013;34:373–385.

27 Olsen BS, Hahnemann JMD, Schwartz M, Østergaard E: Thiamine-responsive megaloblastic anemia: a cause of syndromic diabetes in childhood. Pediatr Diabetes 2007;8:239–241.

28 Borgna-Pignatti C, Azzalli M, Pedretti S: Thiamine-responsive megaloblastic anemia syndrome: long term follow-up. J Pediatr 2009;155:295–297.

29 Ricketts CJ, Minton JA, Samuel J, Ariyawansa I, Wales JK, Lo IF, Barrett TG: Thiamine-responsive megaloblastic anaemia syndrome: long-term follow-up and mutation analysis of seven families. Acta Paediatr 2006;95:99–104.

30 Shaw-Smith C, Flanagan SE, Patch A-M, Grulich-Henn J, Habeb AM, Hussain K, Pomahacova R, Matyka K, Abdullah M, Hattersley AT, Ellard S: Recessive SLC19A2 mutations are a cause of neonatal diabetes mellitus in thiamine-responsive megaloblastic anaemia. Pediatr Diabetes 2012;13:314–321.

31 Fleming JC, Steinkamp MP, Kawatsuji R, Tartaglini E, Pinkus JL, Pinkus GS, Fleming MD, Neufeld EJ: Characterization of a murine high-affinity thiamine transporter, SLC19A2. Mol Genet Metab 2001;74:273–280.

32 Liberman MC, Tartaglini E, Fleming JC, Neufeld EJ: Deletion of SLC19A2, the high affinity thiamine transporter, causes selective inner hair cell loss and an auditory neuropathy phenotype. J Assoc Res Otolaryngol 2006;7:211–217.

33 Poggi V, Longo G, DeVizia B, Andria G, Rindi G, Patrini C, Cassandro E: Thiamin-responsive megaloblastic anemia: a disorder of thiamine transport? J Inherit Metab Dis 1984;7(suppl 2):153–154.

34 Akın L, Kurtoğlu S, Kendirci M, Akın MA, Karakükçü M: Does early treatment prevent deafness in thiamine-responsive megaloblastic anaemia syndrome? J Clin Res Pediatr Endocrinol 2011;3:36–39.

35 Lagarde WH, Underwood LE, Moats-Staats BM, Calikoglu AS: Novel mutation in the SLC19A2 gene in an African-American female with thiamine-responsive anemia syndrome. Am J Med Genet A 2004;125A:299–305.

36 Meire FM, Van Genderen MM, Lemmens K, Ens-Dokkum MH: Thiamine-responsive megaloblastic anemia syndrome (TRMA) with cone rod dystrophy. Ophthalmic Genet 2000;21:243–250.

37 Ach T, Kardorff R, Rohrschneider K: Fundus autofluorescence and optical coherence tomography findings in thiamine responsive megaloblastic anemia. Retin Cases Brief Rep 2015;9:114–116.

Prof. Adriana Franzese
Section of Pediatrics, Department of Translational Sciences
Federico II University of Naples, Via S. Pansini 5
IT–80131 Naples (Italy)
E-Mail franzese@unina.it

Barbetti F, Ghizzoni L, Guaraldi F (eds): Diabetes Associated with Single Gene Defects and Chromosomal Abnormalities. Front Diabetes. Basel, Karger, 2017, vol 25, pp 55–68 (DOI: 10.1159/000454701)

Diabetes Mellitus in Mitochondrial Disease

Yi Shiau Ng · Robert W. Taylor · Andrew M. Schaefer

Wellcome Trust Centre for Mitochondrial Research, Institute of Neuroscience, The Medical School, Newcastle University, Newcastle upon Tyne, UK

Abstract

Mitochondrial diseases arise as a consequence of respiratory chain dysfunction caused by mutations in the mitochondrial genome (mtDNA) or nuclear-encoded mitochondrial genes. Multisystem involvement is a hallmark of many subtypes of mitochondrial disease in which energy-dependent organs including the brain, skeletal muscles, and heart are commonly affected. The most common mitochondrial genotype that causes diabetes mellitus is a single nucleotide substitution (m.3243A>G) in the mitochondrial tRNA$^{Leu(UUR)}$ gene which is linked to a distinctive clinical phenotype – maternally inherited diabetes and deafness. Diabetes mellitus often arises insidiously as part of the clinical presentation associated with mitochondrial disease; however, there are unique clinical features and associated complications compared to other diabetes subtypes. Overall, the treatment of patients with mitochondrial diabetes is similar to those with other causes of diabetes but with additional emphasis on the screening and subsequent management of additional multiorgan involvement.

Mitochondrial disease is a collective term for an ever-increasing number of clinically and genetically heterogeneous disorders that harbour a defect of mitochondrial oxidative phosphorylation (OXPHOS). This occurs as a result of a mutation of either the mitochondrial DNA (mtDNA)- or nuclear DNA-encoded genes responsible for mtDNA maintenance and repair. Multisystem involvement is typical of the mitochondrial disorders, but may not be immediately apparent on first presentation, and is easy to overlook in the early stages of disease. Diabetes mellitus is a common feature of mitochondrial disease, but rarely occurs in isolation; other clinical features depend largely on the underlying mtDNA or nuclear DNA mutation. This association was appreciated in families with either a large-scale mtDNA rearrangement (duplication) or the m.3243A>G mtDNA point mutation over 20 years ago [1, 2]. Subsequently, maternally inherited diabetes and deafness (MIDD) was proposed as a distinct subtype of diabetes mellitus associated with the m.3243A>G mutation [3]. It has since become clear that the m.3243A>G mutation is by far the commonest cause of diabetes amongst the mitochondrial disorders. This is in part because MIDD represents the commonest phenotype associated with the m.3243A>G mutation, but also because prevalence studies of mtDNA-related disease identify the m.3243A>G mutation as by far the most prevalent of all the known pathogenic mutations associated with mitochondrial disease [4, 5].

This chapter begins with an overview of basic mitochondrial biochemistry and the influence exerted by both the mitochondrial and nuclear genomes. We discuss the mechanisms believed to underlie mitochondrial diabetes, how this results in differing diabetic phenotypes, and the role of pattern recognition in diagnosis. The mitochondrial phenotypes associated with diabetes are discussed and best clinical practice considered.

Mitochondrial Biochemistry and Genetics

Mitochondria are cellular organelles found in all nucleated cells, one important role of which is the generation of energy in the form of adenosine triphosphate (ATP) via OXPHOS. The OXPHOS system consists of the mitochondrial respiratory chain (complex I to IV), ATP synthase (complex V), and 2 electron carriers (coenzyme Q10 and cytochrome c). Mitochondria also play important roles in apoptosis, calcium signalling, and iron-sulphur protein biogenesis and haem metabolism.

mtDNA is a double-stranded, small, circular molecule with 16,569 base pairs [6]. mtDNA encodes for 37 genes of which 13 are polypeptides that form the subunits of the OXPHOS system, 22 tRNAs, and 2 rRNAs. It is maternally inherited and present within cells in multiple copies depending on the energy demand of the particular tissue. When all mtDNA copies are identical (i.e., all are wild-type or all harbour mutation), the scenario is referred to as homoplasmy. In contrast, when both mutated and wild-type mtDNA molecules coexist within the same cell or tissue the scenario is described as heteroplasmy [6]. Primary mutations in mtDNA include single nucleotide substitutions (point mutations) and large-scale mtDNA rearrangements which often take the form of single mtDNA deletions. Each individual mtDNA mutation exhibits different thresholds of mtDNA heteroplasmy required to demonstrate significant respiratory chain deficiency, and the same is true of individual tissues which require different heteroplasmic thresholds before disease becomes manifest. The resulting levels of heteroplasmy are determined by segregation of mtDNA through the "genetic bottleneck" and amplification during oogenesis [6]. Heteroplasmic levels of pathogenic mtDNA mutations are broadly correlated with onset of disease and severity, at least in several common point mutations such as the m.3243A>G and m.8344A>G mutations. It is generally accepted that single, large-scale mtDNA deletions arise sporadically and demonstrate a very low risk of transmission [7].

In contrast to the mitochondrial genome that encodes for only a small number of genes, more than 1,300 nuclear gene products are implicated in the mitochondrial proteome, playing various vital roles including encoding most of the subunits for the respiratory chain and all their assembly factors, enzymes involved in mtDNA replication, maintenance, repair, and mitochondrial dynamics, factors involved in mitochondrial protein translation although the function of many genes remain undetermined. Currently, there are more than 200 of these genes established to cause mitochondrial disease [8]. Inheritance patterns are mendelian, with autosomal dominant and autosomal recessive (AR) disease more prevalent than X-linked disorders. For several genes such as *POLG1*, *PEO1*, and *RRM2B*, both dominant and recessive forms of disease exist, with the recessive forms commonly associated with more severe phenotypes. The mtDNA polymerase gamma *(POLG)* gene is the only known gene involved in mtDNA replication and repair, and it is associated with a wide spectrum of clinical phenotypes ranging from early-childhood onset Alpers syndrome to late-adulthood-onset chronic progressive external ophthalmoplegia. Recessive and dominant *POLG* mutations represent one of the commonest nuclear causes of mitochondrial disease, although recent studies have suggested that mutations in the *SPG7* gene may be as prevalent [5].

Pathogenesis of Mitochondrial Diabetes

Plasma glucose levels are tightly regulated in normal individuals. In pancreatic tissue, glucose enters the plasma membrane of β-cells and is phosphorylated by glucokinase to glucose-6-phosphate, which determines the rate of glycolysis and the rate of pyruvate generation. Pyruvate enters the TCA (tricarboxylic acid) or Krebs cycle, and the final product is the generation of ATP in the mitochondria. ATP is exported to the cytosol and causes depolarisation of the plasma membrane by the closure of the ATP-sensitive K^+ channels, and subsequently leads to opening of the Ca^{2+} channel, resulting in an increase in cytosolic calcium and exocytosis of insulin [9]. The net effect of insulin is to normalise blood glucose levels by increasing glucose uptake and protein synthesis in muscle, promoting glycogen synthesis in liver (and meanwhile decreasing the gluconeogenesis) and lipid synthesis in the adipose tissue.

The development of mitochondrial diabetes is not fully understood, but its mechanism appears to be different from the autoimmunity seen in type 1 diabetes and peripheral insulin resistance associated with type 2 diabetes. Insulin secretion is ATP dependent and therefore the respiratory chain dysfunction caused by mitochondrial disease can lead to impaired exocytosis of insulin by pancreatic β-cells. Various clinical studies have supported this notion in m.3243A>G carriers by demonstrating reduced insulin and/or C-peptide secretion, particularly the first-phase response in the intravenous glucose tolerance test [10–12] and oral mixed liquid meal challenge [13]. Postmortem studies of the pancreas have revealed reduction in the islet cell mass, but found no evidence of an autoimmune process. Such findings are consistent with the absence of islet cell antibodies shown in different clinical studies [4, 14, 15]. Surprisingly low heteroplasmy levels were found in individual pancreatic β-cells at autopsy, postulated to represent apoptosis of the most severely affected cells [16]. This hypothesis may also explain the interesting observation that the heteroplasmy levels within pancreatic islets did not show any correlation with the severity of diabetes in those individuals [17]. Most of the early studies have not produced evidence of insulin resistance in patients with MIDD [12, 15]; however, this is a controversial issue because conflicting findings have been reported [18]. A more recent study using PET (positron emission tomography) scans of skeletal muscle demonstrated reduction in glucose uptake among individuals with the m.3243A>G mutation, even among those individuals with normal oral glucose tolerance test compared to healthy controls during euglycaemic hyperinsulinaemia. The insulinogenic index (the marker of insulin secretion) was significantly lower in the diabetic m.3243A>G group compared to control and non-diabetic m.3243A>G groups. The authors suggested that insulin resistance is a contributing factor to the development of diabetes in these patients and that this may precede the impairment of β-cell function [19]. In addition, a further study demonstrated increased gluconeogenesis in both diabetic and non-diabetic m.3243A>G mutation carriers, but also identified the diabetic group as showing evidence of insulin resistance in addition to a relative insulin deficiency (i.e., similar fasting plasma insulin level despite higher plasma glucose levels), suggesting multiple defects in insulin and glucose metabolism are crucial for the development of mitochondrial diabetes [20].

Whilst impaired ATP production is generally accepted as the primary mechanism involved in mitochondrial diabetes, questions remain as to why diabetes tends to develop after other manifestations of disease such as sensorineural deafness [21]. On average, diabetes develops at about 37 or 38 years of age, and rarely presents in childhood even where other signs of disease may be advanced [4, 14]. The mechanisms that account for the progressive nature of impaired insulin secretion in individuals with the m.3243A>G mutation is also poorly understood, with patients typically progressing to insulin requirement within 2 years of the diabetes diagnosis [14]. In well-defined cohorts utilising screening programmes for asymptomatic carriers, early diagnosis of impaired glucose tolerance likely explains the observation of a 4-year delay from the diagnosis of diabetes to insulin dependence [4]. An accelerated ageing process mediated by increased production of reactive oxygen species and apoptosis in the pancreatic β-cells with m.3243A>G mutation seems the most likely hypothesis [10].

Diabetic Phenotypes in Mitochondrial Disease

Multisystem involvement is the hallmark of mitochondrial disease (Fig. 1). Postmitotic tissues with high energy demands such as the brain, heart, skeletal muscles, and endocrine pancreas are frequently affected. Throughout all the known mitochondrial disorders, neurological involvement is most commonly reported, but diabetes

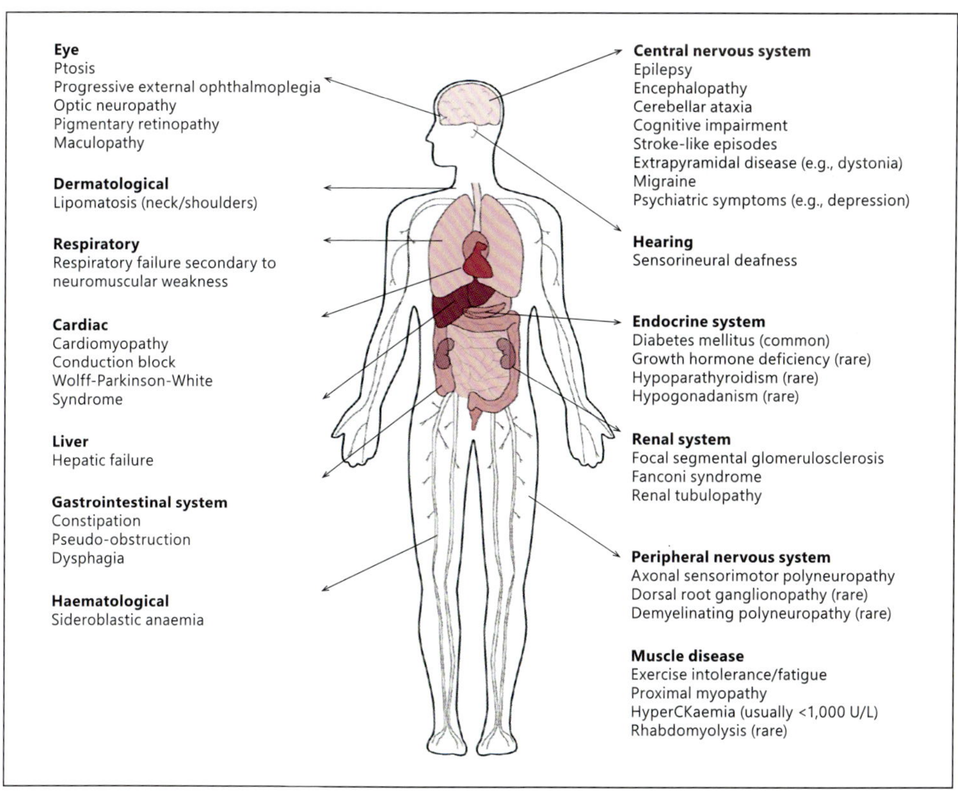

Fig. 1. Multisystem involvement in mitochondrial disease.

mellitus frequently coexists, particularly in the m.3243A>G mtDNA point mutation.

Diabetes mellitus is prevalent and affects approximately 6% of the UK population [22]. Diabetes is also a well-recognised phenotype in mitochondrial disease caused by mtDNA mutations and to a lesser extent mutations of the nuclear genome. The mitochondrial tRNA$^{Leu(UUR)}$ *(MT-TL1)* m.3243A>G point mutation is the most common pathogenic mtDNA mutation [5], and it has been identified in up to 2.8% of unselected diabetic populations [23]. The minimum prevalence of clinically manifest disease due to pathogenic mtDNA mutations alone is reported to be 9.6 per 100,000 in the North East of England [5]. This study highlighted mitochondrial disease to be one of the commonest inherited neuromuscular disorders, but the frequent association of the m.3243A>G mutation with diabetes also confirms mitochondrial disease as a significant cause of monogenic diabetes – albeit a mutation of the mtDNA rather than the nuclear genome. The point prevalence of diabetes mellitus among cohorts with the m.3243A>G mutation has been reported to range from 37 to 42% according to recent case series [4, 24–26]. Other mtDNA point mutations in which diabetes is recognised as part of the clinical phenotype include the m.14709T>C, m.14577T>C, m.8296A>G, and other rarer mutations [10, 27, 28]. More recently, combined data from a cohort study and literature review (n = 321) identified that the point prevalence of diabetes was 6.2% in those carrying the m.8344A>G mutation, which is close to the prevalence within the general population. It therefore seems unlikely that diabetes should be considered an intrinsic component of the clinical phenotype in this mutation [29].

The frequency of diabetes in a single, large-scale mtDNA deletion was reported to range from 11 to 14% [4, 30]. Diabetes appeared more prevalent in those with Kearns-Sayre syndrome compared to more benign chronic progressive external ophthalmoplegia phenotypes in a Japanese study (15 vs. 1%) [31], in keeping with the early multisystem disease seen in Kearns-Sayre syndrome. Many isolated case reports connecting rare mtDNA mutations with diabetes exist but can be difficult to interpret. It is important that the pathogenicity of the reported mtDNA variant has been confirmed previously, has additional supporting evidence from functional analysis, or exhibits cosegregation of disease with the mtDNA mutation in the pedigree.

Although pathogenic mutations have been identified in more than 200 nuclear genes to date [8], only *POLG* mutations show a prevalence of diabetes in excess of that expected for the general population [32]. Case series of patients with *TWNK* [33] or *RRM2B* [34] mutations do not suggest diabetes to be part of the phenotype, with levels of diabetes no greater than background population prevalence. The prevalence of diabetes in less frequently encountered nuclear mutations remains unknown. Anecdotal evidence would suggest that it is much rarer than that seen in mtDNA mutations, but larger case series are required.

Pattern Recognition: Multisystem Involvement and Inheritance

Mitochondrial disease represents a significant diagnostic challenge to clinicians because of its clinical heterogeneity and the absence of a "full house" of clinical features until late in the course of the disease. Individual components of the disease may occur in apparent isolation and can mimic other common disorders. Mitochondrial diabetes rarely occurs in isolation, but may appear so if multisystem involvement is subtle or not specifically sought. Fatigue, irritable bowel symptoms, migraine, and mild hearing impairment are all common in the general population, yet are common features of mitochondrial disease as well. These symptoms are rarely volunteered or looked for if the focus of a consultation is elsewhere, and individually have little predictive value for mitochondrial disease. Together, however, they start to build a case for mitochondrial dysfunction and this case is strengthened by the presence of rarer features such as significant presenile deafness, cardiomyopathy or conduction defects, renal dysfunction, or a family history (in most cases maternal) of similar or other unexpected disorders. Apparent end-organ disease (renal impairment, cardiomyopathy, neuropathy, or retinopathy) should raise suspicion if it appears beyond that expected for the level of glycaemic control.

Pattern Recognition: Diabetic Phenotype in Mitochondrial Disease

Age-At-Onset

The majority of patients with mitochondrial diabetes present insidiously, similar to type 2 diabetes. The mean age of presentation is 37–38 and this finding has been reproduced in both French and UK patient cohorts [4, 14]. Sensorineural hearing loss often precedes the onset of diabetes, but is often either undiagnosed or overlooked as a relevant clinical feature.

Body Mass Index

The majority of patients with mitochondrial diabetes have a mean body mass index (BMI) of less than 20 [14, 35], as compared to typical patients with type 2 diabetes in whom obesity is highly prevalent. Low BMI appears to correlate with the severity of insulin deficiency in the m.3243A>G mutation [14], but it should be noted that a lower BMI is often also associated with a more severe clinical phenotype (e.g., MELAS syndrome) and a higher disease burden in general [21].

Insulin Requirement

The majority of MIDD patients are treated with diet-control or oral hypoglycaemics initially, and only 13–17% of individuals require insulin treatment at the onset [4, 14]. Less than 10% of MIDD patients have ketoacidosis as the initial presentation of their diabetes [36]. It is therefore unusual for mitochondrial diabetes to mimic type 1 diabetes and autoantibodies associated with type 1 diabetes are generally absent. Several studies have suggested that transition to insulin treatment is more rapid in mitochondrial diabetes than type 2 diabetes. On average, insulin is required within 2–4 years, the longer transition period possibly a reflection of very early diagnosis in a UK cohort where diabetes was identified as a result of strict screening programmes in both symptomatic patients and asymptomatic carriers [4].

End-Organ Involvement

Retinopathy

Diabetic retinopathy is relatively uncommon in mitochondrial diabetes. It is observed in less than 10% of patients with a mean duration of diabetes of more than 10 years [37, 38]. It is thought that the reduction in retinal metabolism could lead to decreased production of sorbitol, which plays a role in the pathogenesis of diabetic retinopathy [38]. However, retinal changes characteristic of mtDNA disease are present in between 77 and 86% of patients with the m.3243A>G mutation, and there is a strong association between glucose intolerance and pigmentary retinopathy [14, 39]. These include hyperpigmentation particularly in the macula ("salt and pepper" appearance) and retinal pigment atrophy. The majority of these changes are benign and the prognosis is correlated to the extent of retinal atrophy and involvement of the fovea [40]. Blindness can occur when atrophic changes affect the fovea and mimic age-related macular degeneration [41]. Cataracts appears less prevalent in mitochondrial diabetes. This has been proposed to be due to reduced glucose metabolism by the polyol pathway [39].

Nephropathy
Proteinuria is more prevalent among individuals with mitochondrial diabetes due to the m.3243A>G mutation compared to an age-matched diabetic group with comparable duration of both disease and treatment (54 vs. 29%) [37]. The higher prevalence of renal impairment in MIDD patients compared to other types of diabetes might suggest an increased vulnerability to diabetic microvascular complications due to coexistent respiratory chain deficiencies in renal tissues [4]. Certainly some patients with the m.3243A>G mutation develop kidney disease in the absence of diabetes, suggesting a renal vulnerability to OXPHOS defects as might be expected in a postmitotic tissue. In a minority of patients this rapidly progresses to end-stage renal failure, and renal biopsies have shown focal segmental glomerulosclerosis [37, 42] and less frequently tubulointerstitial changes [42]. The mechanism of underlying kidney disease in mitochondrial disease is perhaps independent of, but worsened by, coexistent diabetic kidney disease as demonstrated by a recent study where abnormalities in the urinary protein and metabolite excretion were observed across different phenotypes in mitochondrial disease and not exclusively confined to those with diabetes [43]. The prevalence of dialysis in diabetic patients with the m.3243A>G mutation has been reported to be approximately 6% in a Japanese study, well above the expected average [44].

Cardiac Disease
Patients with mitochondrial disease, and in particular the m.3243A>G mutation, are at risk of cardiac involvement. Left ventricular hypertrophy is identified in 38–56% of the m.3243A>G patients [45]. Wolff-Parkinson-White syndrome is frequently associated with the m.3243A>G and m.8344A>G mutations, and conduction block is present in a quarter of patients with single mtDNA deletions [31]. The treatment choice for left ventricular hypertrophy is usually an angiotensin-converting enzyme inhibitor or (if intolerant to angiotensin-converting enzyme inhibitors) an angiotensin receptor blocker which is conveniently the same recommendation (at the time of writing) for hypertension and/or microalbuminuria in diabetes [45]. Cardiac autonomic dysfunction appears to be more severe in diabetic patients with the m.3243A>G mutation compared to the ordinary diabetic group as shown in several small case control studies by studying the heart rate variability [46] and cardiac MIBG scintigraphy [47].

Currently, there are limited longitudinal studies examining the risks of coronary artery disease and other macrovascular diseases in patients with mitochondrial disease. According to a multicentre prospective study of diabetic patients with the m.3243A>G mutation (n = 57), coronary artery disease and peripheral vascular disease affected 7 and 3.5% of their patients, suggesting that the prevalence of macrovascular complications is lower in this group compared to the type 2 diabetic population [36].

Neuropathy

The overall prevalence of neuropathy in m.3243A>G cohorts varies from 10 to 27% [4, 24, 25] and where present is almost invariably an axonal sensory motor neuropathy. It should be stressed, however, that the neuropathy is usually very mild or asymptomatic. Among the carriers of the m.3243A>G mutation, neuropathy is more prevalent in those with diabetes when compared to those without diabetes (58 vs. 8%), and the mean interval from the onset of diabetes to the development of neuropathy is 7 years [4]. As we have earlier hypothesised for renal disease, it may be that the metabolic compromise present within peripheral nerves heightens their vulnerability to end-organ disease resulting from poor glycaemic control. When considering the prevalence of the m.3243A>G mutation in diabetic populations, the presence of a sensory neuropathy significantly increased the diagnostic yield (9.8 vs. 1.1%) in a Japanese study, suggesting that neuropathy is one of several examples of multisystem involvement that helps in terms of pattern recognition in mitochondrial disease [48].

Stroke-Like Episodes

Stroke-like episodes are an acute and severe neurological complication strongly associated with the m.3243A>G mutation and to a much lesser extent other mtDNA and nuclear mutations. It rarely presents like an acute thromboembolic stroke and in this sense the term "stroke-like episode" can be misleading. Typically, patients present with obtundation due to insipient encephalopathy, headache, and visual symptoms. The presentation is often more suggestive of migraine than stroke, but positive visual phenomena are often due to non-convulsive status epilepticus involving the occipital lobes. Urgent control of seizures is vital. MRI appearances may vary, but typically show changes which may appear to cross vascular territories and have a predilection for posterior parietal and occipital lobes. In mitochondrial diabetes, it is important to consider the nature of any such events, remembering that not all "stroke-like episodes" will be strokes, but equally that mitochondrial patients are not immune to atherosclerosis.

Diagnosis of Mitochondrial Diseases

Blood-derived DNA has been widely used as a screening and diagnostic tool for several common mtDNA mutations such as m.3243A>G and m.8344A>G mutations. Whilst the mutation load of m.8344A>G can be reliably measured in blood for various age groups, it is important to take into consideration that false-negative results can arise in m.3243A>G mutation because blood mtDNA heteroplasmy levels decrease with age [49]. In addition to that, the nature of tissue segregation of mutation load means that heteroplasmy levels of some mtDNA mutations can only be detected in postmitotic tissues such as skeletal muscle. Measurement of urine heteroplasmy level is advocated as a better non-invasive alternative and has been shown to correlate well with heteroplasmy levels from muscle [50]. In patients who have undergone renal transplantation, however, urine-derived DNA samples are no longer representative and cannot be interpreted reliably (unpublished data). Currently, muscle biopsy remains an integral part of the diagnostic algorithm for mitochondrial disease if screening of common mutations from non-invasive tissues is negative. Investigating mitochondrial disease can remain a laborious process even when respiratory chain dysfunction is detected in the muscle tissue given the potential for screening large numbers of candidate genes. However, the emergence of next-generation and whole-exome sequencing is revolutionizing this field and an increasingly rapid turnaround for diagnostic studies seems inevitable.

Diabetic Screening in Mitochondrial Disease

Diabetic screening is recommended for all asymptomatic mutation carriers by measuring HbA_{1c} annually. For symptomatic patients who display hyperglycaemic symptoms, random glucose and HbA_{1c} should be measured promptly. Patients carrying the m.3243A>G mutation are at higher risk of developing gestational diabetes and oral glucose tolerance should be considered.

Management

Diet and/or oral hypoglycaemic agents are used initially. We recommend a short-acting sulphonylurea initially as occasionally patients are sensitive to sulphonylurea-induced hypoglycaemia. When patients require second-line treatment, newer agents (e.g., DPP-4 inhibitors and GLP-1 analogues) can be considered. Metformin is best avoided in mitochondrial diabetes as there is a risk of exacerbating lactic acidosis. This is not an absolute contraindication, however, as many patients commenced on metformin prior to a formal diagnosis of mitochondrial disease seem to tolerate it well. This is especially true of those with obesity, though this observation does raise the question as to the nature of the diabetes in those individuals. Thiazolidinedione might not be a suitable choice because of its risk profile in heart failure and the high incidence of hypertrophic cardiomyopathy in patients with mtDNA mutations. The transition to insulin therapy from the diagnosis of diabetes appears to be rapid with an average of less than 4 years in m.3243A>G cohorts [4, 35].

Although certain complications such as diabetic retinopathy are less prevalent in mitochondrial diabetes, other micro- and macrovascular complications should be managed similarly to other diabetic groups. Secondary prevention with a statin is generally recommended for diabetic patients. There is a lack of evidence to suggest that patients with mitochondrial myopathy are more susceptible to statin-induced myositis, but such concern is commonly encountered in the clinical setting. We believe that the benefit of risk reduction in atherosclerosis probably outweighs the potential risk in many cases, but caution should be taken. Mild elevation of creatinine kinase (CK <1,000 IU) is often present in patients with mitochondrial disease at baseline and can vary significantly between measurements. We therefore recommend at least one CK measurement prior to commencement of a statin. Any significant rise from the baseline CK level, or new myalgia and/or deteriorating weakness, should prompt review. Alternatively, other lipid-lowering agents such as fibrates and ezetimibe can be used although myositis has also been reported in the latter and similar caution is recommended. Best practice guidelines for the diagnosis and management of mitochondrial diabetes are available online (http://www.newcastle-mitochondria.com/clinical-professional-home-page/clinical-publications/clinical-guidelines/).

Conclusion

Mitochondrial diabetes is a rare but distinctive subtype of diabetes mellitus. The inherent differences in pathogenesis as compared to either type 1 or type 2 diabetes often result in an atypical presentation which may, in its own right, arouse suspicion. Onset is often insidious and in adulthood, like type 2 diabetes, but associated with a low rather than high BMI. Progression to insulin requirements is often rapid. Most commonly a result of the m.3243A>G mutation, awareness of the underlying diagnosis may rely upon recognition of a maternal inheritance pattern or the presence of associated clinical features such as sensorineural deafness, hypertrophic cardiomyopathy, pigmentary retinopathy, and/or other multisystem involvement. The extent of diagnostic investigations are guided by the level of clinical suspicion, but in most cases the m.3243A>G mutation can be reliably excluded using mtDNA extracted from both blood and urine samples. To fully exclude other forms of mitochondrial disease, a skeletal muscle biopsy and/or specialist referral may be required. At the time of writing, there is no known cure or effective disease-modifying treatment for mitochondrial disease itself, and therefore the focus of management centres largely on genetic advice and counselling, supportive care, and treatment of recognised multisystem disease. In family members at risk, or those known to carry pathogenic mtDNA (or nuclear DNA) mutations, we currently recommend annual diabetic screening so that effective treatment can be initiated early in the disease and diabetic complications avoided or minimised. Diabetic care for patients with mitochondrial disease is very similar to care provided for other diabetic patients, with the notable exceptions that

(1) obesity is rarely present, and in fact a low BMI and poor calorific intake is typical; (2) metformin is usually avoided; and (3) additional comorbidities (such as cognitive impairment) may need to be considered when developing a patient-specific management plan. It is important to adopt a multidisciplinary approach to achieve these goals, and close liaison with a specialist centre for the care of patients with mitochondrial disease is recommended.

Acknowledgement

Y.S.N. receives funding for PhD study from the Medical Research Council (UK) Neuromuscular Centre. R.W.T. receives support from the Wellcome Trust Centre for Mitochondrial Research (096919Z/11/Z), the Medical Research Council (UK) Centre for Translational Muscle Disease Research (G0601943), the Medical Research Council (UK) Mitochondrial Disease Patient Cohort (G0800674), the Lily Foundation, and the UK NHS Highly Specialised "Rare Mitochondrial Disorders of Adults and Children" Service.

References

1 Ballinger SW, Shoffner JM, Hedaya EV, Trounce I, Polak MA, Koontz DA, et al: Maternally transmitted diabetes and deafness associated with a 10.4 kb mitochondrial DNA deletion. Nat Genet 1992;1:11–15.

2 van den Ouweland JM, Lemkes HH, Ruitenbeek W, Sandkuijl LA, de Vijlder MF, Struyvenberg PA, et al: Mutation in mitochondrial tRNA(Leu)(UUR) gene in a large pedigree with maternally transmitted type II diabetes mellitus and deafness. Nat Genet 1992;1: 368–371.

3 van den Ouweland JMW, Lemkes HHPJ, Trembath RC, Ross R, Velho G, Cohen D, et al: Maternally inherited diabetes and deafness is a distinct subtype of diabetes and associates with a single point mutation in the mitochondrial tRNA(Leu(UUR)) gene. Diabetes 1994;43:746–751.

4 Whittaker RG, Schaefer AM, McFarland R, Taylor RW, Walker M, Turnbull DM: Prevalence and progression of diabetes in mitochondrial disease. Diabetologia 2007;50:2085–2089.

5 Gorman GS, Schaefer AM, Ng Y, Gomez N, Blakely EL, Alston CL, et al: Prevalence of nuclear and mitochondrial DNA mutations related to adult mitochondrial disease. Ann Neurol 2015;77:753–759.

6 Taylor RW, Turnbull DM: Mitochondrial DNA mutations in human disease. Nat Rev Genet 2005;6: 389–402.

7 Chinnery PF, DiMauro S, Shanske S, Schon EA, Zeviani M, Mariotti C, et al: Risk of developing a mitochondrial DNA deletion disorder. Lancet 2004;364: 592–596.

8 Koopman WJH, Willems PHGM, Smeitink JAM: Monogenic mitochondrial disorders. N Engl J Med 2012;366:1132–1141.

9 Maechler P, Wollheim CB: Mitochondrial function in normal and diabetic beta-cells. Nature 2001;414: 807–812.

10 Maassen JA, 't Hart LM, van Essen E, Heine RJ, Nijpels G, Jahangir Tafrechi RS, et al: Mitochondrial diabetes: molecular mechanisms and clinical presentation. Diabetes 2004;53(suppl 1):S103–S109.

11 Brändle M, Lehmann R, Maly FE, Schmid C, Spinas GA: Diminished insulin secretory response to glucose but normal insulin and glucagon secretory responses to arginine in a family with maternally inherited diabetes and deafness caused by mitochondrial tRNA(LEU(UUR)) gene mutation. Diabetes Care 2001;24:1253–1258.

12 Walker M, Taylor RW, Stewart MW, Bindoff L, Shearing PA, Anyaoku V, et al: Insulin and proinsulin secretion in subjects with abnormal glucose tolerance and a mitochondrial tRNALeu(UUR) mutation. Diabetes Care 1995;18:1507–1509.

13 Salles JE, Kasamatsu TS, Dib SA, Moisés RS: β-cell function in individuals carrying the mitochondrial tRNA(Leu(UUR)) mutation. Pancreas 2007;34:133–137.

14 Guillausseau PJ, Dubois-Laforgue D, Massin P, Laloi-Michelin M, Bellanné-Chantelot C, Gin H, et al: Heterogeneity of diabetes phenotype in patients with 3243 bp mutation of mitochondrial DNA (maternally inherited diabetes and deafness or MIDD). Diabetes Metab 2004;30:181–186.

Ng · Taylor · Schaefer

15 Kadowaki T, Kadowaki H, Mori Y, Tobe K, Sakuta R, Suzuki Y, et al: A subtype of diabetes mellitus associated with a mutation of mitochondrial DNA. N Engl J Med 1994;330:962–968.

16 Lynn S, Borthwick GM, Charnley RM, Walker M, Turnbull DM: Heteroplasmic ratio of the A3243G mitochondrial DNA mutation in single pancreatic beta cells. Diabetologia 2003;46:296–299.

17 Otabe S, Yasuda K, Mori Y, Shimokawa K, Kadowaki H, Jimi A, et al: Molecular and histological evaluation of pancreata from patients with a mitochondrial gene mutation associated with impaired insulin secretion. Biochem Biophys Res Commun 1999;259:149–156.

18 Gebhart SS, Shoffner JM, Koontz D, Kaufman A, Wallace D: Insulin resistance associated with maternally inherited diabetes and deafness. Metabolism 1996;45:526–531.

19 Lindroos MM, Majamaa K, Tura A, Mari A, Kalliokoski KK, Taittonen MT, et al: m.3243A>G mutation in mitochondrial DNA leads to decreased insulin sensitivity in skeletal muscle and to progressive β-cell dysfunction. Diabetes 2009;58:543–549.

20 El-Hattab AW, Emrick LT, Hsu JW, Chanprasert S, Jahoor F, Scaglia F, et al: Glucose metabolism derangements in adults with the MELAS m.3243A>G mutation. Mitochondrion 2014;18:63–69.

21 Schaefer AM, Walker M, Turnbull DM, Taylor RW: Endocrine disorders in mitochondrial disease. Mol Cell Endocrinol 2013;379:2–11.

22 Quality and Outcomes Framework Achievement, Prevalence and Exceptions Data, 2012/13. Leeds, Health and Social Care Information Centre (HSCIC). 2013.

23 Murphy R, Turnbull DM, Walker M, Hattersley AT: Clinical features, diagnosis and management of maternally inherited diabetes and deafness (MIDD) associated with the 3243A>G mitochondrial point mutation. Diabet Med 2008;25:383–399.

24 de Laat P, Koene S, van den Heuvel LP, Rodenburg RJ, Janssen MC, Smeitink JA: Clinical features and heteroplasmy in blood, urine and saliva in 34 Dutch families carrying the m.3243A>G mutation. J Inherit Metab Dis 2012;35:1059–1069.

25 Mancuso M, Orsucci D, Angelini C, Bertini E, Carelli V, Comi G, et al: The m.3243A>G mitochondrial DNA mutation and related phenotypes. A matter of gender? J Neurol 2014;261:504–510.

26 Nesbitt V, Pitceathly RDS, Turnbull DM, Taylor RW, Sweeney MG, Mudanohwo EE, et al: The UK MRC Mitochondrial Disease Patient Cohort Study: clinical phenotypes associated with the m.3243A>G mutation – implications for diagnosis and management. J Neurol Neurosurg Psychiatry 2013;84:936–938.

27 Suzuki S, Hinokio Y, Hirai S, Onoda M, Matsumoto M, Ohtomo M, et al: Diabetes with mitochondrial gene tRNALYS Mutation. Diabetes Care 1994;17:1428–1432.

28 Tsukuda K, Suzuki Y, Kameoka K, Osawa N, Goto Y, Katagiri H, et al: Screening of patients with maternally transmitted diabetes for mitochondrial gene mutations in the tRNA[Leu(UUR)] region. Diabet Med 1997;14:1032–1037.

29 Mancuso M, Orsucci D, Angelini C, Bertini E, Carelli V, Comi GP, et al: Phenotypic heterogeneity of the 8344A>G mtDNA "MERRF" mutation. Neurology 2013;80:2049–2054.

30 Khambatta S, Nguyen DL, Beckman TJ, Wittich CM: Kearns-Sayre syndrome: a case series of 35 adults and children. Int J Gen Med 2014;7:325–332.

31 Yamashita S, Nishino I, Nonaka I, Goto Y: Genotype and phenotype analyses in 136 patients with single large-scale mitochondrial DNA deletions. J Hum Genet 2008;53:598–606.

32 Horvath R, Hudson G, Ferrari G, Futterer N, Ahola S, Lamantea E, et al: Phenotypic spectrum associated with mutations of the mitochondrial polymerase gamma gene. Brain 2006;129:1674–1684.

33 Fratter C, Gorman GS, Stewart JD, Buddles M, Smith C, Evans J, et al: The clinical, histochemical, and molecular spectrum of PEO1 (Twinkle)-linked adPEO. Neurology 2010;74:1619–1626.

34 Pitceathly RDS, Smith C, Fratter C, Alston CL, He L, Craig K, et al: Adults with RRM2B-related mitochondrial disease have distinct clinical and molecular characteristics. Brain 2012;135:3392–3403.

35 Suzuki S, Oka Y, Kadowaki T, Kanatsuka A, Kuzuya T, Kobayashi M, et al: Clinical features of diabetes mellitus with the mitochondrial DNA 3243 (A-G) mutation in Japanese: maternal inheritance and mitochondria-related complications. Diabetes Res Clin Pract 2003;59:207–217.

36 Guillausseau P-J, Massin P, Dubois-LaForgue Dl, Timsit J, Virally M, Gin H, et al: Maternally inherited diabetes and deafness: a multicenter study. Ann Intern Med 2001;134:721–728.

37 Massin P, Dubois-Laforgue D, Meas T, Laloi-Michelin M, Gin H, Bauduceau B, et al: Retinal and renal complications in patients with a mutation of mitochondrial DNA at position 3,243 (maternally inherited diabetes and deafness). A case-control study. Diabetologia 2008;51:1664–1670.

38 Holmes-Walker DJ, Mitchell P, Boyages SC: Does mitochondrial genome mutation in subjects with maternally inherited diabetes and deafness decrease severity of diabetic retinopathy? Diabet Med 1998;15:946–952.

39 Holmes-Walker DJ, Mitchell P, Boyages SC: Does mitochondrial genome mutation in subjects with maternally inherited diabetes and deafness decrease severity of diabetic retinopathy? Diabet Med 1998; 15:946–952.

40 de Laat P, Smeitink JAM, Janssen MCH, Keunen JEE, Boon CJF: Mitochondrial retinal dystrophy associated with the m.3243A>G mutation. Ophthalmology 2013;120:2684–2696.

41 Feigl B, Morris CP: Visual function and risk genotypes in maternally inherited diabetes and deafness. Can J Ophthalmol J 2013;48:e111–e114.

42 Guéry B, Choukroun G, Noël L-H, Clavel P, Rötig A, Lebon S, et al: The spectrum of systemic involvement in adults presenting with renal lesion and mitochondrial tRNA(Leu) gene mutation. J Am Soc Nephrol 2003;14:2099–2108.

43 Hall AM, Vilasi A, Garcia-Perez I, Lapsley M, Alston CL, Pitceathly RD, et al: The urinary proteome and metabonome differ from normal in adults with mitochondrial disease. Kidney Int 2015;87:610–622.

44 Iwasaki N, Babazono T, Tsuchiya K, Tomonaga O, Suzuki A, Togashi M, et al: Prevalence of A-to-G mutation at nucleotide 3243 of the mitochondrial tRNA(Leu(UUR)) gene in Japanese patients with diabetes mellitus and end stage renal disease. J Hum Genet 2001;46:330–334.

45 Bates MG, Bourke JP, Giordano C, d'Amati G, Turnbull DM, Taylor RW: Cardiac involvement in mitochondrial DNA disease: clinical spectrum, diagnosis, and management. Eur Heart J 2012;33:3023–3033.

46 Momiyama Y, Suzuki Y, Ohtomo M, Atsumi Y, Matsuoka K, Ohsuzu F, et al: Cardiac autonomic nervous dysfunction in diabetic patients with a mitochondrial DNA mutation: assessment by heart rate variability. Diabetes Care 2002;25:2308–2313.

47 Ueno H, Shiotani H: Cardiac abnormalities in diabetic patients with mutation in the mitochondrial tRNA(Leu(UUR)) gene. Jpn Circ J 1999;63:877–880.

48 Suzuki Y, Taniyama M, Muramatsu T, Ohta S, Murata C, Atsumi Y, et al: Mitochondrial tRNA(Leu(UUR)) mutation at position 3243 and symptomatic polyneuropathy in type 2 diabetes. Diabetes Care 2003;26:1315–1316.

49 Rahman S, Poulton J, Marchington D, Suomalainen A: Decrease of 3243 A→G mtDNA mutation from blood in MELAS syndrome: a longitudinal study. Am J Hum Genet 2001;68:238–240.

50 Whittaker RG, Blackwood JK, Alston CL, Blakely EL, Elson JL, McFarland R, et al: Urine heteroplasmy is the best predictor of clinical outcome in the m.3243A>G mtDNA mutation. Neurology 2009;72: 568–569.

Prof. Robert W. Taylor or Dr. Andrew M. Schaefer
Wellcome Trust Centre for Mitochondrial Research, Institute of Neuroscience
The Medical School, Newcastle University, Framlington Place
Newcastle upon Tyne NE2 4HH (UK)
E-Mail robert.taylor@newcastle.ac.uk, andrew.schaefer@nuth.nhs.uk

Barbetti F, Ghizzoni L, Guaraldi F (eds): Diabetes Associated with Single Gene Defects and Chromosomal Abnormalities. Front Diabetes. Basel, Karger, 2017, vol 25, pp 69–77 (DOI: 10.1159/000454702)

Diabetes in Wolfram Syndrome: Update of Clinical and Genetic Aspects

Luciana Concetta Rigoli[a] · Giuseppe d'Annunzio[b]

[a]Department of Pediatrics, Medical School, University of Messina, Messina, and [b]Regional Center for Pediatric Diabetes, IRCCS Istituto Giannina Gaslini, Genova, Italy

Abstract

Mutations of the WFS1 (Wolfram syndrome 1) gene cause Wolfram syndrome, which is a rare autosomal recessive disorder characterized by juvenile diabetes mellitus, optic atrophy, deafness, and diabetes insipidus. These clinical characteristics are associated with other variable manifestations. The product encoded by the WFS1 gene, wolframin, could be involved in the endoplasmic reticulum stress response causing β-cell loss through impaired cell cycle progression and increased apoptosis. Recently, another causative gene, CISD2, has been identified from patients with a type of WS (WFS2) resulting in early optic atrophy, diabetes mellitus, deafness, decreased lifespan, and gastrointestinal ulceration, but not diabetes insipidus. The aim of this chapter is to review the current knowledge on these conditions.   © 2017 S. Karger AG, Basel

Wolfram syndrome (WS) (OMIM 222300) is a rare neurodegenerative disease (RN1290) with autosomal recessive inheritance, characterized by early onset of non-autoimmune diabetes mellitus, followed by optic atrophy, leading to blindness, diabetes insipidus, hearing loss, and other neurological, renal, and endocrine dysfunctions [1]. The acronym DIDMOAD (diabetes insipidus, diabetes mellitus, optic atrophy, and deafness) includes the main clinical characteristics of the syndrome. More recently, since urinary dysfunctions (UD) are frequently encountered, the term DIDMOAD has been extended to DIDMOAUD [2].

The prevalence of WS widely ranges among countries (1:68,000 in Lebanon to 1:770,000 in the UK), with a mean estimated frequency in children of 1:550,000. A high rate of consanguinity has been reported, and the carrier frequency is 1 in 354 subjects [3]. Several abnormalities in heterozygous relatives of WS patients have been described, such as glucose abnormalities, subclinical hearing loss, and neuropsychiatric disturbances, including suicidal behavior. Mortality is about 65% before 35 years of age, due to central respiratory failure with brainstem atrophy and renal failure secondary to infections [3].

Clinical Aspects

Diabetes mellitus, due to loss of β-cells, is an invariable finding and the first manifestation. It is characterized by non-autoimmune pathogenesis and an insulin requirement [4]. On the other hand, few case reports have described β-cell autoimmunity in affected adult patients [5]. WS patients usually show lower HbA_{1c} levels, insulin requirement, and frequency of microangiopathic complications as compared to peers with type 1 diabetes [6]. Previous autoptic studies showed loss of β-cells or atrophy of β-pancreatic islets, while the exocrine portion of the gland was normal or with focal areas of fibrosis [7]. Immunohistochemical studies showed absence of cell staining for insulin, but normal cell staining for glucagon, somatostatin, and pancreatic polypeptide, thus indicating selective β-cell loss with a better preservation of the other components of the gland. These findings suggest that WS-associated diabetes mellitus is caused by a functional defect in β-cells and β-cell depletion [7].

Diabetes insipidus has a central origin and is usually diagnosed in the second decade of life. Typical neuroradiological findings include the absence of normal T1 hyperintensity in the posterior pituitary gland with gliosis and atrophy of the paraventricular and supraoptic nuclei of the hypothalamus, associated with their functional defect and loss (fig. 1) [8].

Optic atrophy is usually diagnosed in the first decade of life (Fig. 2a, b). Ophthalmological findings include severe axonal loss and demyelination of the optic nerves and optic chiasma tracts [9]. The pathogenesis of optic atrophy results from the effects of WFS1 gene mutation on the survival of retinal ganglion cells, and leads to anterograde atrophy of retinal axons and shrinkage of the optic nerves [9]. The hypothesis that WFS1 is expressed in glial cells of the optic nerve and in retinal ganglion cells has been tested in cynomolgus monkeys, using affinity-purified antibodies to wolframin. Retinal ganglion cells and optic nerve glial cells were found to be strongly labeled, suggesting that dual dysfunction of wolframin in optic nerve and in retinal ganglion cells might explain the progression of optic atrophy. Uncommon ophthalmological findings have also been reported and include diabetic retinopathy, cataract, glaucoma, nystagmus, and abnormal pupillary light reflexes.

Sensorineural deafness is diagnosed at a median age of 16 years in 60% of cases [10]. Audiometric features consist of severe auditory threshold shift, which is more evident for the medium/high frequencies. As wolframin is expressed in inner ear cells, sensorineural deafness could be a consequence not only of a dysfunction of cochlear neurons and VIII nerve fibers, or of the central nervous pathways in the brainstem and inferior colliculus, but also from a dysfunction of the ear structures themselves.

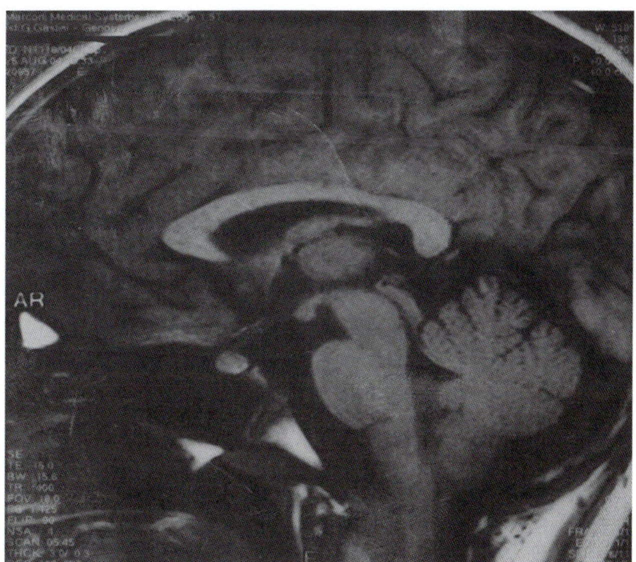

Fig. 1. Brain MRI: absence of posterior pituitary signal (personal observation).

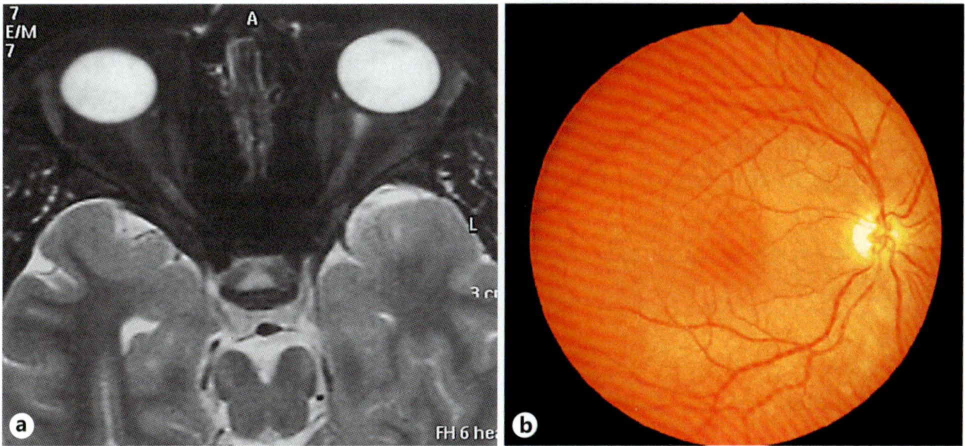

Fig. 2. a Brain MRI: optic nerve and chiasma atrophy (personal observation). **b** Optic atrophy – pale papilla.

Endocrine dysfunctions other than diabetes insipidus include primary and secondary hypogonadism, which typically affect males, while in females menstrual abnormalities are frequently encountered [11]. Anterior pituitary hypofunction seems to have a hypothalamic origin and includes growth hormone deficiency and impaired corticotrophin secretion. Growth velocity and pubertal development deserve attention. Moreover, steroid supplementation in stressful situations needs to be considered.

Urinary tract dysfunctions, previously reported in adulthood, have been recently shown even at a younger age [12]. They include ureterohydronephrosis secondary to bladder dysfunction (as documented by urodynamic testing) and autonomic neuropathy. High-capacity atonic bladder and low-capacity high-pressure bladder have been described [12]. Delayed diagnosis and treatment of urinary tract dysfunctions increase the risk of serious infections of the urinary tract and kidneys, and of acute and chronic renal failure.

Several abnormalities affecting the central nervous system have been described; the most frequently reported include anosmia, ataxia, seizures, nystagmus, gaze palsies, dysarthria, dysphagia, psychiatric disturbances, cognitive impairment, neurogenic bladder, central apnea, neurogenic upper airway collapse, and myoclonus [13]. Severe and progressive neurological impairment is characterized by ataxia, dysarthria, neurogenic bladder, dysphagia, dementia, and gait impairment.

Despite the life-threatening role of neurological involvement in WS, knowledge about the full phenotypic spectrum of the neurological damage is still limited and is based on clinical exams and postmortem neuropathological case studies. These reports describe abnormalities in multiple regions of the brain, in particular the brainstem, cerebellum, thalamus, hypothalamus, pituitary gland, inferior olivary nucleus, lateral geniculate nucleus, and optic nerve. Recently, early brain vulnerability characterized by reduced intracranial volume, preferentially affecting gray matter volume, and white matter microstructural integrity in the brainstem, cerebellum, and optic radiation has been reported [14]. These abnormalities were also observed in the youngest patients, with few clinical symptoms and without an age-dependent trajectory. It has been hypothesized that endothelial reticulum stress due to WFS1 mutations impairs firstly early brain development, followed later by neurodegenerative effects.

Due to the rarity of the disease, a correlation genotype/phenotype is difficult to define [15, 16].

Linkage Studies

Initially, the similarity in phenotype between patients with WS and those with certain types of respiratory chain diseases led to the investigation of mitochondrial DNA mutations in WS patients. However, mitochondrial mutations and deletions in the mitochondrial DNA have been excluded in more than 20 WS patients [17].

Genetic mapping and candidate gene approaches have identified the mutated nuclear gene in WS syndrome, which has been named accordingly wolframin 1 or WFS1. WFS1, spanning approximately 33.4 kb of genomic DNA on chromosome 4p16.1, consists of 8 exons. The start point of translation is in the second exon and produces a peptide product that is 890 amino acids long (wolframin) with an apparent molecular mass of 100 kDa. Wolframin is a hydrophobic and tetrameric protein with 9 transmembrane segments and large hydrophilic regions at both termini [18, 19] (Fig. 3, 4).

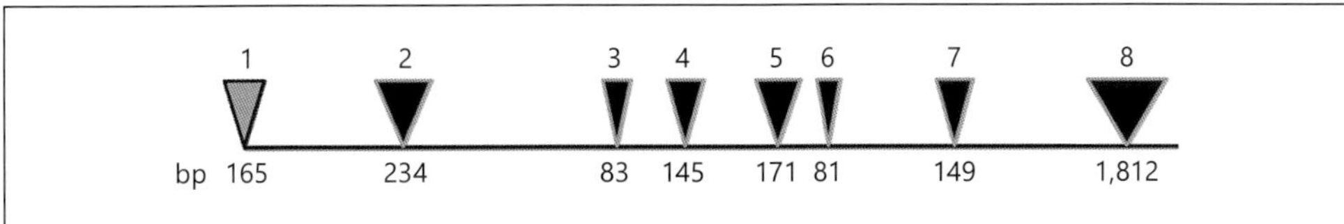

Fig. 3. WFS1 gene structure [3].

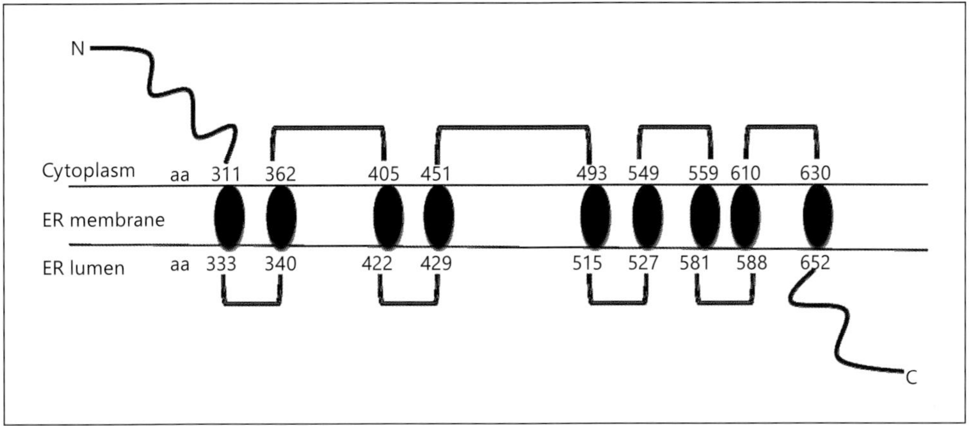

Fig. 4. The structure of wolframin protein [20].

Function of the WFS1 Gene

The wolframin protein is abundantly expressed in the pancreas, brain, heart, muscle, and, to a lesser extent, liver and kidneys. It is a resident component of the endoplasmic reticulum (ER) with a N_{cyt}/C_{lum} orientation in the ER membrane. Some studies have shown that in the ER, wolframin seems to be an integral endoglycosidase H-sensitive membrane glycoprotein [20]. The ER has many roles, which include posttranslational modification, folding, and assembly of newly synthesized proteins such as insulin. When ER function is altered, it causes an imbalance between these processes, leading to accumulation of misfolded and unfolded proteins in the organelle, a state called "ER stress". ER stress induces cellular responses, including apoptosis. Moreover, it activates a network of signaling pathways collectively termed "unfolded protein response" (UPR). The UPR coordinates the temporary downregulation of protein translation, the upregulation of ER chaperones, folding machinery, and ER-associated degradation in order to reduce the workload on the ER protein processing and folding machinery, and prevent the accumulation of misfolded proteins. Within the pancreas, UPR maintains β-cell function and promotes β-cell survival. It has been shown that WFS1 has a crucial role in the negative regulation of a feedback loop of the ER stress signaling network and prevents secretory cells, such as pancreatic β-cells, from death caused by dysregulation of this signaling pathway. Indeed, WFS1 negatively regulates a key transcription factor involved in ER stress signaling, activating transcription factor-6α through the ubiquitin-proteasome pathway [21]. ER localization suggests that wolframin has physiological functions in membrane trafficking, secretion, processing, and/or regulation of ER calcium homeostasis. As wolframin is a calmodulin-binding protein, WFS1 mutations induce calcium regulation dysfunction and it might be responsible for the progression β-cell loss and neuronal degeneration associated with WS [22].

Increasing clinical, experimental, and genetic evidence indicates that ER stress and UPR have a role in β-cell dysfunction and death during progression of type 1, type 2, and genetic forms of diabetes. It is currently believed that UPR regulates the fate of β-cells, behaving like a binary switch between life and death. Wolframin is highly expressed in the pancreas and it may help fold a protein precursor of insulin, proinsulin, into the mature hormone that controls blood glucose levels.

Pancreatic β-cells are the major site of WFS1 expression, which is much greater than in pancreatic exocrine cells. This expression is also found in δ-cells, but not in α-cells. WFS1 expression is transcriptionally upregulated by ER-stress-inducing chemical insults. Accumulating evidence indicates that β-cell death in WS syndrome is due to high levels of ER stress signaling in affected cells [23].

It has been shown that wolframin deficiency in mice leads to progressive loss of β-cells, impaired glucose tolerance, and cell cycle progression, accompanied by the activation of ER stress/UPR pathways and enhanced susceptibility to apoptosis [24]. Thus, WFS1 seems to play a role in the normal function of β-cells, but little is known about its function during embryogenesis.

A close relationship between WFS1 protein and the mesenchymal and/or epithelial interactions in pancreatic development has been found. By immunofluorescence, it has been found that Wfs1 protein is localized to the mesenchyme in the rat pancreas. Thus, Wfs1 could be involved in many aspects of pancreatic development [24].

Genetic analyses in WS have identified a wide spectrum of mutations that appear to be distributed randomly throughout the entire coding sequence of the gene. These mutations are mainly concentrated in the largest exon, exon 8 [25–27].

Several types of loss-of-function gene mutations, such as stop, frame-shift (40% of total), and splice site mutations, have been identified. Missense mutations have been detected in approximately 35% of the cases and they are mainly located in the C-terminal hydrophilic part of the protein. Mutations of the last 7 amino acids also lead to a full-blown disease phenotype, underlining the functional importance of the C-terminus of wolframin [25].

The pathophysiological role of wolframin mutants in WS is still unknown. The stop and frameshift mutations of WFS1 cause complete absence of the wolframin protein rather than synthesis of truncated species [28]. In this case, the nonsense WFS1 transcripts are unstable in vivo and they are recognized and degraded by the cell via a common pathway known as nonsense-mediated mRNA decay [29, 30].

The degradation of nonsense WFS1 transcripts prevents the synthesis of truncation translation products, and this is the molecular mechanism underlying the loss-of-function of wolframin in WS patients. Moreover, some studies have shown that all mutations led to drastically reduced, steady-state levels of WFS1 protein. Indeed, the mutated proteins are rapidly subjected to proteasome degradation at an early stage of biogenesis.

Although no clear genotype-phenotype relationship and no obvious mutation hot spots or clusters have been detected, a molecular screening of WFS1 is required in WS patients. Initially, genetic analysis should target exon 8. Later, if no mutations have been identified, molecular sequencing of the entire gene must be performed.

Wolfram Syndrome 2

In 2000, a second locus, named wolframin syndrome 2 (WFS2), was mapped on chromosome 4q22-q24 following the linkage analysis of 4 consanguineous Jordanian families [17]. WFS2-mutated patients are not affected by diabetes insipidus, but show upper gastrointestinal ulceration even at a young age, due to prolonged bleeding time. Platelet aggregation studies showed absent or impaired aggregation with collagen, but were otherwise normal with adenosine diphosphate, ristocetin, and epinephrine.

WFS2 (MIM 604928) is caused by mutations in CISD2 on chromosome 4q22 [18]. Like wolframin, the *CISD2*-encoded protein, ERIS (endoplasmic reticulum intermembrane small protein), also localizes to ER, and is expressed in numerous tissues, including the brain and pancreas. ERIS has a molecular mass of 15.3 kD and contains a predicted transmembrane domain and a C-terminal CDGSH domain. ERIS plays a role in Ca^{2+} homeostasis, as well as wolframin [29]. Therefore, both genes, WFS1 and CISD2, could be part of the same pathway, although CISD2 does not interact directly with wolframin. Each gene probably has a specific mechanism that leads to nerve and pancreatic degeneration.

Conclusions

As the function of WFS1 is unknown and it is difficult to assess or predict the effect of these mutations on protein function and, hence, their biological relevance, the diagnosis of WS remains essentially clinical. However, the recognized association between WS and WFS1 mutations, as well as of other interacting genes is important for the identification of treatable complications in WS patients, and for their parents, since genetic counselling is possible. Moreover, the identifications of precise functions of the WFS1 gene could enable researchers to seek novel therapeutic approaches.

References

1   Barrett TG, Bundey SE: Wolfram (DIDMOAD) syndrome. J Med Genet 1997;34:838–841.

2   Kumar S: Wolfram syndrome: important implications for pediatricians and pediatric endocrinologists. Pediatr Diabetes 2010;11:28–37.

3   Inoue H, Tanizawa Y, Wasson J, Behn P, Kalidas K, Bernal-Mizrachi E, Mueckler M, Marshall H, Donis-Keller H, Crock P, Rogers D, Mikuni M, Kumashiro H, Higashi K, Sobue G, Oka Y, Permutt MA: A gene encoding a transmembrane protein is mutated in patients with diabetes mellitus and optic atrophy (Wolfram syndrome). Nat Genet 1998;20:143–148.

4   Riggs AC, Bernal-Mizrachi E, Ohsugi M, Wasson J, Fatrai S, Welling C, Murray J, Schmidt RE, Herrera PL, Permutt MA: Mice conditionally lacking the Wolfram gene in pancreatic islet beta cells exhibit diabetes as a result of enhanced endoplasmic reticulum stress and apoptosis. Diabetologia 2005;48:2313–2321.

5   Nakamura A, Shimizu C, Nagai S, Taniguchi S, Umetsu M, Atsumi T, Wada N, Yoshioka N, Ono Y, Tanizawa Y, Koike T: A novel mutation of WFS1 gene in a Japanese man of Wolfram syndrome with positive diabetes-related antibodies. Diabetes Res Clin Pract 2006;73:215–217.

6   Cano A, Molines L, Valero R, Simonin G, Paquis-Flucklinger V, Vialettes B; The French Group of Wolfram Syndrome: Microvascular diabetes complications in Wolfram syndrome (diabetes insipidus, diabetes mellitus, optic atrophy, and deafness [DIDMOAD]): an age- and duration-matched comparison with common type 1 diabetes. Diabetes Care 2007;30:2327–2330.

7   Karasik A, O'Hara C, Srikanta S, Swift M, Soeldner JS, Kahn CR, Herskowitz RD: Genetically programmed selective islet beta-cell loss in diabetic subjects with Wolfram's syndrome. Diabetes Care 1989;12:135–138.

8   Pandemirli E, Karabulut N, Bir LS, Sermez Y: Cranial magnetic resonance imaging of Wolfram (DIDMOAD) syndrome. Australas Radiol 2005;49:189–191.

9   Medlej R, Wasson J, Baz P, Azar S, Salti I, Loiselet J, Permutt A, Halaby G: Diabetes mellitus and optic atrophy: a study of Wolfram syndrome in the Lebanese population. J Clin Endocrinol Metab 2004;89:1656–1661.

10   Megighian D Savastano M: Wolfram syndrome. Int J Ped Otorhinolaryngol 2004;68:243–247.

11   Boutzios G, Livadas S, MarinakisE, Opie N, Economou F, Diamanti-Kandarakis E: Endocrine and metabolic aspects of the Wolfram syndrome. Endocrine 2011;40:10–13.

12   Tekgul S, Oge O, Simsek E, Yordam N, Kendi S: Urological manifestations of the Wolfram syndrome: observations in 14 patients. J Urol 1999;161:616–617.

13   Chaussenot A, Bannwarth S, Rouzier C, Vialettes B, Mkadem SA, Chabrol B, Cano A, Labauge P, Paquis-Flucklinger V: Neurologic features and genotype-phenotype correlation in Wolfram syndrome. Ann Neurol 2011;69:501–508.

14   Hershey T, Lugar HM, Shimony JS, Rutlin J, Koller JM, Perantie DC, Paciorkowski AR, Eisenstein SA, Permutt MA; Washington University Wolfram Study Group: Early brain vulnerability in Wolfram syndrome. PLoS One 2012;7:e40604.

15   d'Annunzio G, Minuto N, D'Amato E, de Toni T, Lombardo F, Pasquali L, Lorini R. Wolfram syndrome (diabetes insipidus, diabetes, optic atrophy, and deafness): clinical and genetic study. Diabetes Care 2008;31:1743–1745.

16   Aloi C, Salina A, Pasquali L, Lugani F, Perri K, Russo C, Tallone R, Ghiggeri GM, Lorini R, d'Annunzio G: Wolfram syndrome: new mutations, different phenotype. PLoS One 2012;7:e29150.

17   Ajlouni K, Jarrah N, El-Khateeb M, El-Zaheri M, El Shanti H, Lidral A: Wolfram syndrome: identification of a phenotypic and genotypic variant from Jordan. Am J Med Genet 2002;115:61–65.

18   Mozzillo E, Delvecchio M, Carella M, Grandone E, Palumbo P, Salina A, Aloi C, Buono P, Izzo A, D'Annunzio G, Vecchione G, Orrico A, Genesio R, Simonelli F, Franzese A: A novel CISD2 intragenic deletion, optic neuropathy and platelet aggregation defect in Wolfram syndrome type 2. BMC Med Genet 2014;15:88.

19   Rigoli L, Arrigo T, Corigliano G, Degiorgi G, Franzese A, Giorgetti R, Lasco A, Lucentini L, Marietti G, Martinucci ME, Parrillo M, Picco P, Iafusco D, Deluca F, Cucinotta D: Mitochondrial DNA studies and clinical findings in Wolfram syndrome: an Italian multicenter survey. Diab Nutr Metab 1998;11:114–120.

20   Strom TM, Hörtnagel K, Hofmann S, Gekeler F, Scharfe C, Rabl W, Gerbitz KD, Meitinger T: Diabetes insipidus, diabetes mellitus, optic atrophy and deafness (DIDMOAD) caused by mutations in a novel gene (wolframin) coding for a predicted transmembrane protein. Hum Mol Genet 1998;7:2021–2028.

21   Hofmann S, Philbrook C, Gerbitz KD, Bauer MF: Wolfram syndrome: structural and functional analyses of mutant and wild-type wolframin, the WFS1 gene product. Hum Mol Genet 2003;12:2003–2012.

Rigoli · d'Annunzio

22 Fonseca SG, Ishigaki S, Oslowski CM, Lu S, Lipson KL, Ghosh R, Hayashi E, Ishihara H, Oka Y, Permutt MA, Urano F: Wolfram syndrome 1 gene negatively regulates ER stress signaling in rodent and human cells. J Clin Invest 2010;120:744–755.

23 Osman AA, Saito M, Makepeace C, Permutt MA, Schlesinger P, Mueckler M: Wolframin expression induces novel ion channel activity in endoplasmic reticulum membranes and increases intracellular calcium. J Biol Chem 2003;278:52755–52762.

24 Fonseca SG, Fukuma M, Lipson KL, Nguyen LX, Allen JR, Oka Y, Urano F: WFS1 is a novel component of the unfolded protein response and maintains homeostasis of the endoplasmic reticulum in pancreatic beta-cells. J Biol Chem 2005;280:39609–39615.

25 Ishihara H, Takeda S, Tamura A, Takahashi R, Yamaguchi S, Takei D, Yamada T, Inoue H, Soga H, Katagiri H, Tanizawa Y, Oka Y: Disruption of the Wfs1 gene in mice causes progressive beta-cell loss and impaired stimulus-secretion coupling in insulin secretion. Hum Mol Genet 2004;13:1159–1170.

26 Rigoli L, Lombardo F, Di Bella C: Wolfram syndrome and WFS1 gene. Clin Genet 2011;79:103–117.

27 Lombardo F, Salzano G, Di Bella C, Aversa T, Pugliatti F, Cara S, Valenzise M, De Luca F, Rigoli L: Phenotypical and genotypical expression of Wolfram syndrome in 12 patients from a Sicilian district where this syndrome might not be so infrequent as generally expected. J Endocrinol Invest 2014;37:195–202.

28 Rigoli L, Lombardo F, Salzano G, Di Bella C, Messina MF, De Luca F, Iafusco D: Identification of one novel causative mutation in exon 4 of WFS1 gene in two Italian siblings with classical DIDMOAD syndrome phenotype. Gene 2013;526:487–489.

29 Rigoli L, Di Bella C: Wolfram syndrome 1 and Wolfram syndrome 2. Curr Opin Pediatr 2012;24:512–517.

30 Frischmeyer PA, Dietz HC: Nonsense-mediated mRNA decay in health and disease. Hum Mol Genet 1999;8:1893–1900.

Luciana Concetta Rigoli, MD
Department of Pediatrics, Medical School, University of Messina
Via Consolare Valeria, IT–98125 Messina (Italy)
E-Mail luciana.rigoli@unime.it

Barbetti F, Ghizzoni L, Guaraldi F (eds): Diabetes Associated with Single Gene Defects and Chromosomal Abnormalities. Front Diabetes. Basel, Karger, 2017, vol 25, pp 78–90 (DOI: 10.1159/000454703)

Type 1 Diabetes Mellitus in Monogenic Autoimmune Diseases

Rosa Bacchetta[a] · Maria Elena Maccari[b]

[a]Division of Stem Cell Transplantation and Regenerative Medicine, Department of Pediatrics, Stanford University School of Medicine, Stanford, CA, USA; [b]San Raffaele Telethon Institute for Gene Therapy (HSR-TIGET), Division of Regenerative Medicine, Stem Cells, and Gene Therapy, San Raffaele Scientific Institute, Milan, Italy

Abstract

Immune dysregulation-polyendocrinopathy-enteropathy-X-linked syndrome (IPEX) is a rare monogenic X-linked autoimmune disorder caused by mutations in the transcription factor forkhead box p3 (*FOXP3*) gene. The pathogenesis of the disease is due to defective function of T-regulatory cells (Tregs), whose normal function is to maintain immunological tolerance. Similar to other primary defects of the immune system, IPEX clinical manifestations occur during early infancy. Of these, type 1 diabetes mellitus (T1D) together with enteropathy and eczema are common signs of the typical forms of IPEX. Less frequently, patients with *FOXP3* mutations present with different autoimmune manifestations with or without T1D. Patients with atypical IPEX have recently posed a strong diagnostic challenge. Quantitative or qualitative alterations of Tregs have been recently associated with mutations in genes other than *FOXP3*, causing immunodysfunctional syndromes, termed "IPEX-like syndromes", in which T1D presents with less frequency. In this chapter we discuss the main clinical and immunogenetic features of IPEX and similar immunodysregulatory Treg deficiencies, highlighting the presence of T1D, as either a constant or a rare clinical manifestation.

© 2017 S. Karger AG, Basel

Immune dysregulation-polyendocrinopathy-enteropathy-X-linked syndrome (IPEX) (OMIM ID: 304790) is a rare monogenic disorder caused by mutations in the *FOXP3* gene. *FOXP3* encodes for the forkhead box protein 3 and maps on Xp11.23 [1]. Since the disease is X-linked, only males are affected, and healthy mothers are disease-carriers. The 3 main clinical features are autoimmune enteropathy, type 1 diabetes mellitus (T1D), and cutaneous manifestations; less frequently, other autoimmune disorders can occur [2]. Less than 150 cases have been reported to date, but the disease has probably been underdiagnosed in the past because of lack of awareness and early morbidity. Indeed, most cases have been diagnosed only in the past few years, including those with atypical presentation. Unlike polygenic autoimmunity, which has a clear geographic distribution, IPEX has been sporadically diagnosed in many diverse geographic areas, indicating a strong penetrance and predominance of the genetic flaw over, for example, environmental factors. Currently, the exact prevalence of the disease is unknown.

FOXP3 Gene and T-Regulatory Cells in Immunological Tolerance

Immunological tolerance is established by multiple mechanisms that cooperate to maintain the physiological balance between all immune cell types and to prevent reaction against self-antigens. Impairment of one of these regulatory functions can lead to the development of autoimmune disorders. Tolerance "checkpoints" are present in both T- and B-cell development [3]. The common essential principle upon which all these mechanisms are based is the correct determination of autoreactive cells and nonautoreactive ones, not only during their development, but also later on in life in the periphery.

The first step in T cell-mediated tolerance is represented by central tolerance, which is mainly achieved by removing immature self-reactive lymphocytes through negative selection in the thymus. Thanks to central tolerance, the vast majority of autoreactive T cells are deleted in the thymus. In this process, the autoimmune regulator gene (*AIRE*) is crucial and its mutation leads to the development of APECED syndrome (autoimmune polyendocrinopathy candidiasis ectodermal dystrophy).

Despite the efficiency of clonal deletion in the thymus, some autoreactive T cells escape and are present in healthy individuals in the periphery. These autoreactive T cells remain harmless thanks to peripheral tolerance, another important arm of immunological tolerance that acts through anergy, deletion, or active suppression by regulatory cells. T-cell anergy is when lymphocytes are functionally inactivated following an antigen encounter, but remain alive in a hyporesponsive state. Deletion refers to the apoptosis of autoreactive T cells. Suppression is an active process, mediated by a specific subset of lymphocytes, named T-regulatory cells (Tregs).

Several types of Tregs exist, each characterized by unique features, although there is often shared common mechanisms of action. CD4+CD25+FOXP3+ Tregs are so far the best characterized [4]. Tregs are generated in the thymus. Several models, focused on affinity of the self-reactive T-cell receptor, have been proposed to explain the generation of Tregs in the thymus, although the precise mechanism of origin is still a matter of debate. Essential for regulatory function of Tregs is the key transcription factor *FOXP3*. The specific function of Tregs resides in their capacity to efficiently suppress effector T cells as well as antigen-presenting cells via different mechanisms that are also common to other types of Tregs. This regulatory function is an activation-dependent process that requires cell-cell interactions [5]. The induction of FOXP3 transcription is strictly dependent on phosphorylation of the signal transducer and activator of transcription 5 (STAT5) [6], which is regulated by T-cell receptor activation and costimulatory molecules and cytokines, such as IL-2, IL-7, or IL-15 [7]. Moreover, FOXP3 expression is also epigenetically regulated [8]. Studies of the specific methylation/demethylation patterns of Tregs have allowed the identification of the Treg-specific demethylated region (TSDR). This CpG region in the FOXP3 promoter is completely and persistently demethylated exclusively on Tregs, while it is completely methylated on naïve T cells [9]. The demethylated status of the TSDR influences FOXP3 expression, which is markedly diminished when the region is methylated. Reduced levels of TSDR indicate a quantitative reduction in Tregs, recently associated with some IPEX-like syndromes [10].

FOXP3 regulates the expression of many genes that are fundamental in maintaining phenotypic and functional Treg characteristics. FOXP3 promotes the expression of CD25 while downregulating IL-2 production. This is important considering that the typical low levels of Treg proliferation (anergy) correlate with the rapid response to changes in levels of IL-2. The influence of FOXP3 on IL-2 homeostasis is evident also by its interaction with other transcription factors involved in the pathway, such as AP-1 (activator protein 1) and RUNX1 (runt-related transcription factor 1). Moreover, FOXP3 upregulates CTLA-4, an important inhibitory Treg surface molecule counterpart of CD28. While CD28 signaling promotes T-cell activation, CTLA-4 has an immunoregulatory function, suppressing the T-cell response [11]. Intact high FOXP3 expression in Tregs is therefore essential for their function. However, FOXP3 operates in a complex molecular network that can be disrupted because of mutations in other genes involved in the FOXP3-dependent pathway of regulation within Tregs. Wild-type FOXP3 expression can be indirectly altered, and Tregs become dysfunctional because of different mutations underlying diseases that are often similar to IPEX, as discussed below.

FOXP3 Mutations Lead to IPEX Syndrome

Mutations in *FOXP3* are associated with IPEX. According to the Human Gene Mutation Database, 64 mutations in *FOXP3* had been described as of 2014. The majority of these are missense mutations, located in the C-terminal forkhead DNA-binding domain of the protein. In nearly all cases, the genetic alteration leads to impaired FOXP3 transcriptional activity [12]. However, a precise genotype-phenotype correlation is not apparent: patients carrying the same *FOXP3* mutation present a broad clinical heterogeneity, thus suggesting a multilayer FOXP3 genetic and epigenetic regulation [13].

Since *FOXP3* mutations do not often alter the protein expression, Tregs develop normally and a reduction in this T-cell subset is not evident in IPEX patients. However, IPEX patients present an impairment in Treg function, detected by in vitro studies of Treg-suppressive function [14]. In addition to this dysfunctional regulatory activity, IPEX patients present a dysregulated effector T-cell compartment, represented for example by an increase in IL-17-producing cells [15]. Among the consequences of *FOXP3* mutations, there are not only T-cell alterations but also B-cell impairments. Indeed, in the presence of dysfunctional Tregs, there is an accumulation of autoreactive B cells and a homeostatic expansion of mature B cells, thus highlighting the importance of Tregs in peripheral B cell tolerance [16].

Clinical and Immunological features of IPEX

The main clinical features of IPEX are intractable diarrhea, T1D, and eczema. Frequently, these signs and symptoms occur in patients in their first months of life and can be lethal if not adequately treated; however, some cases with an unusual and late-onset presentation have been recently described [17].

Interestingly, a recent paper has highlighted the diagnostic importance of a detailed family history, often characterized by multiple spontaneous abortions in the maternal family [18]. FOXP3 mutations have been detected in fetuses with hydrops occurring within the second trimester of pregnancy [19].

Autoimmune enteropathy is the most common clinical manifestation of IPEX: the onset is in the neonatal period with acute, watery diarrhea. Less frequently, the presentation is mucoid or bloody diarrhea. At onset, the main differential diagnosis is therefore with infectious diseases. Unlike other forms of persistent diarrhea (e.g., food-sensitive enteropathies, anatomical or transport defects, and malabsorption disorders), diarrhea in IPEX patients typically persists despite dietary exclusions and bowel rest with parenteral nutrition. The result is severe malabsorption and significant failure to thrive. In addition to diarrhea, other gastrointestinal manifestations can occur, such as vomiting, gastritis, ileus, and colitis [2]. A gastrointestinal biopsy can be useful for diagnosis and differential diagnosis since it highlights mucosal lymphocytic and eosinophilic infiltration with villous atrophy, according to the immune-mediated origin of the enteropathy.

T1D can precede or follow enteritis. It is present in the majority (65%) of patients including newborns [13].

Cutaneous manifestations appear in the first months of life and are often severe, with poor response to classical topical treatments. Dermatitis can be eczematiform but also ichthyosiform or psoriasiform. Frequent complications are represented by bacterial infections.

Less common clinical manifestations include severe allergies to food or other allergens, alopecia or onychodystrophy, thyroiditis, cytopenia, and renal diseases [13].

An increased number of infectious episodes, mainly respiratory, likely caused by long-standing immunosuppression, are often observed in patients with IPEX and can worsen their clinical condition. Not surprisingly, gastrointestinal infections can lead, in some cases, to life-threatening sepsis.

Laboratory tests can be normal at onset. Lymphocytosis can be present without alterations of the main lymphocyte subpopulations (CD3, CD4, CD8, CD16, and CD19). The CD4/CD8 ratio is normal or slightly increased. The T-cell repertoire is polyclonal. Naïve and memory T cells are normally distributed. An elevated IgE and eosinophil count are found in many patients [20]. IgA, IgG, and IgM are generally normal but can be reduced due to the protein-losing enteropathy. As described earlier, B cells present an expansion in the mature B-cell compartment. Treg frequency, assessed through TSDR analysis, is quantitatively normal or elevated. However, FOXP3 expression can be reduced or, less frequently, abrogated depending on the effect of the specific mutation. A reduced expression can also depend on the ongoing immunosuppressive therapy. Autoantibodies, associated with the target organs, such as pancreatic antigens or thyroid antigens can be detected. Interestingly, recent studies have identified anti-enterocyte antibodies in IPEX patients. The 2 main antigens against which these antibodies are directed are villin and harmonin. Harmonin was previously described as an autoimmune enteropathy-related 75-kDa antigen [21]. Both of the antigens are expressed in the brush border of the small intestine and in the proximal renal tubules. Anti-harmonin and anti-villin antibodies have been quantitatively evaluated in IPEX patients and have been found to be highly specific for this disease, being absent both in healthy subjects and in patients who suffer from other forms of enteropathy [22]. Another antigen against which sera from IPEX patients has been shown to react is keratin 14, a skin protein and potential target for autoreactive cells.

The acute onset of IPEX can be life-threatening. Therefore, treatment firstly includes replacement (insulin and/or thyroid hormones, and/or intravenous immunoglobulins) and supportive therapy, such as fluids and/or parenteral nutrition. Prompt antibiotic management of infectious complications is another important therapeutic measure. In order to control immune dysregulation symptoms, immunosuppressive therapy has been used: glucocorticoids represent the first-line therapy; cyclosporine, azathioprine, or tacrolimus usually have to be added if the first-line therapy fails [13]. Recently, sirolimus has been shown to have a good clinical effect [23], probably related to the biologic function of rapamycin that targets effector cells without affecting Treg survival [24]. All of these immunosuppressive drugs must be adequately tailored in order to minimize adverse effects, worsened by the young age of the patients at the beginning of the treatment. Hematopoietic stem cell transplantation is the only curative treatment for IPEX [25]. When performed early, it leads to a better limiting of the autoimmune damage and to a better prevention of the side effects related to immunosuppressive drugs. Nonmyeloablative conditioning is often attempted in order to allow better tolerability. Moreover, complete donor engraftment, more likely reachable with myeloablative conditioning, is not necessary to achieve a cure since the preferential engraftment of donor Tregs is sufficient. Novel therapeutic strategies, including Treg-based immunotherapy, gene therapy, and genome editing, are currently under investigation and could become the gold standard curative approach for IPEX patients in the future [26].

IPEX and Type 1 Diabetes Mellitus

The onset of permanent T1D in the neonatal age is considered a rare event. When it occurs, a monogenic form of diabetes should be primarily suspected since the polyautoimmune form is uncommon. This is confirmed by the fact that newborns diagnosed with T1D do not often harbor HLA haplotypes predisposing to T1D and associated with the polyautoimmune form [27]. However, T1D is the second most common clinical manifestation of IPEX patients and therefore IPEX must be considered in the differential diagnosis of T1D with neonatal onset, especially when other immune dysregulation phenomena coexist. Autoantibodies against insulin, pancreatic islet cells, or glutamate decarboxylase can be detectable in IPEX patients within the first 3–4 months of life, but detectable autoantibodies in the first days of life are not uncommon [28]. There have been rare cases presenting with diabetes mellitus without known autoantibodies [29]. This suggests that the main pathogenic mechanism could be T-cell mediated but the presence of autoantibodies against unknown antigens could not be excluded. Interestingly, the histological examination of twin male fetuses with a *FOXP3* mutation, dead at 21 weeks of gestation due to hydrops, revealed the presence of CD3 lymphocytes infiltrating the pancreas [18]. Although the Langerhans islets were preserved, the histological patterns were suggestive of the initial stage of diabetes development.

Imaging studies or autopsy and histological examination of several IPEX cases have indeed revealed that the pancreatic damage is associated with a large lymphocytic infiltrate, suggesting that the pathogenesis should be immune mediated [20, 29]. The possible absence of autoantibodies and the T-cell infiltrates suggest a specific role for T cells. However, a defect in Treg function has been shown to also affect B-cell tolerance, resulting in an accumulation of autoreactive B cells in the periphery that, in turn, could give rise to organ-specific autoantibodies. Moreover, the increased T-cell activation and the predominant effector phenotype could favor the expansion of these autoreactive B cells [16]. The damage could therefore be T-cell driven but subsequently also expanded by the B-cell compartment.

Of note, in the milder cases of IPEX described to date, T1D is less frequently diagnosed [17]. This observation is difficult to interpret as we do not yet understand the mechanism that leads to IPEX mainly targeting the pancreas and gut.

T1D in IPEX patients is treated with normal insulin replacement therapy, which often needs to be adequately tailored to allow good glycometabolic control [13]. Importantly, the extensive pancreatic damage can also lead to a reduction in exocrine function, which in turn can worsen the gastrointestinal symptoms and nutritional status. As a result, management and treatment can become more difficult [29].

IPEX patients who had T1D and were treated with hematopoietic stem cell transplantation did not experience remission of the diabetes since the islet cells had already been destroyed [25]. It would be interesting to analyze the course of the disease in those patients who present a very early stage of T1D development at the time of the transplantation.

Many IPEX-like syndromes of known monogenic origin can resemble IPEX clinical manifestations in the absence of *FOXP3* mutations, and can present T1D (Fig. 1, 2). Here, we briefly describe them from a clinical and immunological point of view. Many other cases of autoimmune diseases characterized by very early onset and coexistence of multiple autoimmune manifestations still lack precise evidence of a monogenic origin. However, in these cases, a monogenic origin should always be suspected and specific genetic and immunological analyses (e.g., whole-genome sequencing and functional immunological tests) aimed at unraveling the etiology and pathogenesis should always be performed.

CD25 deficiency was first described in 1997 [30]. It is an autosomal recessive disease caused by mutations in the *CD25* gene, encoding for the α-chain of the IL-2 receptor. Unlike IPEX, female patients can also be affected. The clinical manifestations are similar to IPEX, but this syndrome is characterized by a more evident susceptibility to infections, particularly of viral origin, indicating the important role played by IL-2 in T-cell immunity. In fact, CD25 is not only constitutively expressed by Tregs, where it promotes FOXP3 transcription through a STAT5-dependent pathway, but it is also fundamental in effector T-cell activation and expansion after an antigenic stimulus. Although diarrhea and cutaneous manifestations are frequent, there is only 1 documented case of a *CD25* mutation associated with T1D, which developed at 6 weeks of age [31]. The male patient presented with severe diarrhea and insulin-dependent diabetes, complicated by lung CMV infection. No data are reported regarding the diabetes-specific autoantibodies. Subsequently, he developed eczema and other autoimmune manifestations, such as cytopenia and thyroiditis, while still suffering from frequent respiratory tract infections. After ruling out a *FOXP3* mutation, a compound heterozygous *CD25* mutation was found that led to a CD4 T-cell proliferative defect. Similar to IPEX, no quantitative defect in Tregs was found and no data regarding Treg regulatory function were reported. A more recent *CD25* mutation report [32] confirmed the presence of Tregs, suggesting normal development while highlighting a reduction in the bona fide Treg, evaluated through the analysis of the TSDR of *FOXP3* [10]. This indicates the presence of a quantitative reduction of regulatory elements, associated with impaired peripheral survival and compromised IL-2 responsiveness through STAT5 signaling. Moreover, in all CD25-deficient patients described to date, a defect in antigen-specific immune response was demonstrated. This is consistent with the increased susceptibility to infections.

De novo germline-activating *STAT3* mutations, which were recently described in 5 individuals [33], cause early-onset autoimmunity, including T1D. All the genetic alterations reported lead to enhanced STAT3 activity, unlike what happens in the case of inactivating *STAT3* mutations, which are responsible for hyper-IgE syndrome. Four out of 5 patients presented with very-early-onset (0–43 weeks) T1D, and in 3 of these 4 T1D autoantibodies were detected. Probands also showed intrauterine growth

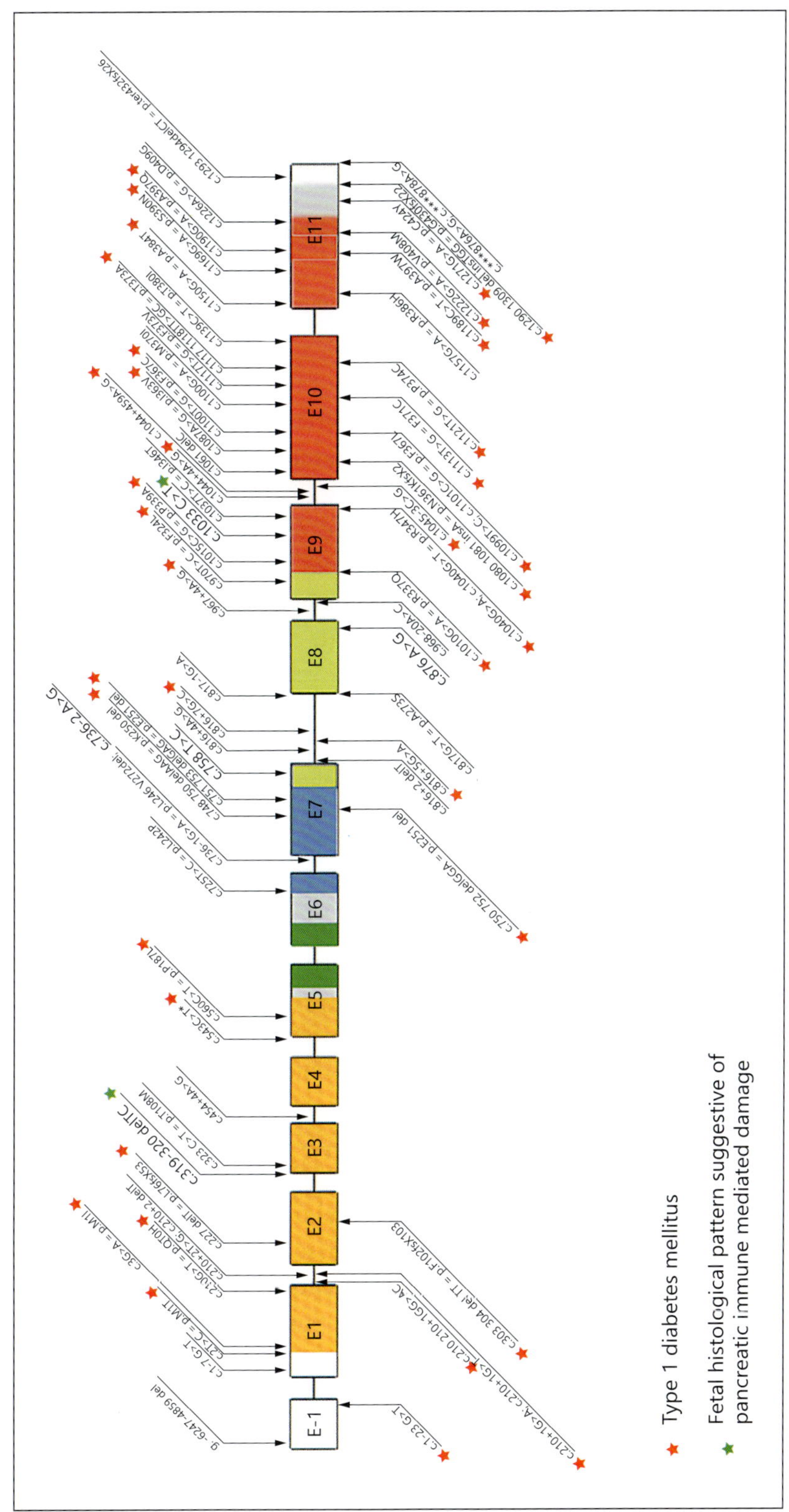

Fig. 1. *FOXP3* gene reporting the currently reported mutations with highlighted the cases in which type 1 diabetes was present. Annotations refer to both the coding sequence and protein, when applicable (www.ncbi.nlm.nih.gov/CCDS, accession No. CCDS14323.1).c543C>T is a polymorphism. E, exon. Color code: orange, N-terminal domain; green, zinc finger domain; blue, Leucin zipper domain; yellow, prolin rich domain; red, forkhead domain. Modified from Barzaghi et al. [2].

Type 1 Diabetes Mellitus in Monogenic Autoimmune Diseases

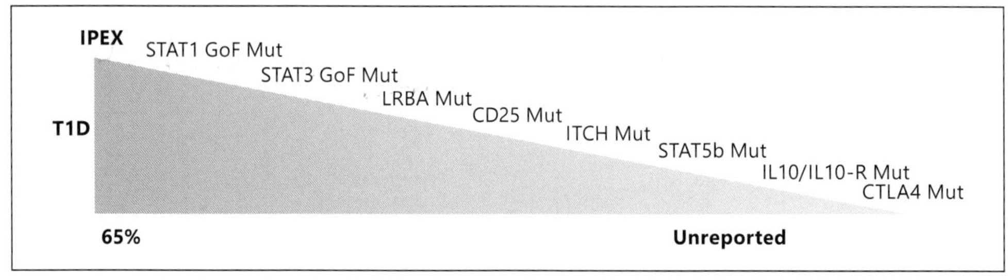

Fig. 2. Overview of type 1 diabetes (T1D) occurrence in different immunodeficiencies with autoimmunity.

retardation due to severe impairment in fetal insulin secretion, a common feature in different subtypes of neonatal diabetes. Other autoimmune manifestations included autoimmune enteropathy, autoimmune interstitial lung disease, and juvenile-onset arthritis. All the patients presented short stature and eczema. The immunological analyses performed in 2 affected individuals revealed not only a reduction in Treg levels and an increase in CD4 T-cell cytokine production, but also hypogammaglobulinemia with terminal B-cell maturation arrest, dendritic cell deficiency, peripheral eosinopenia, increased double-negative (CD4–CD8–) T cells, and decreased natural killer cells [34]. It has been hypothesized that a *STAT3* activation mutation could determine Treg deficiency through a shift to an effector phenotype, represented for example by an increase in Th17. In support of this hypothesis is the fact that, unlike *STAT3* gain of function mutation, germline dominant-negative *STAT3* mutations in individuals with hyper-IgE syndrome cause a primary immunodeficiency disorder characterized by elevated serum IgE levels and recurrent staphylococcal infections resulting from a deficiency in Th17 cells. However, the *STAT3* patients described by Haapaniemi et al. [34] presented reduced frequency of Th17 cells and reduced IL-17 production.

Interestingly, 13 other individuals with heterozygous activating *STAT3* mutations have been described [28]. Of these patients, only 2 presented T1D, and enteropathy was not predominant. The most common autoimmune manifestations were represented by autoimmune cytopenia. Many patients also presented lymphadenopathy and short stature. Cases of arthritis, lymphocytic interstitial pneumonia, hepatitis, atopic dermatitis, and alopecia were also present. Several patients also had recurrent and severe infections (mainly of fungal origin), often associated with hypogammaglobulinemia. Notably, 2 relatives of the described patients presented *STAT3* mutations associated with a much milder clinical phenotype, thus suggesting the presence of incomplete penetrance, in addition to clinical heterogeneity.

Immunological studies revealed increased STAT3 transcriptional activity, which was not associated with a constitutively phosphorylation but, more likely, with a delayed phosphorylation kinetics. Of note, the reduction in Tregs was confirmed and a possible mechanism of this reduction was provided: a major downstream STAT3 target, *SOCS3*, also upregulated, can suppress Treg function. Moreover, STAT5 phosphorylation appeared persistently decreased in response to IL-2. In addition, STAT1 phosphorylation was decreased. Interestingly, Milner et al. [28] also provide information regarding the therapeutic management of these patients that can involve, for example, anti-IL-6R monoclonal antibody therapy (tocilizumab). IL-6 is in fact one of the primary cytokines that utilizes STAT3 for signal transduction. The patient treated presented a severe form of arthritis and scleroderma-like skin changes that significantly improved with anti-IL-6 therapy. The clinical improvement was accompanied by a decrease in Th17 frequency. The curative approach remains hematopoietic stem cell transplantation, which was performed in 2 patients: in one case, the patient is alive and well and presents a complete remission of the autoimmune manifestations; in the other, a severe graft-versus-host disease associated with disseminated adenoviral infection led to the patient's death.

Heterozygous *STAT1* gain-of-function mutations can cause an IPEX-like syndrome, which has been characterized by enteropathy, growth failure, eczema, and T1D in 3 cases out of the 5 described up to now [35]. Interestingly, only 1 patient had antiglutamate decarboxylase antibodies. Moreover, 4 patients presented chronic mucocutaneous candidiasis (in the absence of anti-IL-17 or IL-22 antibodies), and all of them had frequent respiratory tract infections. Two patients presented autoimmune thyroiditis. Three patients had cardiac or vascular defects. CD4 T-cell lymphopenia, reduced memory B cells, and defective vaccine responses were common among the patients and progressed with age. Gain-of-function mutations determine STAT1 hyperphosphorylation and abnormal dephosphorylation. Patients presented normal Treg percentages in the CD4 T-cell compartment, with normal suppressive function, and reduced Th17 cells, in contrast with what has been seen in IPEX patients. A possible pathogenic mechanism could reside in the increase in STAT1-related cytokines that in turn would alter regulatory functions, although this hypothesis has not yet been demonstrated.

STAT5b deficiency is an autosomal recessive syndrome characterized by chronic diarrhea, failure to thrive, growth hormone insensitivity, recurrent infections, and eczema [36]. Less than 10 cases have been described in the literature. Rare cases of arthritis, thyroiditis, and thrombocytopenic purpura have been reported but, interestingly, no cases of T1D have been described.

Similarly to CD25 deficiency, Tregs are quantitatively normal or slightly reduced. The increased susceptibility to infections is explained by the fact that STAT5 is part of IL-2 signaling. The milder presentation, when compared to CD25 deficiency, can be due to the fact that *STAT5a*, the homologous gene of *STAT5b*, can replace some of the functions.

The analysis of several members of a highly consanguineous Amish family presenting with organomegaly, failure to thrive, developmental delay, dysmorphic features, and autoimmune inflammatory cell infiltration of the lungs, liver, and gut revealed a homozygous *ITCH* mutation [37]. Out of 10 patients, only 1 was diagnosed with T1D;

autoantibodies were not measured. *ITCH* encodes for an E3 ubiquitin ligase that attaches ubiquitin to substrate proteins and, therefore, catalyzes the final steps of protein degradation. In T cells, this role can, for example, affect the downregulation of the T-cell receptor. An inactivating homologous mutation in *ITCH* can therefore lead to indiscriminate T-cell activation and loss of tolerance to self-antigens. In mice, mutations of the E3 ligase *Itch* cause fatal autoimmune disease characterized by histiocyte and lymphocyte multiorgan infiltration. Human ITCH deficiency causes disease beyond the immune system, consistent with the role of protein ubiquitination in cell trafficking, functional activation, proteosomal degradation, and programmed cell death.

A recent report has described an IPEX-like syndrome caused by loss-of-function mutations in *LRBA* (LPS-responsive beige-like anchor) [38], previously reported as causative in cases of CVID with autoimmunity. One of the 6 affected patients suffered from intractable diarrhea, early-onset T1D (within 4 months), autoimmune hypothyroidism, autoimmune anemia, and recurrent sepsis. In the other affected individuals, recurrent infections and lymphoproliferation were the main clinical features. Moreover, immunological analyses performed in a large cohort of *LRBA*-mutated patients revealed Treg deficiency, impaired Treg-suppressive function, and increased levels of autoantibodies against autologous antigens.

The possible pathogenic mechanism could be related to an LRBA-mediated mTOR impairment responsible for altered metabolic sensing in Tregs.

As recently reported in 4 patients from unrelated families [39], germline heterozygous *CTLA-4* mutations cause a severe form of immune dysregulation, characterized by lymphocytic infiltration of organs, such as intestine, brain, and lung, lymphadenopathy, hepatosplenomegaly, and autoimmune cytopenia. Immunologically, these patients present hypogammaglobulinemia, reduced naïve T cells, and mature B cells. CTLA-4 is an inhibitory receptor constitutively expressed by Tregs, conferring suppressive functions. Tregs of affected patients were quantitatively normal, but expressed reduced levels of FOXP3 and CD25 and presented impaired suppressive functions. On the other hand, the patients' T cells were hyperproliferative. The simultaneous presence of lymphopenia could be due to increased apoptotic mechanisms. B cells appeared altered with an increase in autoreactive cell populations, thus highlighting the possible role of Tregs in promoting B-cell tolerance. Interestingly, 3 relatives harboring *CTLA-4* mutations were healthy and did not present clinical or immunological findings consistent with the disease, thus leading to the possibility of incomplete penetrance. Despite the reported Treg dysfunction, T1D or other endocrinopathies were not reported.

A last possible cause of an IPEX-like syndrome with severe inflammatory bowel disease is represented by loss-of-function alterations in the *IL10* or *IL10-R* genes [40]. In the reported patients, however, no association between enteropathy and T1D was found. In addition, no clear overlap is evident between *IL10/IL10-R*-deficient patients and *STAT3*-mutated patients (neither activating nor inactivating) although they share the same signaling pathway, with IL-10 eliciting STAT3 phosphorylation.

Conclusions

Monogenic diseases have shed light onto the pathogenesis of immune-mediated diseases, such as T1D. The discovery of new forms of monogenic autoimmune syndromes has revealed an ever more complex network of common pathogenic pathways. The study of these mechanisms can improve the understanding of the pathogenesis of polygenic forms of diabetes, in which the role of Treg dysfunction is still controversial.

The elucidation of the immunological alterations responsible for both the monogenic and polygenic forms of diseases will allow the development of therapies that will potentially correct or prevent the actual origin of the disease, substituting immunosuppressive and replacement treatments.

References

1 Wildin RS, et al: X-linked neonatal diabetes mellitus, enteropathy and endocrinopathy syndrome is the human equivalent of mouse scurfy. Nat Genet 2001; 27:18–20.

2 Barzaghi F, Passerini L, Bacchetta R: Immune dysregulation, polyendocrinopathy, enteropathy, X-linked syndrome: a paradigm of immunodeficiency with autoimmunity. Front Immunol 2012;3:211.

3 von Boehmer H, Melchers F: Checkpoints in lymphocyte development and autoimmune disease. Nat Immunol 2010;11:14–20.

4 Sakaguchi S: Naturally arising CD4+ regulatory t cells for immunologic self-tolerance and negative control of immune responses. Annu Rev Immunol 2004;22:531–562.

5 Schmetterer KG, Neunkirchner A, Pickl WF: Naturally occurring regulatory T cells: markers, mechanisms, and manipulation. FASEB J 2012;26:2253–2276.

6 Burchill MA, et al: IL-2 receptor beta-dependent STAT5 activation is required for the development of Foxp3+ regulatory T cells. J Immunol 2007;178:280–290.

7 Passerini L, et al: STAT5-signaling cytokines regulate the expression of FOXP3 in CD4+CD25+ regulatory T cells and CD4+CD25– effector T cells. Int Immunol 2008;20:421–431.

8 Lal G, et al: Epigenetic regulation of Foxp3 expression in regulatory T cells by DNA methylation. J Immunol 2009;182:259–273.

9 Baron U, et al: DNA demethylation in the human FOXP3 locus discriminates regulatory T cells from activated FOXP3(+) conventional T cells. Eur J Immunol 2007;37:2378–2389.

10 Barzaghi F, et al: Demethylation analysis of the FOXP3 locus shows quantitative defects of regulatory T cells in IPEX-like syndrome. J Autoimmun 2012;38:49–58.

11 Walker LS: Treg and CTLA-4: two intertwining pathways to immune tolerance. J Autoimmun 2013; 45:49–57.

12 d'Hennezel E, et al: The immunogenetics of immune dysregulation, polyendocrinopathy, enteropathy, X linked (IPEX) syndrome. J Med Genet 2012;49:291–302.

13 Gambineri E, et al: Clinical and molecular profile of a new series of patients with immune dysregulation, polyendocrinopathy, enteropathy, X-linked syndrome: inconsistent correlation between forkhead box protein 3 expression and disease severity. J Allergy Clin Immunol 2008;122:1105–1112.e1.

14 Bacchetta R, et al: Defective regulatory and effector T cell functions in patients with FOXP3 mutations. J Clin Invest 2006;116:1713–1722.

15 Passerini L, et al: Forkhead box protein 3 (FOXP3) mutations lead to increased Th17 cell numbers and regulatory T-cell instability. J Allergy Clin Immunol 2011;128:1376–1379.e1.

16 Kinnunen T, et al: Accumulation of peripheral autoreactive B cells in the absence of functional human regulatory T cells. Blood 2013;121:1595–1603.

17 Zama D, et al: Late-onset of immunodysregulation, polyendocrinopathy, enteropathy, X-linked syndrome (IPEX) with intractable diarrhea. Ital J Pediatr 2014;40:68.

18 Xavier-da-Silva MM, et al: Fetal-onset IPEX: report of two families and review of literature. Clin Immunol 2015;156:131–140.

19 Vasiljevic A, et al: Immune dysregulation, polyendo-crinopathy, enteropathy, X-linked syndrome and re-current intrauterine fetal death. Lancet 2015;385:2120.

20 Wildin RS, Smyk-Pearson S, Filipovich AH: Clinical and molecular features of the immunodysregulation, polyendocrinopathy, enteropathy, X linked (IPEX) syndrome. J Med Genet 2002;39:537–545.

21 Kobayashi I, et al: Autoantibodies to villin occur fre-quently in IPEX, a severe immune dysregulation, syndrome caused by mutation of FOXP3. Clin Im-munol 2011;141:83–89.

22 Lampasona V, et al: Autoantibodies to harmonin and villin are diagnostic markers in children with IPEX syndrome. PLoS One 2013;8:e78664.

23 Yong PL, Russo P, Sullivan KE: Use of sirolimus in IPEX and IPEX-like children. J Clin Immunol 2008; 28:581–587.

24 Battaglia M, et al: Rapamycin promotes expansion of functional CD4+CD25+FOXP3+ regulatory T cells of both healthy subjects and type 1 diabetic patients. J Immunol 2006;177:8338–8347.

25 Burroughs LM, et al: Stable hematopoietic cell en-graftment after low-intensity nonmyeloablative con-ditioning in patients with immune dysregulation, polyendocrinopathy, enteropathy, X-linked syn-drome. J Allergy Clin Immunol 2010;126:1000–1005.

26 Passerini L, et al: Gene/cell therapy approaches for immune dysregulation polyendocrinopathy enter-opathy X-linked syndrome. Curr Gene Ther 2014; 14:422–428.

27 Edghill EL, et al: HLA genotyping supports a nonau-toimmune etiology in patients diagnosed with diabe-tes under the age of 6 months. Diabetes 2006;55: 1895–1898.

28 Milner JD, et al: Early-onset lymphoproliferation and autoimmunity caused by germline STAT3 gain-of-function mutations. Blood 2015;125:591–599.

29 Rubio-Cabezas O, et al: Clinical heterogeneity in pa-tients with FOXP3 mutations presenting with per-manent neonatal diabetes. Diabetes Care 2009;32: 111–116.

30 Sharfe N, et al: Human immune disorder arising from mutation of the alpha chain of the interleukin-2 re-ceptor. Proc Natl Acad Sci U S A 1997;94:3168–3171.

31 Caudy AA, et al: CD25 deficiency causes an immune dysregulation, polyendocrinopathy, enteropathy, X-linked-like syndrome, and defective IL-10 expres-sion from CD4 lymphocytes. J Allergy Clin Immunol 2007;119:482–487.

32 Goudy K, et al: Human IL2RA null mutation mediates immunodeficiency with lymphoproliferation and au-toimmunity. Clin Immunol 2013;146:248–261.

33 Flanagan SE, et al: Activating germline mutations in STAT3 cause early-onset multi-organ autoimmune disease. Nat Genet 2014;46:812–814.

34 Haapaniemi EM, et al: Autoimmunity, hypogamma-globulinemia, lymphoproliferation, and mycobacte-rial disease in patients with activating mutations in STAT3. Blood 2015;125:639–648.

35 Uzel G, et al: Dominant gain-of-function STAT1 mutations in FOXP3 wild-type immune dysregula-tion-polyendocrinopathy-enteropathy-X-linked-like syndrome. J Allergy Clin Immunol 2013;131: 1611–1623.

36 Nadeau K, Hwa V, Rosenfeld RG: STAT5b deficien-cy: an unsuspected cause of growth failure, immuno-deficiency, and severe pulmonary disease. J Pediatr 2011;158:701–708.

37 Lohr NJ, et al: Human ITCH E3 ubiquitin ligase de-ficiency causes syndromic multisystem autoimmune disease. Am J Hum Genet 2010;86:447–453.

38 Charbonnier LM, et al: Regulatory T-cell deficiency and immune dysregulation, polyendocrinopathy, enteropathy, X-linked-like disorder caused by loss-of-function mutations in LRBA. J Allergy Clin Im-munol 2015;135:217–227.

39 Kuehn HS, et al: Immune dysregulation in human subjects with heterozygous germline mutations in CTLA4. Science 2014;345:1623–1627.

40 Beser OF, et al: Clinical features of interleukin 10 re-ceptor gene mutations in children with very early-onset inflammatory bowel disease. J Pediatr Gastro-enterol Nutr 2015;60:332–338.

Rosa Bacchetta, MD
Division of Stem Cell Transplantation and Regenerative Medicine
Department of Pediatrics, Stanford University School of Medicine
Lorry I. Lokey Stem Cell Research Building
265 Campus Drive West, Room G3015, Stanford, CA 94305-5461 (USA)
E-Mail rosab@stanford.edu

Barbetti F, Ghizzoni L, Guaraldi F (eds): Diabetes Associated with Single Gene Defects and Chromosomal Abnormalities. Front Diabetes. Basel, Karger, 2017, vol 25, pp 91–103 (DOI: 10.1159/000454704)

Genetic and Immunological Features of Insulin-Dependent Diabetes Mellitus as a Clinical Manifestation of Type 1 Autoimmune Polyglandular Syndrome

Alessandra Fierabracci · Benedetta Russo

Infectivology and Clinical Trials Area, Bambino Gesù Children's Hospital, IRCCS, Rome, Italy

Abstract

Type 1 autoimmune polyglandular syndrome (APS1) is a rare autosomal recessive disease caused by mutations in the autoimmune regulator gene (AIRE). The fundamental pathogenetic mechanism appears to be mediated by T cells since the translated Aire protein is involved in the transcriptional regulation of the expression of organ-specific antigens within the thymus. While a high prevalence of this monogenic disease is reported in Finland and Scandinavia (Norway), there are also clusters of similar patients in continental Italy and Sardinia, among Iranian Jews, and in other countries. Criteria for the diagnosis of the syndrome are the presence of at least 2 of the following disorders: chronic mucocutaneous candidiasis, hypoparathyroidism, and Addison disease. Other endocrine or non-endocrine autoimmune conditions can be associated with it, including insulin-dependent diabetes mellitus (type 1 diabetes). Type 1 diabetes has been rarely reported in different series of patients affected by the syndrome and especially among Finnish patients. In this chapter we discuss the relevant studies that highlight the peculiar genetic and immunological features that in addition to the effect of *AIRE* gene mutations are responsible for the occurrence of type 1 diabetes within the APS1 population in different countries. © 2017 S. Karger AG, Basel

Type 1 autoimmune polyglandular syndrome (APS1) (OMIM ID: 240300), also known as autoimmune polyendocrinopathy-candidiasis-ectodermal dystrophy syndrome or Whitaker's syndrome, was first reported by Leonard in 1929 (reviewed in [1]) and is an inherited rare autosomal recessive disorder, characterized by a broad spectrum of endocrine deficiencies (reviewed in [2]). While a high prevalence of this monogenic disease is reported in Finland (1:25,000) and Scandinavia (Norway) [3], there are also clusters of similar patients in continental Italy [4] and Sardinia (1:14,000) [5], among Iranian Jews (1:9,000) [3, 6], and in other countries as well [7–9].

Criteria for the diagnosis of APS1 are the presence of at least 2 of the following disorders: chronic mucocutaneous candidiasis (CMC), hypoparathyroidism, and primary adrenal insufficiency (Addison disease). Other endocrine or non-endocrine autoimmune conditions can be associated (vide infra). The locus for APS1, the *AIRE* (autoimmune regulator) gene has been mapped on chromosome 21q22.3 [2]. This monogenic disease has offered a unique possibility to gain new knowledge on the immune system, especially on the function of the translated Aire protein which is affected by *AIRE* mutations. Several molecular studies and in vitro experiments have documented that this protein is involved in the transcriptional regulation of the expression of organ-specific antigens within the thymus [2]. This envisages its relevant role for the establishment of T-cell tolerance and regulating the negative selection of autoreactive T-cell clones. In light of this, APS1 has certainly worked as a powerful model to address the question of how a tolerant state is achieved or maintained and to explore how it gets lost in the context of autoimmunity.

To date, over 60 mutations of the *AIRE* gene have been discovered, which helps to facilitate the genetic diagnosis of APS1 in different groups of patients together with testing anti-interferon-ω (IFNω) autoantibodies [2]. Mutation c.769 C>T (p.Arg257X) was demonstrated to be responsible for 82% of APS1 alleles in Finnish patients, while the c.254A>G (A374G, p.Tyr85Cys) mutation was prevalent in Iranian Jewish patients [10]. In Sardinia, the c.415C>T (p.Arg139X) mutation was common in APS1 patients [5]. A 964del13 mutation in the *AIRE* gene encoding a p.Cys322fsX372 change was present in 71% of British and 56% of United States APS1 patients (reviewed in [10]). All APS1 patients from 15 Irish families carried a c.967_979del (p.L323_L327>SfsX51) mutation (reviewed in [10]). Despite the known monogenic etiology, there are no known genotype/phenotype correlations in different populations, except for the missense mutation 6 c.682T>G (p.Gly228Trp) identified in an Italian family with APS1, closely cosegregating with hypothyroid autoimmune thyroiditis [11].

Immunological Features of Type 1 Autoimmune Polyglandular Syndrome

APS1 patients develop autoantibodies against affected organs, i.e., autoantibodies against the steroidogenic enzymes P450scc, P450c17, and P450c21 in patients with Addison disease and/or gonadal failure [12], diabetes-related autoantibody specificities including insulin, proinsulin, glutamic acid decarboxylase isoform 65 (GAD65), aromatic L-amino acid decarboxylase (AADC) (vide infra), the insulinoma-associated antigen/tyrosine-phosphatase-like molecule (IA-2), IA-2β or phogrin, thyroid-related autoantibodies, antithyroglobulin and antithyroperoxidase, celiac disease-related antitransglutaminase antibodies, autoimmune enteropathy-related specificities against tryptophan hydroxylase, and parathyroid autoantigen NACHT leucine-rich-repeat protein 5 (NALP5) [13]. Mostly organ-specific autoantibodies are directed

Table 1. Incidence of clinical manifestations in representative type 1 autoimmune polyglandular syndrome series

Author	Patients, n	Population	CMC, %	Adrenal failure, %	Parathyroid insufficiency, %	T1D, %	Ovarian failure, %	Malabsorption intestinal dysfunction, %	Alopecia, %	Parietal cell atrophy, %	Keratopathy, %	Hepatitis, %
Ahonen et al. [3], 1990	68	Finnish	100	72	79	12	60	18	29	13	35	12
Zlotogora and Shapiro [6], 1992	23	Iranian	17	22	96	4	38		22		0	
Faiyaz-Ul-Haque et al. [7], 2009	14	Arab	78	42.8	100	14.2			57		7.1	
Cihakova et al. [26], 2001	27	Eastern European	85	88.8	92.6	3.7		18.5	40.7	11 gastritis	37 ectodermal dystrophy keratoconjunctivitis	14.8
Collins et al. [27], 2006	18	Irish	100	72	77.7	11	18		33		11	16.6
Meloni et al. [38], 2012	22	Sardinian	95.4	68	77	4.5	61	50 intestinal dysfunction	45.4	31.8	63.6 dental enamel defects/ nail dystrophy/ keratoconjunctivitis	27

against enzymes that play a role in hormonogenesis within the intracellular compartment. Therefore, they appear to have no pathogenic role. Another immunological feature is the presence of circulating neutralizing antibodies to cytokines in the peripheral blood of APS1 patients. These specificities are rare in healthy controls and can block class I IFN secretion in vivo and in vitro [14]. Neutralizing autoantibodies to Th17 cytokines, i.e., IL-17A, IL-17F, and IL-22, are also present in the peripheral blood of patients, causing defective antifungal responses as putative contributors to the occurrence of CMC in APS1 [15].

The fundamental pathogenetic mechanisms in APS1 appear to be T-cell mediated. Regarding the T-cell phenotype, CD8+ effector T cells were reported to circulate at increased frequency [16]. Contradictory reports refer to the CD4+ T-cell population, with Perniola et al. [17] observing an increased frequency of CD4+CD25+ lymphocytes and Kekäläinen et al. [18] a reduction of the FoxP3$^+$Treg population.

Clinical Manifestations of APS1
APS1 is a complex syndrome of associated autoimmune and immunodeficiency manifestations (vide supra). Clinically, APS1 patients present the sequential occurrence of a variety of different disorders with different degrees of severity and at different time lapses from the occurrence of the first manifestation (Table 1) [19]. The number of disease components in the same individual can vary from 0 to 9 and the age of the first clinical manifestation from some months to adulthood [19]. Also the sequence in which disease components present can be different and variations within the same

family suggest that factors other than specific *AIRE* mutations may contribute. Generally, patients develop CMC in early infancy or during childhood [20] with the only R257X genotype reported as a frequent association.

CMC has a prevalence of 100% in Finnish APS1 patients, while it is rarely reported in Iranian Jews [6]. Usually, APS1 patients subsequently develop autoimmune hypoparathyroidism and Addison disease. Hypoparathyroidism is the most common autoimmune component in APS1. When hypoparathyroidism occurs without any known cause, the differential diagnosis with APS1 should be considered. Addison disease is the second most frequent autoimmune disorder. In a large series of Finnish APS1 patients [3] it was reported in 72% of cases. Gonadal failure is a common autoimmune component, especially in females. Ovarian insufficiency was reported as the third most frequent autoimmune component, reaching up to 65% of APS1 women [21]. It can manifest as primary amenorrhea with failure of arrested pubertal development. Insulin-dependent diabetes (type 1 diabetes [T1D]), alopecia areata, vitiligo, ectodermal dystrophy, non-infectious nail dysplasia, enamel dysplasia, transient skin rash during fever episodes, and ocular symptoms [22] are other rare associated diseases. APS1 patients may also develop celiac disease and other intestinal dysfunctions including chronic diarrhea, constipation and malabsorption, chronic atrophic gastritis with or without pernicious anemia (Biermer disease), and chronic active hepatitis. Rarely, APS1 patients may be affected by tubule-interstitial nephritis or organized pneumonitis, autoimmune thyroid disease, and pernicious anemia [20]. Hyposplenism/asplenia, probably due to an autoimmune mechanism, may occur [20].

Some population-based differences were reported for peculiar phenotypic manifestations. For example, Addison disease is less common in Iranian Jewish patients, whereas in Finnish patients diabetes mellitus is more common than in other ethnic groups [6, 23].

In this chapter we review the incidence of T1D in APS1 patients of different geographical distribution. We also highlight the peculiar immunological features of the disorder when developed in the context of this syndrome.

Insulin-Dependent Diabetes Mellitus as a Clinical Manifestation in APS1

T1D is a multifactorial autoimmune disease with a strong genetic component. The disorder occurs in HLA genetically predisposed individuals as a consequence of organ-specific immune destruction of the insulin-producing β-cells in the islets of Langerhans within the pancreas [24]. In the genetic background, dominant loci predisposing to the disease were recognized within the major histocompatibility complex and the human leukocyte antigen (HLA) region. In both Europeans and North Americans of European ancestry, susceptibility loci within the HLA complex DRB1 0401, DRB1 0402, DRB1 0405, DQA1 0301, DQB1 0302, or DQB1 0201 alleles were identified. In contrast, certain HLA alleles, DRB1 1501, 1401, or 0701 and DQB1 0602, 0503, or 0303, confer strong protection [24].

The disorder develops as a consequence of a combination of genetic predisposition, still unknown environmental factors, and stochastic events [24]. From a pathogenetic point of view, the disease is the result of a breakdown in immune regulation that leads to expansion of autoreactive CD4+ and CD8+ T cells, autoantibody-producing B lymphocytes, and activation of the innate immune system.

T1D has been reported as occurring in different series of APS1 patients with a frequency that varies from 1 to 18% of cases [1, 3, 23]. Several studies have demonstrated that the prevalence of T1D in Finnish APS1 patients is considerably elevated [3]. A series of 68 APS1 patients documented to have APS1 in Finland between 1910 and 1988, recruited from 54 families, was followed up by Ahonen et al. [3]. The age of patients varied from 10 months to 60 years. All patients developed candidiasis during their life. Oral candidiasis was observed as the first symptom in 60% of patients, while malabsorption was observed in 9% and keratopathy in 3%. Eight patients (12%) developed T1D with an age of disease onset varying from 4.1 to 37 years. In a subsequent series of Finnish APS1 patients published by Perheentupa and Miettinen [23], T1D appeared in 18% of 78 patients at the age of 4.1 to 45 years. The highest incidence for T1D was 0.014 cases per patient/year at 15–20 years of age; the highest incidence was 0.03 in the age range between 40 and 50 years. In a subsequent investigation, 8 out of 47 patients were affected by T1D [25].

Cihakova et al. [26] investigated 27 APS1 patients of Eastern and Central European origin. Only 1 patient in this APS1 series was affected by T1D as a secondary manifestation.

An Irish APS1 case series including 18 patients from 15 families was reported by Collins et al. [27] with a mean age at diagnosis of 6 years (range: 8 months to 18 years). In this series only 2 patients were affected by T1D.

APS1 has not been fully investigated in Arab countries. Faiyaz-Ul-Haque et al. [7] reported 7 Arab families in which 18 patients were affected by the syndrome. In addition to the main components, T1D was diagnosed in only 2 patients.

Genetic Factors Predisposing to Type 1 Diabetes in APS1 Patients

From epidemiological studies, APS1 is seen as occurring sporadically or among siblings [1]. In unraveling factors that may predispose APS1 patients to peculiar immunological disorders, we have to point out that in early studies no association was reported between APS1 and HLA class I or II [1, 28]. Further studies demonstrated that the HLA-A28 haplotype was more frequent in APS1 patients than in healthy controls [1, 29]; the same studies reported the HLA-A3 is more frequent in APS1 patients with ovarian failure than in APS1 patients with normal ovarian function. In the series of Betterle et al. [1], the examination of HLA class I antigens in 17 patients did not show significant differences compared to normal controls, while when analyzing HLA class II (DR genes) an increased frequency of DR3 and DR5 was detected.

Subsequently, the discovery that APS1 is a monogenic disorder due to mutations in the *AIRE* gene led to the hypothesis that allelic variants of the *AIRE* gene are involved in autoimmunity in general. In particular, the high incidence of T1D in APS1 patients from Finland led to the idea that *AIRE* variants could underlie the pathogenesis of general T1D. It has been suggested that genetic variability in the *AIRE* locus and in particular heterozygous loss-of-function mutations might favor development of certain organ-specific autoimmune disorders by affecting the presentation of self-antigens in the thymus and borderline tolerance [30]. According to a modern view, predisposition to develop autoimmunity can also be enhanced by sequence polymorphisms in the coding sequence of *AIRE* [30]. Of note in parents of APS1 patients harboring heterozygous *AIRE* mutations, immunological dysregulation was detected in the peripheral blood, demonstrated by elevated levels of IgA and activated T lymphocytes [31]. Thus, the possibility remains that more detailed analysis of *AIRE* may show that genetic variability of the gene affects the predisposition to non-APS1 autoimmunity [21].

The insulin (*INS*) gene has repeatedly been associated with T1D [32]. This association was probably reported as due to the locus IDDM2, mapped within the upstream region of the *INS* gene and corresponding to a minisatellite polymorphism of VNTR (variable number of tandem repeats) of the chromosome 11p15.5 [33]. VNTR affects the ectopic expression of insulin in the thymus, thus inducing susceptibility to T1D [34].

In light of this, Turunen et al. [33] explored the potential interaction of *AIRE* and *INS* genes in the development of T1D in Finnish APS1 patients. They failed to detect an association of any of 5 common *AIRE* SNPs selected from the public database (dsSNP) (rs2776377, rs878081, rs1800520, rs933150, and rs1800522) or the corresponding *AIRE* haplotypes in T1D when examining 733 Finnish patients and 735 controls. Instead, as expected, the –23*Hph*I polymorphism in the *INS* gene was significantly associated with T1D in the Finnish population ($p = 6.8 \times 10^{-12}$) [32].

A subsequent genetic study was conducted by Paquette et al. [35] to ascertain the risk of autoimmune diabetes among APS1 patients in Finland. It is known that the most important susceptibility locus for T1D called IDDM is found within the major histocompatibility complex class II region of chromosome 6p21.31. In addition, protective alleles for T1D such as DRB1*15 and DQB1*0602 are also protective in APS1, and alleles predisposing to Addison disease (DRB1*03) and alopecia (DRB1*0302, DRB1*04) in patients without APS1 are also predisposing to these conditions in APS1 patients [19]. Paquette et al. [35] investigated the locus IDDM2 of the chromosome 11p15 as predisposing to T1D. The authors had previously reported 2 APS1 siblings, members of a French Canadian Family, who in spite of having the same *AIRE* mutation were discordant for T1D [36]. The affected sibling was found to possess a 5′ INS VNTR I/I genotype, while the unaffected sibling had a I/III genotype, suggesting the involvement of this locus in APS1-associated T1D. Therefore, the 5′ INS VNTR locus was genotyped together with several flanking 11p15.5 markers in a cohort of 50 Finnish APS1 patients. They found that *IDDM2* is more prevalent in the diabetic Finnish APS1 patients than in the non-diabetic ones, adding evidence that loss of Aire function is not exclusively involved in the development of T1D in APS1.

A similar study was conducted by Adamson et al. [37] in the UK, where APS1 is a rare disease with an estimated prevalence of 2–3 cases per million. They investigated a cohort of 33 patients with APS1, representing a substantial sample of all the APS1 patients in the UK population. The mean age was 23.5 years and 24% of them had T1D. The patients were genotyped for the HPhI polymorphism, which is in high linkage disequilibrium with the insulin gene VNTR alleles. They found an association between the occurrence of T1D and homozygosity for the T1D susceptibility locus class I/INS VNTR allele in APS1 patients.

In the study by Halonen et al. [19], the association of *AIRE* mutations and HLA class II genotypes was evaluated in a series of APS1 patients from different countries. The only genotype-phenotype correlation was found for the R257X mutation and the high frequency of MC (vide supra). They discovered that individual HLA class II genotypes may modify the APS1 phenotype since interesting associations with some alleles were found for Addison disease, alopecia, and T1D. These associated alleles were those established for these disorders in the absence of APS1. The DB1*03 allele had a higher prevalence of Addison disease. Alopecia showed a strong association with the DRB1*04 allele. DRB1*15-DQB1*0602, the major protective haplotype for T1D, was also found to be protective in APS1 patients. In addition, an association between HLA alleles and the presence of serum antibodies was found; however, only a tendency toward an association was observed, suggesting that HLA alleles do not have a strong influence on autoantibody formation. This result appeared in contrast with what was described for isolated diseases in which peculiar HLA alleles are frequently associated with the presence of circulating autoantibodies.

The clinical features of 22 pediatric Sardinian APS1 patients were examined prospectively within a follow-up of 25 years [38]. Their symptoms were correlated with *AIRE* and HLA class II genotypes. In this sample population, the female/male ratio was 1.44 with an age range between 1.8 and 46 years. Age of disease onset was 0.3–10 years with a median of 3.6 years. Besides the classical triad components, autoimmune hepatitis occurred in 27% of cases, with a higher incidence in females (5:1). Only 1 patient developed T1D. The most represented *AIRE* nonsense mutation was R139X, which was found in 93% of mutant *AIRE* alleles while serum anti-IFNω antibodies were detected in all patients – even in the preclinical period at 4 months of age in 1 sibling. HLA alleles appear to influence the phenotype. In particular, the association of autoimmune hepatitis with the HLA-DRB1*0301-DQB1*0201 allele and the presence of liver-kidney microsomal antibodies was evident.

The rare incidence of T1D in APS1 patients was interpreted as due not only to the absence of genetic haplotypes predisposing to the disease [1], but also to predisposing markers of pancreatic autoimmunity.

Major autoantigens in T1D include insulin, GAD65 and GAD67, IA-2, IA-2β or phogrin, and proinsulin [39]. GAD65 antibodies are present in the serum of 80% of T1D patients at diagnosis, while GAD67 antibodies are less frequent and are probably the result of reactivity against epitopes shared with GAD65 [25, 40].

As reported by Björk et al. [40], elevated titers of GADA and ICA were detected although clinical T1D is a rare entity in APS1 patients. However, APS1 patients have antibodies reactive with epitopes within the GAD65 molecule that are different from those of non-APS1 T1D patients, and the autoantigenic molecule can be presented to the immune system through different pathogenetic mechanisms. In their experimental setup, the different reactivity of anti-GAD containing sera from patients with recent-onset T1D, stiff-man syndrome (SMS), and APS1 was investigated. All 3 types of pathological samples immunoprecipitated GAD from $[^{35}S]$-methionine-labeled rat islet lysates. Sera from SMS and APS1 patients, but not from T1D patients, recognized the human GAD conformation on Western blot. Inhibition of the GAD enzymatic activity was obtained with APS1 and SMS sera, but not with T1D sera. These data led some authors to hypothesize that GAD antibody specificities can simply represent an epiphenomenon of an inflammatory process within the pancreas that does not lead to clinical disease manifestations [25].

Ronkainen et al. [41] also evaluated the human autoimmune response to the main autoantigen GAD65 found both in T1D and APS1 patients. They further unraveled whether the difference in the T1D incidence was associated with a different humoral response to GAD65. The sera of 20 APS1 patients and 20 T1D patients were analyzed for the presence of epitope and isotope-specific GAD65 antibodies. In contrast to the study by Björk et al. [40], GAD65 antibodies were found to target both the middle carboxy-terminal and less frequently the amino-terminal region of GAD65 in both categories of patients. These antibodies were especially of the IgG1 subclass and less frequently of the IgG2 and IgG4 subclasses. However, human IgG2-GAD65 antibodies were more frequently associated with T1D.

In the series of patients followed-up by Betterle et al. [1] only 1 patient had T1D, and in this patient the serum ICA tested negative. Circulating ICA were detectable in the series of 12 out of 40 patients with T1D (30%), especially in association with antibodies to GAD65 (GADA). Nevertheless, positivity for 51-kDa protein antibodies was found in 10 out of 15 APS1 patients (66%) without any correlation with ICA or GADA positivity. Five patients were followed up for a mean period of 8 years, but T1D clinical onset was not reported.

In the paper by Gylling et al. [42], β-cell autoantibodies directed against GAD65, ICA, IA2, and anti-insulin (IAA) together with HLA II alleles were investigated in 60 Finnish patients with APS1. Out of the 60 patients, 12 developed T1D, and 36% of the patients for whom prediabetic samples were available had IA2 antibodies and IAA. Of the non-diabetics, none had IAA and only 4% had IA2 antibodies. Furthermore, these specificities persisted in the circulation for years without development of clinical T1D. The authors concluded that IA2 or IAA antibodies have a low sensitivity (36%), but that they are nevertheless highly specific (96 and 100%, respectively). Overall, their predictive value is 67% for T1D development in APS1 patients. Prior to this study, no positive or negative association with human leukocyte II antigens was reported for any disease component. Instead, Gylling et al. [42] reported data available by examining 59 patients, including 11 with T1D and 8 additional non-diabetic patients. No T1D patients had the protective DQB1*0602 allele, while 15 out of 56 non-diabetic patients and 24 out of 93 individuals of the control group possessed it.

In the Finnish study by Perheentupa and Miettinen [23], out of 47 patients, 5 were diabetic and only 1 was ICA positive in repeated serum samples. In a subsequent investigation, 8 out of 47 patients were affected by T1D [43]. Of these, 6 tested positive for GAD65 antibodies, 1 for GAD67 antibodies, and 4 for ICA. Two samples tested negative for all these specificities. Conversely, out of the 39 non-diabetic patients, 16 had circulating GAD65 antibodies, 11 had GAD67 antibodies, and 11 had ICA; 20 had at least 1 antibody specificity. There was no difference in the age of onset of GAD65 antibodies among patients who did or did not develop T1D. Antibody positivity persisted for 10.1 years in patients who did not develop T1D, while it persisted for 4.4 years in patients who developed the disease. An in vitro proliferative response of peripheral blood lymphocytes was observed in 15 out of 44 patients versus 3 out of 28 normal controls. An increased secretion of IFNγ was detected in the supernatants of GAD65-stimulated peripheral blood lymphocytes of 16 out of 28 patients, and in 19% of normal controls. Cellular responses and levels of IFNγ secretion correlated negatively with antibody levels. A parallel tendency was only observed in 4 patients, indicating a reciprocal control of humoral and cellular immunity [44]. Furthermore, the proliferative response to GAD65 was significantly associated with the HLA diabetes risk genotype HLA DQB1*0201, but the humoral response was not associated with a particular allele. Interestingly, in GAD65 antibody-positive non-diabetics, a lower frequency of diabetes predisposing alleles HLA DQ and HLADR was found than in the GAD65 antibody-negative non-diabetics, justifying the lower incidence of T1D in GAD65 antibody-positive patients.

The L-Amino Acid Decarboxylase Autoantigen
Velloso et al. [45] investigated the autoimmune response against the pancreatic β-cells in 6 APS1 patients. All of the patients were affected by the classical main symptoms of mucocutaneous candidiasis. All of the patients had high titers of islet cell antibodies. Five out of 6 sera had reactivity against GAD65. All sera from APS1 patients immunoprecipitated the 51-KDa antigen from [^{35}S]-methionine-labelled rat islet cell lysates. The control sera of 9 T1D patients, 7 patients with Addison disease, 4 patients

with autoimmune gastritis, 5 patients with Graves disease, and 2 patients with SMS showed similar reactivity. This novel autoantigen was not detectable in tissue homogenates of other endocrine and non-endocrine organs. However, the antigen was detectable in the RINm5F rat insulinoma cell line, but not in the SV-40 transformed monkey kidney cell line COS. This antigen was found unrelated to GAD since depletion from the islet lysate with GAD did not affect the amount of the 51-KDa autoantigen [45]. Nonetheless, in the study by Velloso et al. [45], APS1 patients did not show clinical T1D or had an altered insulin response to the glucose challenge test, suggesting that they have an autoimmune response against the islets, which is different from that causing the classical T1D. Subsequently, the 51-KDa antigen was characterized as AADC (reviewed in [46]).

In the study by Husebye et al. [46], the presence of AADC antibodies was assessed in APS1 patients and in patients affected by T1D. These specificities were detected in 51% of APS1 patients, but in none of the 138 T1D patients or in the healthy controls. AADC antibodies were more frequent in APS1 patients with autoimmune hepatitis than in those without hepatitis. Eighty percent of APS1 patients with vitiligo had these antibodies compared to 43% of those without vitiligo. Out of 9 APS1 patients with diabetes, 5 had both AADC antibodies and GADA, 2 only AADC, and 2 only GADA. The authors concluded that AADC antibodies are especially involved in the pathogenesis of autoimmune chronic active hepatitis and vitiligo in APS1 patients, whereas the role of these specificities in the development of T1D in APS1 patients remains to be unraveled.

Conclusions

APS1 is a rare disease, and the incidence of T1D reported in APS1 population studies where the disorder has been mainly investigated, such as Finland, the UK, and Sardinia, is also rare. The rarity of APS1 has generally caused difficulties in recruiting biological samples to unravel the relevant disease-related immunological features and even more for the diabetic APS1 population. So far, the different humoral response to GAD65 in the diabetic APS1 patients compared to the non-APS1 diabetics has not been ascertained, such as the relevance of the AADC antibody specificities. No *AIRE* SNP association has been found with T1D in APS1 patients as for other diseases except for the R257X genotype frequently associated with candidiasis. Studies have pointed to the involvement of the *INS*-23HphI variant or IDDM2 in diabetic Finnish APS1 in comparison to non-diabetics. As far as how studies on the pathogenetic events that influence the disease development and clinical features of APS1 will progress, new knowledge will be gained also regarding the factors leading to T1D clinical onset in APS1 patients. These studies will help to predict with more accuracy the T1D onset and outcome in APS1 patients in reference to other clinical manifestations.

References

1 Betterle C, Greggio NA, Volpato M: Clinical review 93: autoimmune polyglandular syndrome type 1. J Clin Endocrinol Metab 1998;83:1049–1055.

2 Fierabracci A: Recent insights into the role and molecular mechanisms of the autoimmune regulator (AIRE) gene in autoimmunity. Autoimmun Rev 2011;10:137–143.

3 Ahonen P, Myllärniemi S, Sipilä I, Perheentupa J: Clinical variation of autoimmune polyendocrinopathy-candidiasis-ectodermal dystrophy (APECED) in a series of 68 patients. N Engl J Med 1990;322:1829–1836.

4 Scott HS, Heino M, Peterson P, Mittaz L, Lalioti MD, Betterle C, Cohen A, Seri M, Lerone M, Romeo G, Collin P, Salo M, Metcalfe R, Weetman A, Papasavvas MP, Rossier C, Nagamine K, Kudoh J, Shimizu N, Krohn KJ, Antonarakis SE: Common mutations in autoimmune polyendocrinopathy-candidiasis-ectodermal dystrophy patients of different origins. Mol Endocrinol 1998;12:1112–1119.

5 Rosatelli MC, Meloni A, Meloni A, Devoto M, Cao A, Scott HS, Peterson P, Heino M, Krohn KJ, Nagamine K, Kudoh J, Shimizu N, Antonarakis SE: A common mutation in Sardinian autoimmune polyendocrinopathy-candidiasis-ectodermal dystrophy patients. Hum Genet 1998;103:428–434.

6 Zlotogora J, Shapiro MS: Polyglandular autoimmune syndrome type I among Iranian Jews. J Med Genet 1992;29:824–826.

7 Faiyaz-Ul-Haque M, Bin-Abbas B, Al-Abdullatif A, Abdullah Abalkhail H, Toulimat M, Al-Gazlan S, Al-mutawa AM, Al-Sagheir A, Peltekova I, Al-Dayel F, Zaidi SH: Novel and recurrent mutations in the AIRE gene of autoimmune polyendocrinopathy syndrome type 1 (APS1) patients. Clin Genet 2009;76:431–440.

8 Bin-Abbas BS, Faiyaz-Ul-Haque M, Al-Fares AH, Al-Gazlan SS, Bhuiyan JA, Al-Muhsen SZ: Autoimmune polyglandular syndrome type 1 in Saudi children. Saudi Med J 2010;31:788–792.

9 Orlova EM, Bukina AM, Kuznetsova ES, Kareva MA, Zakharova EU, Peterkova VA, Dedov II: Autoimmune polyglandular syndrome type 1 in Russian patients: clinical variants and autoimmune regulator mutations. Horm Res Paediatr 2010;73:449–457.

10 Björses P, Halonen M, Palvimo JJ, Kolmer M, Aaltonen J, Ellonen P, Perheentupa J, Ulmanen I, Peltonen L: Mutations in the AIRE gene: effects on subcellular location and transactivation function of the autoimmune polyendocrinopathy-candidiasis-ectodermal dystrophy protein. Am J Hum Genet 2000;66:378–392.

11 Cetani F, Barbesino G, Borsari S, Pardi E, Cinferotti L, Pinchera A, Marcocci C: A novel mutation of the autoimmune regulator gene in an Italian kindred with autoimmune polyendocrinopathy-candidiasis-ectodermal dystrophy, acting in a dominant fashion and strongly cosegregating with hypothyroid autoimmune thyroiditis. J Clin Endocrinol Metab 2001;86:4747–4752.

12 Uibo R, Aavik E, Peterson P, Perheentupa J, Aranko S, Pelkonen R, Krohn KJ: Autoantibodies to cytochrome P450 enzymes P450scc, P450c17 and P450c21 in autoimmune polyglandular disease types I and II and in isolated Addison's disease. J Clin Endocrinol Metab 1994;78:323–328.

13 Alimohammadi M, Björklund P, Hallgren A, Pöntynen N, Szinnai G, Shikama N, Keller MP, Ekwall O, Kinkel SA, Husebye ES, Gustafsson J, Rorsman F, Peltonen L, Betterle C, Perheentupa J, Akerström G, Westin G, Scott HS, Holländer GA, Kämpe O: Autoimmune polyendocrine syndrome type 1 and NALP5, a parathyroid autoantigen. N Engl J Med 2008;358:1018–1028.

14 Meloni A, Furcas M, Cetani F, Marcocci C, Falorni A, Perniola R, Pura M, Bøe Wolff AS, Husebye ES, Lilic D, Ryan KR, Gennery AR, Cant AJ, Abinun M, Spickett GP, Arkwright PD, Denning D, Costigan C, Dominguez M, McConnell V, Willcox N, Meager A: Autoantibodies against type I interferons as an additional diagnostic criterion for autoimmune polyendocrine syndrome type I. J Clin Endocrinol Metab 2008;93:4389–4389.

15 Puel A, Döffinger R, Natividad A, Chrabieh M, Barcenas-Morales G, Picard C, Cobat A, Ouachée-Chardin M, Toulon A, Bustamante J, Al-Muhsen S, Al-Owain M, Arkwright PD, Costigan C, McConnell V, Cant AJ, Abinun M, Polak M, Bougnères PF, Kumararatne D, Marodi L, Nahum A, Roifman C, Blanche S, Fischer A, Bodemer C, Abel L, Lilic D, Casanova JL: Autoantibodies against IL-17A, IL-17F, and IL-22 in patients with chronic mucocutaneous candidiasis and autoimmune polyendocrine syndrome type I. J Exp Med 2010;207:291–297.

16 Laakso SM, Kekäläinen E, Rossi LH, Laurinolli TT, Mannerström H, Heikkilä N, Lehtoviita A, Perheentupa J, Jarva H, Arstila TP: IL-7 dysregulation and loss of CD8+ T cell homeostasis in the monogenic human disease autoimmune polyendocrinopathy-candidiasis-ectodermal dystrophy. J Immunol 2011;187:2023–2030.

17 Perniola R, Lobreglio G, Rosatelli MC, Pitotti E, Accogli E, De Rinaldis C: Immunophenotypic characterisation of peripheral blood lymphocytes in autoimmune polyglandular syndrome type 1: clinical study and review of the literature. J Pediatr Endocrinol Metab 2005;18:155–164.

18 Kekäläinen E, Tuovinen H, Joensuu J, Gylling M, Franssila R, Pöntynen N, Talvensaari K, Perheentupa J, Miettinen A, Arstila TP: A defect of regulatory T cells in patients with autoimmune polyendocrinopathy-candidiasis-ectodermal dystrophy. J Immunol 2007;178:1208–1215.

19 Halonen M, Eskelin P, Myhre AG, Perheentupa J, Husebye ES, Kämpe O, Rorsman F, Peltonen L, Ulmanen I, Partanen J: AIRE mutations and human leukocyte antigen genotypes as determinants of the autoimmune polyendocrinopathy-candidiasis-ectodermal dystrophy phenotype. J Clin Endocrinol Metab 2002;87:2568–2574.

20 Kluger N, Ranki A, Krohn K: APECED: is this a model for failure of T cell and B cell tolerance? Front Immunol 2012;3:232.

21 Arstila TP, Jarva H: Human APECED; a sick thymus syndrome? Front Immunol 2013;4:313.

22 Merenmies L, Tarkkanen A: Chronic bilateral keratitis in autoimmune polyendocrinopathy-candidiadis-ectodermal dystrophy (APECED). A long-term follow-up and visual prognosis. Acta Ophthalmol Scand 2000;78:532–535.

23 Perheentupa J, Miettinen A: Autoimmune polyendocrine syndrome type I (APECED); in Eisenbarth GS (ed): Endocrine and Organ Specific Autoimmunity. Austin, RG Landes Company, 1999, pp 19–40.

24 Bluestone JA, Herold K, Eisenbarth G: Genetics, pathogenesis and clinical interventions in type 1 diabetes. Nature 2010;464:1293–1300.

25 Tuomi T, Björses P, Falorni A, Partanen J, Perheentupa J, Lernmark A, Miettinen A: Antibodies to glutamic acid decarboxylase and insulin-dependent diabetes in patients with autoimmune polyendocrine syndrome type I. J Clin Endocrinol Metab 1996;81:1488–1494.

26 Cihakova D, Trebusak K, Heino M, Fadeyev V, Tiulpakov A, Battelino T, Tar A, Halász Z, Blümel P, Tawfik S, Krohn K, Lebl J, Peterson P: Novel AIRE mutations and P450 cytochrome autoantibodies in Central and Eastern European patients with APECED. Hum Mutat 2001;18:225–232.

27 Collins SM, Dominguez M, Ilmarinen T, Costigan C, Irvine AD: Dermatological manifestations of autoimmune polyendocrinopathy-candidiasis-ectodermal dystrophy syndrome. Br J Dermatol 2006;154:1088–1093

28 Maclaren NK, Riley WJ: Inherited susceptibility to autoimmune Addison's disease is linked to human leukocyte antigens-DR3 and or DR4, except when associated with type I autoimmune polyglandular syndrome. J Clin Endocrinol Metab 1986;62:455–459.

29 Ahonen P, Koskimies S, Lokki ML, Tiilikainen A, Perheentupa Y: The expression of autoimmune polyglandular disease type I appears associated with several HLA-A antigens but not with HLA-DR. J Clin Endocrinol Metab 1998;66:1152–1157.

30 Fierabracci A: The role of heterozygous mutations of the autoimmune regulator gene (AIRE) in non-APECED autoimmunity: a comment on recent findings. Clin Endocrinol (Oxf) 2011;74:532–533.

31 Sedivá A, Ciháková D, Lebl J: Immunological findings in patients with autoimmune polyendocrinopathy-candidiasis-ectodermal dystrophy (APECED) and their family members: are heterozygotes subclinically affected? J Pediatr Endocrinol Metab 2002;15:1491–1496.

32 Hirschhorn JN: Genetic epidemiology of type 1 diabetes. Pediatr Diabetes 2003;4:87–100.

33 Turunen JA, Wessman M, Forsblom C, Kilpikari R, Parkkonen M, Pöntynen N, Ilmarinen T, Ulmanen I, Peltonen L, Groop PH: Association analysis of the AIRE and insulin genes in Finnish type 1 diabetic patients. Immunogenetics 2006;58:331–338.

34 Vafiadis P, Ounissi-Benkalha H, Palumbo M, Grabs R, Rousseau M, Goodyer CG, Polychronakos C: Class III alleles of the variable number of tandem repeat insulin polymorphism associated with silencing of thymic insulin predispose to type 1 diabetes. J Clin Endocrinol Metab 2001;86:3705–3710.

35 Paquette J, Varin DS, Hamelin CE, Hallgren A, Kämpe O, Carel JC, Perheentupa J, Deal CL: Risk of autoimmune diabetes in APECED: association with short alleles of the 5′insulin VNTR. Genes Immun 2010;11:590–597.

36 Ward L, Paquette J, Seidman E, Huot C, Alvarez F, Crock P, Delvin E, Kämpe O, Deal C: Severe autoimmune polyendocrinopathy-candidiasis-ectodermal dystrophy in an adolescent girl with a novel AIRE mutation: response to immunosuppressive therapy. J Clin Endocrinol Metab 1999;84:844–852.

37 Adamson KA, Cheetham TD, Kendall-Taylor P, Seckl JR, Pearce SH: The role of the IDDM2 locus in the susceptibility of UK APS1 subjects to type 1 diabetes mellitus. Int J Immunogenet 2007;34:17–21.

38 Meloni A, Willcox N, Meager A, Atzeni M, Wolff AS, Husebye ES, Furcas M, Rosatelli MC, Cao A, Congia M: Autoimmune polyendocrine syndrome type 1: an extensive longitudinal study in Sardinian patients. J Clin Endocrinol Metab 2012;97:1114–1124.

39 Fierabracci A: The potential of multimer technologies in type 1 diabetes prediction strategies. Diabetes Metab Res Rev 2011;27:216–229.

40 Björk E, Velloso LA, Kämpe O, Karlsson FA: GAD autoantibodies in IDDM, stiff-man syndrome, and autoimmune polyendocrine syndrome type I recognize different epitopes. Diabetes 1994;43:161–165.

41 Ronkainen MS, Härkönen T, Perheentupa J, Knip M: Characterization of the humoral immune response to glutamic acid decarboxylase in patients with autoimmune polyendocrinopathy-candidiasis-ectodermal dystrophy (APECED) and/or type 1 diabetes. Eur J Endocrinol 2005;153:901–906.

42 Gylling M, Tuomi T, Björses P, Kontiainen S, Partanen J, Christie MR, Knip M, Perheentupa J, Miettinen A: ss-cell autoantibodies, human leukocyte antigen II alleles, and type 1 diabetes in autoimmune polyendocrinopathy-candidiasis-ectodermal dystrophy. J Clin Endocrinol Metab 2000;85:4434–4440.

43 Perheentupa J: APS-I/APECED: the clinical disease and therapy. Endocrinol Metab Clin North Am 2002;31:295–320.

44 Harrison LC, Honeyman MC, DeAizpurua HJ, Schmidli RS, Colman PG, Tait BD, Cram DS: Inverse relation between humoral and cellular immunity to glutamic acid decarboxylase in subjects at risk of insulin-dependent diabetes. Lancet 1993;341:1365–1369.

45 Velloso LA, Winqvist O, Gustafsson J, Kämpe O, Karlsson FA: Autoantibodies against a novel 51 kDa islet antigen and glutamate decarboxylase isoforms in autoimmune polyendocrine syndrome type I. Diabetologia 1994;37:61–69.

46 Husebye ES, Gebre-Medhin G, Tuomi T, Perheentupa J, Landin-Olsson M, Gustafsson J, Rorsman F, Kämpe O: Autoantibodies against aromatic L-amino acid decarboxylase in autoimmune polyendocrine syndrome type I. J Clin Endocrinol Metab 1997;82:147–150.

Alessandra Fierabracci, MD, PhD
Infectivology and Clinical Trials Area
Bambino Gesù Children's Hospital, IRCCS
Viale S. Paolo 15, IT–00146 Rome (Italy)
E-Mail alessandra.fierabracci@opbg.net

Barbetti F, Ghizzoni L, Guaraldi F (eds): Diabetes Associated with Single Gene Defects and Chromosomal Abnormalities. Front Diabetes. Basel, Karger, 2017, vol 25, pp 104–118 (DOI: 10.1159/000454738)

Syndromes Associated with Mutations in the Insulin Signalling Pathway

Sarah M. Leiter · Robert K. Semple

University of Cambridge Metabolic Research Laboratories, Wellcome Trust-MRC Institute of Metabolic Science, Addenbrooke's Hospital, Cambridge, UK

Abstract

Insulin resistance is a common feature of type 2 diabetes mellitus and the metabolic syndrome, in which it is believed to be a key pathogenic factor. In such common diseases, insulin resistance is likely to have an oligogenic or polygenic aetiology. It may also more rarely be caused by monogenic defects affecting components of the insulin signalling pathway. The most commonly identified mutations, first described in 1988, lie in the *INSR* gene, encoding the insulin receptor. These may lead to either extreme infantile insulin resistance with autosomal recessive inheritance, or to autosomal dominant insulin resistance presenting peripubertally. Insulin receptor defects may present with hyperinsulinaemic hypoglycaemia and concomitant postprandial hyperglycaemia, but by the time of diagnosis insulin-resistant diabetes is more common. Frequently, however, the syndromes are recognised first by severe clinical hyperandrogenism in peripubertal girls, or by growth disorders including impaired linear growth, acanthosis nigricans, and pseudoacromegaly. Since 2004, several other genetic defects in the canonical insulin signalling pathway have been identified, affecting *PIK3R1*, *AKT2*, or *TBC1D4*. An overview of the genetic, metabolic, and syndromic features of the resulting forms of severe insulin resistance is given.

© 2017 S. Karger AG, Basel

The purification and first therapeutic use of insulin in 1922 has led to more than a century of intensive investigation to date aimed at elucidating the mechanisms by which insulin acts on its target tissues in health, and the mechanisms whereby its action goes awry in pandemic diseases. Insulin resistance (IR) is generally defined in terms of attenuation of the hypoglycaemic actions of insulin, and was noted first in the 1930s in the condition that has later come to be described, somewhat loosely, as type 2 diabetes [1]. IR is well recognised as a precursor of diabetes, is present in almost 90% of patients with established type 2 diabetes, and is moreover a key component of the metabolic syndrome [2, 3]. It is especially seen in older, obese patients with a family history of diabetes, and has been linked to non-alcoholic fatty liver disease, dyslipidaemia, ovarian dysfunction, and cancer as well as to diabetes itself [4–6]. IR may also sometimes be "physiological", such as during puberty and pregnancy, where it reflects modulation of the relative anabolic and catabolic actions of insulin on different tissues, such that metabolism is remodelled to allow efficient channelling of energy to growing tissues.

Elucidating the pathophysiological mechanisms underlying common IR has proved a thorny challenge. No individual factor is identified as being causative in most cases. Instead, IR is usually considered to reflect interaction between an oligogenic or polygenic diathesis and a series of environmental stressors, principal among which is obesity. Since at least the 1950s, however, small numbers of patients with early onset and severe resistance to insulin have been described, and in the past 30 years many such patients have been shown to harbour single gene pathogenic mutations underlying their extreme metabolic phenotype. In this chapter we will discuss the clinical and genetic features of severe IR associated with monogenic defects in the insulin signalling pathway. Severe IR caused by failure of adipocyte development or function is discussed in the following chapter [Leiter and Semple, this vol., pp. 119–133].

Biochemical Diagnosis of Severe Insulin Resistance

Insulin sensitivity is a continuous variable. In other words, it runs as a spectrum across the population, and so numerical thresholds used to define different severities of IR are arbitrary. This problem is rendered more complex still by variation in insulin sensitivity across the lifespan and according to environmental factors. As an approximate guideline, in lean patients with fully functional β-cells, concentrations of postprandial insulin (>1,500 pmol/L) or elevated fasting insulin (>150 pmol/L) may be operationally regarded as diagnostic for severe IR. In the face of obesity, puberty, or pregnancy, however, insulin concentrations should ideally be viewed in the context of a reference range from appropriately matched patients. Where there is absolute β-cell failure and dependence upon exogenous insulin, conversely, insulin requirements in excess of 3 U/kg/day suggests severe resistance to insulin. In most patients, however, there is some degree of dysglycaemia, and usually relative insulin deficiency, complicating interpretation of biochemical parameters.

Syndromes of severe IR may pose further diagnostic challenges: abnormal glucose homeostasis is usually present long before presentation with signs and symptoms of hyperglycaemia, and, for reasons which are not fully understood, hypoglycaemia, which may be occur postprandially or in the fasting state, is fairly frequent early in the disease course before β-cell decompensation occurs [7–9]. Screening using fasting blood glucose alone for severe IR is thus potentially highly misleading, and often oral glucose tolerance testing with determination of glucose and insulin is needed to demonstrate severe hyperinsulinaemia unequivocally. All these considerations mean that a clinical assessment taking into account the history and clinical features of severe IR is of critical importance.

General Clinical Features of Severe Insulin Resistance

Acanthosis nigricans (AN) denotes hyperpigmented, velvety thickening of the skin, usually in skin folds such as in the axillae, groin, and submammary and nuchal regions. In very severe cases it may also occur on the face (e.g., periocular, perioral, and in nasolabial folds), perianally, or even on planar surfaces. Histological appearances are somewhat bland, with evidence of dermal and epidermal hyperproliferation. It is often seen together with skin tags (acrochordons), and is a cardinal clinical feature of severe IR, at least before β-cell deficiency supervenes. Indeed, although it may very rarely be seen in isolation as a familial condition, observed as a paraneoplastic phenomenon, or seen in complex syndromes, for example with craniosynostosis, it is a visible sign of IR in the vast majority of cases [10].

AN is a particularly valuable clinical sign as it is easily observable in any clinical setting, irrespective of ready access to facilities for insulin assay and other biochemical evaluations. Moreover, although frequently not volunteered by patients or their families, it is not uncommon for those with congenital severe IR to remember regularly having their neck scrubbed by their mothers in childhood because of "having a dirty neck". While AN is a reliable clinical correlate of IR, it is not specific to monogenic severe IR, most commonly being seen in more prevalent, obesity-related IR, meaning that it occurs at relatively high prevalence in obese populations [11]. There is also considerable interindividual variability in the clinical expression of AN. Nevertheless, it is a key clinical sign of potential monogenic severe IR when seen in lean individuals.

The occurrence of AN in all known genetic forms of IR, whether affecting the receptor or distal signalling molecules, and the common observation that it fades gradually as β-cell decompensation appears and hyperglycaemia worsens, strongly implicates hyperinsulinaemia in the pathogenesis of AN. It is most likely that increased signalling through another trophic receptor by very elevated levels of plasma insulin mediates this association, and the IGF-1 receptor is the most likely candidate receptor by virtue of its ability to bind and be activated by insulin, albeit with less potency than the cognate ligand, IGF-1. Some of the increased IGF-1 signalling may relate to changes in IGF-1R expression, or to paracrine alterations in IGF-1 production or bioavailability.

Perhaps the commonest reasons for presentation to medical attention of severe IR are clinical features of androgen excess in young women, coupled with oligomenorrhoea or amenorrhoea, which may even be primary in severe cases. In effect, the presentation is with a severe form of "polycystic ovary syndrome", and indeed the ovarian morphology and histological appearances in severe IR is indistinguishable from that described in prevalent polycystic ovary syndrome. SIR-associated hyperandrogenism can sometimes correspond to testosterone levels in excess of 10 nmol/L, in the normal male range, commonly triggering a search for virilising tumours.

Ovarian enlargement and hyperandrogenism is seen in infants with few or no functional insulin receptors [12, 13], and may appear acutely and reversibly appear upon development of anti-insulin receptor antibodies in later life [14]. The trophic effects of hyperinsulinaemia on the ovary appear to require synergy with gonadotrophin action, and unpublished experience suggests that suppressive use of GnRH agonists may be an effective treatment for severe hyperandrogenism in the context of severe or extreme IR. As for AN, the most plausible mechanism proposed for the actions of very high levels of insulin on the ovary involve excessive stimulation of the IGF-1 receptor by a combination of direct agonism of high insulin levels at the receptor itself, and also possibly perturbation of levels of the IGF-1 receptor and/or its binding proteins [15]. Hyperinsulinism also commonly leads to decreased circulating levels of sex hormone-binding globulin, potentially increasing the bioavailability of testosterone, thereby exacerbating the clinical problem, although hyperandrogenism is still seen in cases of insulin receptoropathy, where sex hormone-binding globulin is often preserved or frankly elevated [16].

Specific Monogenic Forms of Severe Insulin Resistance

Syndromes due to Mutation of the Insulin Receptor

Painstaking biochemical studies led in 1985 to identification and sequencing of the cellular receptor for insulin, which was shown to be a transmembrane receptor tyrosine kinase [17]. The insulin receptor (INSR) is now known to be a heterotetrameric receptor consisting of 2 extracellular α-subunits as well as 2 transmembrane β-subunits. Both α- and β-subunits are encoded by the same gene located on chromosome 19 and are proteolytically cleaved following translation [18]. Interstitial insulin binds to the extracellular domain of the insulin receptor leading to a conformational change and the activation of the kinase domains within the β-subunit causing transphosphorylation between the subunits. These phosphorylation events bring about the recruitment of receptor substrates, in particular members of the insulin receptor substrate (IRS) family, and induce activation of a signalling network in responsive tissues that is simply schematised in Figure 1.

Rare and extreme forms of IR had already been described clinically in the 1950s [19, 20], although biochemical proof of IR in these and further syndromes had to wait for development of radioimmunoassays [21], and was forthcoming in the 1970s. Following publication of the sequence of the human insulin receptor gene [17], attention quickly turned to sequencing the gene in patients with severe IR and

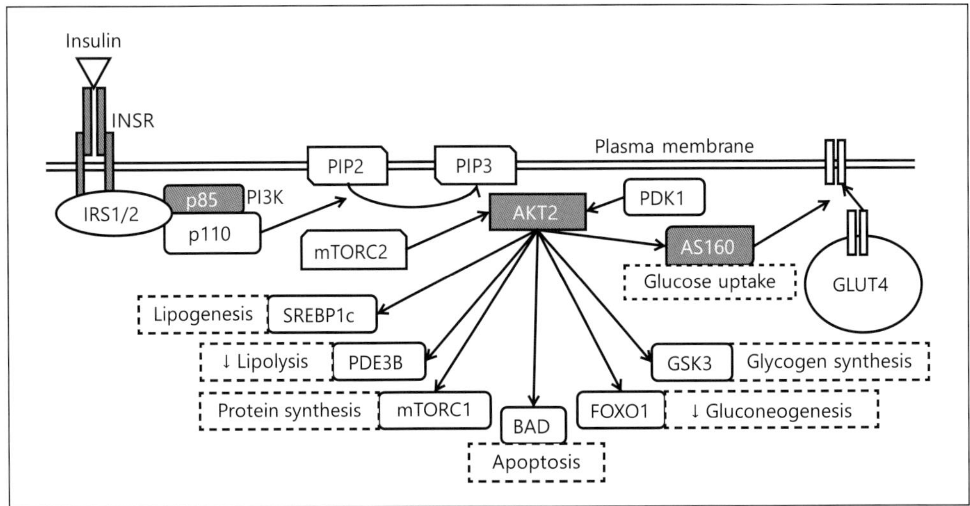

Fig. 1. Overview over the canonical insulin signalling pathway. Grey proteins are those known to cause monogenic forms of severe insulin resistance. INSR, insulin receptor; IRS1/2, insulin receptor substrate 1/2; PI3K, phosphoinositide-3-kinase; p85 and p110, regulatory and catalytic subunits of PI3K, respectively; PIP2, phosphatidylinositol-4,5-bisphosphate; PIP3, phosphatidylinositol-3,4,5-trisphosphate; AKT2, protein kinase B β (PKBβ); mTORC2, mammalian target of rapamycin complex 2; PDK1, 3-phosphoinositide dependent protein kinase-1; AS160, AKT substrate of 160 kDa; GLUT4, glucose transporter type 4; SREBP1c, sterol regulatory element-binding protein 1; PDE3B, phosphodiesterase 3B; mTORC1, mammalian target of rapamycin complex 2; BAD, Bcl-2-associated death promoter; FOXO1, forkhead box protein O1; GSK3, glycogen synthase kinase.

reduced cellular insulin binding. In 1988, the first papers describing pathogenic loss-of-function mutations in the human insulin receptor were duly published [22, 23], and since then over 150 different mutations have been described, including missense, nonsense, and splice site mutations, as well as small and large insertion-deletion mutations [24].

Pathogenic mutations in the insulin receptor have been classified according to the nature of the deficit in receptor expression or function (Table 1) [25]. The most important division of the mutations clinically, however, is between those which lead to loss-of-function of the receptor coded by the mutant allele without interfering with the coexpressed wild-type allele, and those which not only impair function of the mutant itself, but also have the ability to interfere with the wild-type allele [24]. The latter class of mutations invariably fall in the intracellular domains of the receptor, and confer autosomal dominant severe IR, whereas the former types of mutation confer severe IR with autosomal recessive inheritance (Fig. 2). From a clinical point of view, syndromes due to genetic alterations in the insulin receptor are best divided into extreme infantile forms, almost invariably with recessive inheritance, or less extreme forms, most commonly diagnosed peripubertally, which are most commonly inherited as dominant traits.

Table 1. Classification of loss-of-function mutations in the insulin receptor gene *INSR* (adapted from [25])

Class	Mechanism	Examples of mutations	Comments
I	Decreased mRNA levels	R372X, R897X	Reduced mRNA levels without *INSR* mutations have been observed suggesting the presence of unproven *cis*-acting promotor mutations
II	Defects in post-translational processing or transport	G31R, L62P, L93Q, H209R, G359S	Commonly also result in abnormal receptor function
III	Impairment in ligand binding	L233P, R252C, S323L, L460E	
IV	Reduction in tyrosine kinase activity	A1135E, R1164Q, R1174Q, P1178L	Most frequent class of mutations in "type A" insulin resistance
V	Increase in receptor degradation	K460E, N462S	

Recessive Extreme Insulin Receptoropathy

The most extreme forms of congenital IR were first described in the 1950s based on the dysmorphic features of the conditions [19, 20], but it was more than 30 years until they were proven to be accounted for by *INSR* mutations [22]. These syndromes form a continuum of severity, ranging from those caused by complete absence of functional receptors, generally lethal in the first year of life, and those where small residual amounts of receptor expression are retained, and in which survival until the third decade of life is possible. The term "leprechaunism" was once widely used to describe the most severe cases, but is now increasingly avoided in favour of "Donohue syndrome" (DS) in the most severe cases or "Rabson-Mendenhall syndrome" (RMS) in those with more prolonged survival [19, 20].

Donohue Syndrome

Patients with DS may be recognised during gestation due to intrauterine growth retardation, with birth weight commonly in the range of 1–1.5 kg. As well as severely impaired linear growth, severely decreased or absent INSR signalling leads to poor development of skeletal muscle and adipose tissue. In contrast, however, many non-classically insulin-responsive tissues show marked overgrowth, seen as thick lips, enlarged ears, and a generally coarse facial appearance, hypertrichosis, AN, and generalised organomegaly (Fig. 3) [26]. Ovarian enlargement may be severe and sufficient to compromise ventilation in severe cases, and development of granulosa cell tumours has been described [12, 27]. Nephrocalcinosis is also extremely common [28, 29], sometimes in association with a renal tubulopathy resembling Bartter syndrome [29, 30], while enlarged livers are reported at postmortem to be green and bile engorged [31, 32]. Cardiac hypertrophy is also commonly

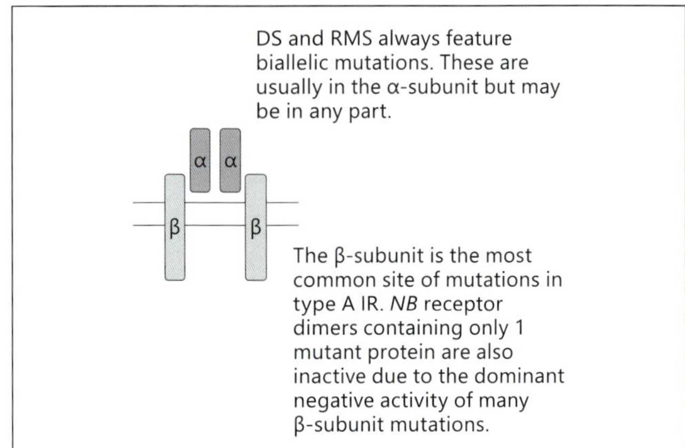

Fig. 2. INSR genotype-phenotype correlations. DM, Donohue syndrome; RMS, Rabson-Mendenhall syndrome.

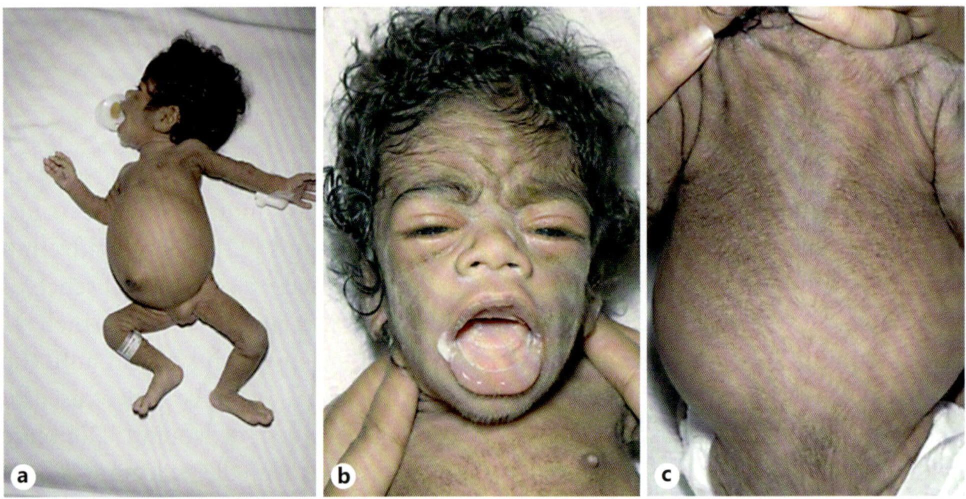

Fig. 3. Characteristic appearance of Donohue syndrome. **a** Abdominal distension, inguinal hernia, large hands and feet, clitoromegaly, and lipohypotrophy. **b** Gum and lip hypertrophy, triangular facies, hirsutism, prominent eyes with infraorbital creases, and nipple hypertrophy. **c** Hypertrichosis and acanthosis nigricans. Reproduced with permission from [26].

described [30, 33], and overgrowth of colonic mucosa, sometimes with rectal prolapse, may be seen.

DS usually presents with fasting hypoglycaemia and postprandial hyperglycaemia as well as extreme hyperinsulinaemia, with blood insulin concentrations commonly in excess of 10,000 pmol/L. Severe glycaemic fluctuations between fed and fasted states pose a major therapeutic challenge. Surprisingly, neonates and infants with DS do not exhibit diabetic ketoacidosis [34], which is at odds with mice deficient in the Insr, which die neonatally of rampant acidosis [35]. The reasons for this protection are not fully understood, but growth hormone suppression due to central IGF-1-like feedback by extreme hyperinsulinaemia with attendant loss of lipolytic drive, paucity of stored triglyceride, and persistence of foetal hepatic IGF-1R expression have all been mooted to play an important role [34].

Current therapy for DS is suboptimal, with no evidence beyond case series and expert opinion guiding practice. Vicissitudes in blood glucose may be mitigated by continuous feeding, but while use of insulin-sensitising agents including metformin and glitazones has a theoretical basis, little evidence for efficacy exists. Recombinant human IGF-1 is often used and is able to exert an acute glucose-lowering effect in DS. It has also been associated with improved longevity in some case series; however, no controlled trials have been undertaken, and assessing its value is extremely difficult in the face of the rarity of DS and a variety of different reported dosing regimens, ranging from multiple daily subcutaneous dosing to continuous subcutaneous infusion [36]. Given the extensive soft tissue overgrowth reported in DS, concern remains about potential actions of IGF-1 to exacerbate this, and more rigorous trials are required [12, 37]. The prognosis in DS remains generally very poor, with death most frequent within the first 2 years of life due to intercurrent infection and associated refractory metabolic derangement.

Rabson-Mendenhall Syndrome
The distinction between DS and RMS is one of degree, and is arbitrary. RMS is most commonly used to describe patients with recessive insulin receptoropathy who survive beyond the first 5 years of life, commonly into their second or third decade. Linear growth retardation coupled with soft tissue overgrowth, in a broadly similar, though less severe, pattern to that of DS, is often what leads to clinical recognition of RMS, with premature eruption of disorganised carious dentition an additional common feature. Enlargement of the pineal gland was prominently reported in early cases [20], and was even suspected to hold clues to the pathogenesis of the syndrome before the insulin receptor was known, but this is most likely to represent one more feature of the general soft tissue overgrowth rather than a functionally important component of the syndrome. Severe IR with hyperinsulinaemia is congenital in RMS; however, β-cell failure and diabetes mellitus may not occur until several years have passed. Unlike DS, RMS features a high rate of microvascular complications of chronic hyperglycaemia, and these are the most common mode of death reported [38]. Diabetic ketoacidosis also poses a major challenge, often requiring prolonged intensive therapy. Clinical experience suggests that ketoacidosis starts to complicate RMS towards the end of the first decade; however, the time of transition from the protection from ketoacidosis seen in infancy is not precisely described, nor are the mechanisms underlying it clear.

As for DS, no controlled trial evidence exists to guide management of RMS. Insulin sensitisers, high-dose insulin, and recombinant human IGF-1 are all sometimes used, as in DS, while recombinant human leptin has also been suggested to give some benefit [39].

Extreme Congenital Insulin Resistance without INSR Mutations

In rare cases, babies and infants with convincing DS and RMS on phenotypic and biochemical grounds are identified without *INSR* mutations. Where cells are available to study, expression of the INSR is usually found to be extremely low, leading to the inference of the presence of mutations acting in *cis* or *trans* to impair receptor expression. Many such mutations are likely to lie in regulatory sequences of the *INSR* gene, but in some patients mutations of the transcription factor *HMGA1* gene have been reported to lead to severely impaired INSR expression and extreme IR [40]. In one further case, extreme IR was reported in association with haploinsufficiency for both the *INSR* and *CHN2* genes [41], suggesting that some digenic cases may also exist.

"Type A" Insulin Resistance and "HAIR-AN"

Both DS and RMS are extremely rare. Much more commonly, pathogenic *INSR* mutations give rise to severe IR that does not present to clinical attention until the peripubertal period. In a large majority of cases the causative mutations fall in the intracellular domain of the INSR, exert a dominant negative mutation on the other, wild-type allele, and so transmit severe IR as an autosomal dominant trait (Fig. 2). Females are far more likely to present to clinical attention than males, usually being referred for evaluation of oligomenorrhoea and hirsutism despite being lean, with AN and dysglycaemia noted on subsequent evaluation. In males the significance of AN is often not appreciated, and so the underlying severe IR is commonly not diagnosed until much later in life when diabetes develops. As previously mentioned, postprandial hypoglycaemia may also be prominent before diabetes develops, and may sometimes be the reason for presentation [7–9].

The nomenclature is somewhat confusing for monogenic severe IR presenting peripubertally. It was designated "type A" IR in the 1970s to discriminate it from a "type B" form of severe or extreme IR associated with autoantibodies against the insulin receptor [42]. This label has stuck, being used fairly generally to denote severe IR in lean women, although the clinical features are not specific to *INSR* mutations. "HAIR-AN" ("hyperandrogenism, insulin resistance, and acanthosis nigricans") is another commonly used term [43]. However, as will be appreciated from the foregoing discussion, this simply describes the general clinical features of severe IR in women, and does not imply a precise aetiology.

INSR mutations are only identified in around 10–20% of patients with type A IR when ascertained purely by phenotypic features and biochemical confirmation of severe IR. However, patients with receptoropathies have recently been shown to exhibit a distinct subphenotype of severe IR, with a characteristically normal lipid profile [44], preserved or elevated plasma adiponectin levels [45], and sometimes elevated IGFBP1 and sex hormone-binding globulin [46]. These markers can be used to refine biochemical triage for patients with type A IR for genetic testing, leading to very high rates of positive mutational analysis of the *INSR* gene.

As for other insulin receptoropathies, no specific treatments for type A IR have been proven. However, a strong emphasis on use of lifestyle interventions coupled to insulin sensitisers is rational. A major concern of patients is often the severity of the associated clinical hyperandrogenism, and ovarian suppression using GnRH analogues, with add-back hormonal therapies, is an approach that holds promise, though no systematic studies have been reported. Where insulin therapy is required, high doses may be needed, using the concentrated U-500 formulation when the total daily dose exceeds around 300 units [47].

Downstream Insulin Signalling Mutations
The key components of the signalling pathways downstream from the insulin receptor were delineated in the 1990s, and many investigators anticipated that most of the cases of familial severe IR not accounted for by receptor mutations would be attributable to defects in the corresponding genes. In fact, few gene variants in bona fide insulin signalling genes were revealed in this period, and often those that were described showed only equivocal cosegregation with the metabolic derangement. Instead, as discussed in the next chapter [Leiter and Semple, this vol., pp. 119–133], genetic defects with a primary effect to impair adipose tissue development or function (the so-called lipodystrophies) have proved to constitute by far the largest group of single gene IR, and most of the causative genes play no direct role in insulin signalling.

Nevertheless, in this century several convincing examples of severe IR due to defects in canonical insulin signalling genes have been reported, although in some of these, too, abnormal adipose development is seen. These will be described in order of their appearance in the signalling pathway.

SHORT Syndrome
SHORT syndrome was described clinically in the mid-1970s based on its characteristic gestalt, the acronym denoting short stature, joint hyperextensibility or hernias, ocular depression, Rieger anomaly (a developmental anomaly of the anterior chamber of the eye), and delayed tooth eruption. Several additional features of the syndrome have subsequently been highlighted including dysmorphic triangular facies, nephrocalcinosis, and sometimes glaucoma. In the early 1990s, the frequent occurrence of insulin-resistant diabetes, often with a paucity of adipose tissue in the face, hands, and gluteal region, was highlighted [48].

SHORT syndrome may either be sporadic or show autosomal dominant inheritance, with a significant number of de novo mutations. In 2013, three groups independently used exome-wide sequencing to identify causal mutations in the *PIK3R1* gene, which encodes 3 regulatory subunits of phosphatidylinositol-3-kinase (PI3K) [49–51]. These mutations are concentrated within the C-terminal SH2 domain of the protein, with one mutation – p.Arg649Trp – accounting for around 50% of cases [52]. These mutations are believed to impair interaction of PI3K with phosphorylated insulin receptor substrate proteins.

Since identification of the causal mutations, meta-analysis of known cases with a molecular diagnosis has led to refinement of the clinical criteria for clinical diagnosis, and while IR is not universal in SHORT syndrome [52], it has been shown often to be severe, associated with marked ovarian hyperandrogenism in women, and, like insulin receptoropathies, not to feature an abnormal lipid profile.

Fascinatingly, a distinct genotype-phenotype correlation has been demonstrated for mutations in the *PIK3R1* gene, with either genetic loss of the longest protein product of the gene, p85α [53], or inheritance of activating mutations in the gene [54], both shown to produce immunodeficiency due to effects on lymphocyte development, but without any features of SHORT syndrome or other metabolic or growth defects.

A Loss-of-Function Mutation in AKT2

AKT2 is a serine-threonine kinase 2 steps downstream from PI3K in the insulin signalling pathway, is dependent on the activation of PI3K, and is known to play a critical role in mediating many of the metabolic actions of insulin. A missense mutation in *AKT2* was reported in 2004 in a single family to cause severe IR, early-onset diabetes mellitus, and lipodystrophy transmitted as an autosomal dominant trait [55], and was the first example of highly penetrant defect in a postreceptor signalling gene in the insulin signalling cascade. The mutation lies within the highly conserved catalytic domain of the enzyme, and hyperinsulinaemic-euglycaemic clamp studies confirmed severe IR in liver and muscle tissue of the female proband, who also exhibited marked reduction in subcutaneous adipose tissue. Like *PIK3R1*, *AKT2* is known to have a key role in adipocyte differentiation as well as in acute metabolic actions of insulin, which may account for this abnormal adipose topography, yet unlike patients with SHORT syndrome, the patients carrying the *AKT2* mutation also showed severe fatty liver and metabolic dyslipidaemia [55].

Loss-of-Function of TBC1D4/AS160

Once activated, AKT2 phosphorylates many downstream targets to alter diverse aspects of cell growth and metabolism, for example suppressing hepatic gluconeogenesis, promoting hepatic lipogenesis, and driving translocation of the GLUT4 glucose transporter to the cell surface of skeletal muscle and fat cells, thereby stimulating glucose uptake (Fig. 1). This effect on GLUT4 is mediated by the small Rab-GTPase AS160 encoded by *TBC1D4*, also commonly known as *AS160*. A single family with a premature stop mutation and reduced expression of AS160 has been reported [56]. The index patient showed marked AN, and selective postprandial hyperinsulinaemia, while functional studies in mouse preadipocytes showed increased basal GLUT4 translocation as well as reduced insulin-stimulated cell membrane expression of the glucose transporter. Although this *TBC1D4* mutation was reported in only 1 family, subsequently a population-wide study in Greenland showed a different prevalent stop mutation in *TBC1D4* to make a significant contribution population wide to IR and

Table 2. Overview of genetic syndromes of severe insulin resistance caused by mutations within the insulin signalling pathway and associated clinical features

Name of syndrome	Underlying genetic cause	Metabolic phenotype	Additional clinical features
Donohue syndrome	Biallelic *INSR* mutations; little/no residual INSR signalling	Congenital IR with very high serum insulin	IUGR, linear growth retardation, decreased muscle and adipose tissue, soft-tissue overgrowth, organomegaly, precocious development of genitalia, acanthosis nigricans, death usual by 1–2 years during infection
Rabson-Mendenhall syndrome	Biallelic *INSR* mutations; small amount of residual INSR signalling	Congenital IR decompensating to diabetes usually by age 10 years	IUGR, linear growth retardation, acanthosis nigricans, hypertrichosis, premature carious dentation, overgrowth of sex-hormone responsive and soft tissues, death commonly during 2nd/3rd decade from microvascular complications or diabetic ketoacidosis
Type A insulin resistance	Usually monoallelic dominant negative *INSR* mutations; more rarely biallelic with milder loss-of-function alleles than seen in infantile syndromes	Sometimes early hypoglycaemia with features of IR presenting peripubertally in females; later in males, often when diabetes occurs in mid-life	Hyperandrogenism (most notable in females): precocious puberty, oligomenorrhea, PCOS, hirsutism, acne, acanthosis nigricans
SHORT syndrome	Heterozygous C terminal *PIK3R1* mutations	IR presentation variable: childhood to 30's/40's	SHORT, triangular face, speech delay, partial lipodystrophy (face, hands, buttocks), acanthosis nigricans
N/A	*AKT2* R274H point mutation	Severe IR with fatty liver and dyslipidaemia	Acanthosis nigricans, hypertension, lipodystrophy
N/A	AS160 *(TBC1D4)*	Postprandial IR in adolescence	Acanthosis nigricans

INSR, insulin receptor; IR, insulin resistance; IUGR, intrauterine growth restriction; PCOS, polycystic ovary syndrome; SHORT, short stature, hyperextensibility, ocular depression, Rieger anomaly, delayed tooth eruption syndrome; *PIK3R1*, gene encoding p85α regulatory subunit of phosphoinositol-3 kinase; *AKT2*, gene encoding protein kinase B β (PKBβ); AS160, AKT substrate of 160kDa; *TBC1D4*, TBC1 domain family member 4 gene.

other metabolic traits [57]. This illustrates the value of "sentinel" findings even in single patients or kindreds.

Known human genetic defects in insulin signalling genes are summarised in Table 2.

Conclusion

Over the past 28 years, study of the genetics of severe IR syndromes has identified many mutations within genes of the insulin signalling pathway. Affected patients can be stratified for genetic testing based on syndromic and biochemical assessment. Current treatment strategies are limited to high-dose concentrated insulin and, in some cases, insulin sensitizers, but practice is currently guided only by small case series and expert opinion. As current large-scale efforts to apply genomics in a health care context develop, there is a major opportunity for collaborative identification of patients for the purposes of more formal clinical trials of different treatment strategies and agents.

Acknowledgement

R.K.S. is supported by a Senior Research Fellowship from the Wellcome Trust (Grant WT098498). S.M.L. is supported by the Rosetrees Trust.

Disclosure Statement

R.K.S. has received speaker fees from Novo Nordisk and Sandoz.

References

1 Himsworth HP: Insulin deficiency and insulin inefficiency. Br Med J 1940;1:719–722.

2 Hanson RL, Imperatore G, Bennett PH, Knowler WC: Components of the "metabolic syndrome" and incidence of type 2 diabetes. Diabetes 2002;51:3120–3127.

3 Resnick HE, Jones K, Ruotolo G, Jain AK, Henderson J, Lu W, Howard BV: Insulin resistance, the metabolic syndrome, and risk of incident cardiovascular disease in nondiabetic American Indians: the Strong Heart Study. Diabetes Care 2003;26:861–867.

4 Utzschneider KM, Kahn SE: Review: the role of insulin resistance in nonalcoholic fatty liver disease. J Clin Endocrinol Metab 2006;91:4753–4761.

5 Pollak M: Insulin, insulin-like growth factors and neoplasia. Best Pract Res Clin Endocrinol Metab 2008;22:625–638.

6 Poretsky L, Cataldo NA, Rosenwaks Z, Giudice LC: The insulin-related ovarian regulatory system in health and disease. Endocr Rev 1999;20:535–582.

7 Huang Z, Li Y, Tang T, Xu W, Liao Z, Yao B, Hu G, Weng J: Hyperinsulinaemic hypoglycaemia associated with a heterozygous missense mutation of R1174W in the insulin receptor (IR) gene. Clin Endocrinol (Oxf) 2009;71:659–665.

8 Højlund K, Hansen T, Lajer M, Henriksen JE, Levin K, Lindholm J, Pedersen O, Beck-Nielsen H: A novel syndrome of autosomal-dominant hyperinsulinemic hypoglycemia linked to a mutation in the human insulin receptor gene. Diabetes 2004;53:1592–1598.

9 Kuroda Y, Iwahashi H, Mineo I, Fukui K, Fukuhara A, Iwamoto R, Imagawa A, Shimomura I: Hyperinsulinemic hypoglycemia syndrome associated with mutations in the human insulin receptor gene: report of two cases. Endocr J 2015;62:353–362.

10 Torley D, Bellus GA, Munro CS: Genes, growth factors and acanthosis nigricans. Br J Dermatol 2002;147:1096–1101.

11 Stuart CA, Pate CJ, Peters EJ: Prevalence of acanthosis nigricans in an unselected population. Am J Med 1989;87:269–272.

12 Weber DR, Stanescu DE, Semple R, Holland C, Magge SN: Continuous subcutaneous IGF-1 therapy via insulin pump in a patient with Donohue syndrome. J Pediatr Endocrinol Metab 2014;27:1237–1241.

13 de Kerdanet M, Caron-Debarle M, Nivot S, Gaillot T, Lascols O, Fremont B, Bonaure M, Gie S, Massart C, Capeau J: Ten-year improvement of insulin resistance and growth with recombinant human insulin-like growth factor 1 in a patient with insulin receptor mutations resulting in leprechaunism. Diabetes Metab 2015;41:331–337.

14 Arioglu E, Andewelt A, Diabo C, Bell M, Taylor SI, Gorden P: Clinical course of the syndrome of autoantibodies to the insulin receptor (type B insulin resistance): a 28-year perspective. Medicine (Baltimore) 2002;81:87–100.

15 Biddinger SB, Hernandez-Ono A, Rask-Madsen C, Haas JT, Alemán JO, Suzuki R, Scapa EF, Agarwal C, Carey MC, Stephanopoulos G, Cohen DE, King GL, Ginsberg HN, Kahn CR: Hepatic insulin resistance is sufficient to produce dyslipidemia and susceptibility to atherosclerosis. Cell Metab 2008;7:125–134.

16 Semple RK, Cochran EK, Soos MA, Burling KA, Savage DB, Gorden P, O'Rahilly S: Plasma adiponectin as a marker of insulin receptor dysfunction. Diabetes Care 2008;31:977–979.

17 Ullrich A, Bell R, Chen EY, Herrera R, Petruzzelli LM, Dull TJ, Gray A, Coussens L, Liao Y-C, Tsubokawa M, Mason A, Seeburg PH, Grunfeld C, Rosen OM, Ramachandran J: Human insulin receptor and its relationship to the tyrosine kinase family of oncogenes. Nature 1985;313:756–761.

18 De Meyts P: The insulin receptor: a prototype for dimeric, allosteric membrane receptors? Trends Biochem Sci 2008;33:376–384.

19 Donohue W, Uchida I: Leprechaunism: a euphemism for a rare familial disorder. J Pediatr 1954;45:505–519.

20 Rabson SM, Mendenhall EN: Familial hypertrophy of pineal body, hyperplasia of adrenal cortex and diabetes mellitus; report of 3 cases. Am J Clin Pathol 1956;26:283–290.

21 Yalow RS, Berson SA: Immunoassay of endogenous plasma insulin in man. J Clin Invest 1960;39:1157–1175.

22 Kadowaki T, Bevins CL, Cama A, Ojamaa K, Marcus-Samuels B, Kadowaki H, Beitz L, McKeon C, Taylor SI: Two mutant alleles of the insulin receptor gene in a patient with extreme insulin resistance. Science 1988;240:787–790.

23 Yoshimasa Y, Seino S, Whittaker J, Kakehi T, Kosaki A, Kuzuya H, Imura H, Bell GI, Steiner DF, Napier JR, Mus B, Hist N, Vrba ES, Robinson JT, Mus AT, Whrrraker J, Kosaiu A, Yoshimasa Y, Seino S, Whrrraker J, Kakehi T, Kosaiu A, Kuzuya H, Imura H: Insulin-resistant diabetes due to a point mutation that prevents insulin prorecepter processing. Science 1988;240:784–787.

24 Semple RK, Savage DB, Brierley GV, O'Rahilly S: Syndromes of severe insulin resistance and/or lipodystrophy; in Weiss RE, Refetoff S (eds): Genetic Diagnosis of Endocrine Disorders, ed 2. Amsterdam, Elsevier, 2016, pp 307–324.

25 Taylor SI, Cama A, Accili D, Barbetti F, Quon MJ, de la Luz Sierra M, Suzuki Y, Koller E, Levy-Toledano R, Wertheimer E: Mutations in the insulin receptor gene. Endocr Rev 1992;13:566–595.

26 De Bock M, Hayes I, Semple R: Donohue syndrome. J Clin Endocrinol Metab 2012;97:1416–1417.

27 Brisigotti M, Fabbretti G, Pesce F, Gatti R, Cohen A, Parenti G, Callea F: Congenital bilateral juvenile granulosa cell tumor of the ovary in leprechaunism: a case report. Pediatr Pathol 1993;13:549–558.

28 Simpkin A, Cochran E, Cameron F, Dattani M, de Bock M, Dunger DB, Forsander G, Guran T, Harris J, Isaac I, Hussain K, Kleta R, Peters C, Tasic V, Williams R, Yap Kok Peng F, O'Rahilly S, Gorden P, Semple RK, Bockenhauer D: Insulin receptor and the kidney: nephrocalcinosis in patients with recessive INSR mutations. Nephron Physiol 2014;128:55–61.

29 Grasso V, Colombo C, Favalli V, Galderisi A, Rabbone I, Gombos S, Bonora E, Massa O, Meschi F, Cerutti F, Iafusco D, Bonfanti R, Monciotti C, Barbetti F: Six cases with severe insulin resistance (SIR) associated with mutations of insulin receptor: Is a Bartter-like syndrome a feature of congenital SIR? Acta Diabetol 2013;50:951–957.

30 Hovnik T, Bratanič N, Podkrajšek KT, Kovač J, Paro D, Podnar T, Bratina N, Battelino T: Severe progressive obstructive cardiomyopathy and renal tubular dysfunction in Donohue syndrome with decreased insulin receptor autophosphorylation due to a novel INSR mutation. Eur J Pediatr 2013;172:1125–1129.

31 Furste HO, Bohm N, Pringsheim W: Leprechaunism (Donohue's syndrome). Clinical and pathologico-anatomical findings. Helv Paediatr Acta 1984;39:95–104.

32 Gurgey A, Gogus S, Saatci U, Bilginturan N, Yordam N, Coskun T, Ozkutlu S, Sahin N: Leprechaunism in two Turkish patients. Turk J Pediatr 1997;39:387–393.

33 Nobile S, Semple RK, Carnielli VP: A novel mutation of the insulin receptor gene in a preterm infant with Donohue syndrome and heart failure. J Pediatr Endocrinol Metab 2012;25:363–366.

34 Ogilvy-Stuart AL, Soos MA, Hands SJ, Anthony MY, Dunger DB, O'Rahilly S: Hypoglycemia and resistance to ketoacidosis in a subject without functional insulin receptors. J Clin Endocrinol Metab 2001;86:3319–3326.

35 Accili D, Drago J, Lee EJ, Johnson MD, Cool MH, Salvatore P, Asico LD, José PA, Taylor SI, Westphal H: Early neonatal death in mice homozygous for a null allele of the insulin receptor gene. Nat Genet 1996;12:106–109.

36 McDonald A, Williams RM, Regan FM, Semple RK, Dunger DB: IGF-I treatment of insulin resistance. Eur J Endocrinol 2007;157:51–56.

37 Semple RK, Williams RM, Dunger DB: What is the best management strategy for patients with severe insulin resistance? Clin Endocrinol (Oxf) 2010;73:286–290.

38 Musso C, Cochran E, Moran SA, Skarulis MC, Oral EA, Taylor S, Gorden P: Clinical course of genetic diseases of the insulin receptor (type A and Rabson-Mendenhall syndromes): a 30-year prospective. Medicine (Baltimore) 2004;83:209–222.

39 Brown RJ, Cochran E, Gorden P: Metreleptin improves blood glucose in patients with insulin receptor mutations. J Clin Endocrinol Metab 2013;98:E1749–E1756.

40 Foti D, Chiefari E, Fedele M, Iuliano R, Brunetti L, Paonessa F, Manfioletti G, Barbetti F, Brunetti A, Croce CM, Fusco A, Brunetti A: Lack of the architectural factor HMGA1 causes insulin resistance and diabetes in humans and mice. Nat Med 2005;11:765–773.

41 Suliman SGI, Stanik J, McCulloch LJ, Wilson N, Edghill EL, Misovicova N, Gasperikova D, Sandrikova V, Elliott KS, Barak L, Ellard S, Volpi EV, Klimes I, Gloyn AL: Severe insulin resistance and intrauterine growth deficiency associated with haploinsufficiency for INSR and CHN2: new insights into synergistic pathways involved in growth and metabolism. Diabetes 2009;58:2954–2961.

42 Kahn CR, Flier JS, Bar RS, Archer JA, Gorden P, Martin MM, Roth J: The syndromes of insulin resistance and acanthosis nigricans. N Engl J Med 1974;294:739–745.

43 Barbieri RL, Ryan KJ: Hyperandrogenism, insulin resistance, and acanthosis nigricans syndrome: a common endocrinopathy with distinct pathophysiologic features. Am J Obstet Gynecol 1983;147:90–101.

44 Semple RK, Sleigh A, Murgatroyd PR, Adams CA, Bluck L, Jackson S, Vottero A, Kanabar D, Charlton-Menys V, Durrington P, Soos MA, Carpenter TA, Lomas DJ, Cochran EK, Gorden P, O'Rahilly S, Savage DB: Postreceptor insulin resistance contributes to human dyslipidemia and hepatic steatosis. J Clin Invest 2009;119:315–322.

45 Semple RK, Soos MA, Luan J, Mitchell CS, Wilson JC, Gurnell M, Cochran EK, Gorden P, Chatterjee VKK, Wareham NJ, O'Rahilly S: Elevated plasma adiponectin in humans with genetically defective insulin receptors. J Clin Endocrinol Metab 2006;91:3219–3223.

46 Hattori Y, Hirama N, Suzuki K, Hattori S, Kasai K: Elevated plasma adiponectin and leptin levels in sisters with genetically defective insulin receptors. Diabetes Care 2007;30:2007.

47 Cochran E, Musso C, Gorden P: The of use of U-500 in patients with extreme insulin resistance. Diabetes Care 2005;28:1240–1244.

48 Schwingshandl J, Mache CJ, Rath K, Borkenstein MH: SHORT syndrome and insulin resistance. Am J Med Genet 1993;47:907–909.

49 Dyment DA, Smith AC, Alcantara D, Schwartzentruber JA, Basel-Vanagaite L, Curry CJ, Temple IK, Reardon W, Mansour S, Haq MR, Gilbert R, Lehmann OJ, Vanstone MR, Beaulieu CL, Majewski J, Bulman DE, O'Driscoll M, Boycott KM, Innes AM: Mutations in PIK3R1 cause SHORT syndrome. Am J Hum Genet 2013;93:158–166.

50 Chudasama KK, Winnay J, Johansson S, Claudi T, König R, Haldorsen I, Johansson B, Woo JR, Aarskog D, Sagen J V, Kahn CR, Molven A, Njølstad PR: SHORT syndrome with partial lipodystrophy due to impaired phosphatidylinositol 3 kinase signaling. Am J Hum Genet 2013;93:150–157.

51 Thauvin-Robinet C, Auclair M, Duplomb L, Caron-Debarle M, Avila M, St-Onge J, Le Merrer M, Le Luyer B, Héron D, Mathieu-Dramard M, Bitoun P, Petit J-M, Odent S, Amiel J, Picot D, Carmignac V, Thevenon J, Callier P, Laville M, Reznik Y, Fagour C, Nunes M-L, Capeau J, Lascols O, Huet F, Faivre L, Vigouroux C, Rivière J-B: PIK3R1 mutations cause syndromic insulin resistance with lipoatrophy. Am J Hum Genet 2013;93:141–149.

52 Avila M, Dyment DA, Sagen JV, St-Onge J, Moog U, Chung BHY, Mo S, Mansour S, Albanese A, Garcia S, Martin DO, Lopez AA, Claudi T, König R, White SM, Sawyer SL, Bernstein JA, Slattery L, Jobling RK, Yoon G, Curry CJ, Merrer ML, Luyer BL, Héron D, Mathieu-Dramard M, Bitoun P, Odent S, Amiel J, Kuentz P, Thevenon J, Laville M, Reznik Y, Fagour C, Nunes ML, Delesalle D, Manouvrier S, Lascols O, Huet F, Binquet C, Faivre L, Rivière JB, Vigouroux C, Njølstad PR, Innes AM, Thauvin-Robinet C: Clinical reappraisal of SHORT syndrome with PIK3R1 mutations: Toward recommendation for molecular testing and management. Clin Genet 2015, DOI: 10.1111/cge.12688.

53 Conley ME, Dobbs AK, Quintana AM, Bosompem A, Wang Y-D, Coustan-Smith E, Smith AM, Perez EE, Murray PJ: Agammaglobulinemia and absent B lineage cells in a patient lacking the p85 subunit of PI3K. J Exp Med 2012;209:463–470.

54 Deau M, Heurtier L, Frange P, Suarez F, Bole-Feysot C, Nitschke P, Cavazzana M, Picard C, Durandy A, Fischer A, Kracker S: A human immunodeficiency caused by mutations in the PIK3R1 gene. J Clin Invest 2014;124:3923–3928.

55 George S, Rochford JJ, Wolfrum C, Gray SL, Schinner S, Wilson JC, Soos MA, Murgatroyd PR, Williams RM, Carlo L, Dunger DB, Barford D, Umpleby AM, Wareham NJ, Davies HA, Schafer AJ, Stoffel M, O'Rahilly S: A Family with severe insulin resistance and diabetes mellitus due to a missense mutation in AKT2. Science 2004;304:1325–1328.

56 Dash S, Sano H, Rochford JJ, Semple RK, Yeo G, Hyden CSS, Soos MA, Clark J, Rodin A, Langenberg C, Druet C, Fawcett KA, Tung YCL, Wareham NJ, Barroso I, Lienhard GE, O'Rahilly S, Savage DB: A truncation mutation in TBC1D4 in a family with acanthosis nigricans and postprandial hyperinsulinemia. Proc Natl Acad Sci U S A 2009;106:9350–9355.

57 Moltke I, Grarup N, Jørgensen ME, Bjerregaard P, Treebak JT, Fumagalli M, Korneliussen TS, Andersen MA, Nielsen TS, Krarup NT, Gjesing AP, Zierath JR, Linneberg A, Wu X, Sun G, Jin X, Al-Aama J, Wang J, Borch-Johnsen K, Pedersen O, Nielsen R, Albrechtsen A, Hansen T: A common Greenlandic TBC1D4 variant confers muscle insulin resistance and type 2 diabetes. Nature 2014;512:190–193.

Dr. Robert K. Semple
University of Cambridge Metabolic Research Laboratories, Level 4
Wellcome Trust-MRC Institute of Metabolic Science
Box 289, Addenbrooke's Hospital
Hills Road, Cambridge CB2 0QQ (UK)
E-Mail rks16@cam.ac.uk

Barbetti F, Ghizzoni L, Guaraldi F (eds): Diabetes Associated with Single Gene Defects and Chromosomal Abnormalities. Front Diabetes. Basel, Karger, 2017, vol 25, pp 119–133 (DOI: 10.1159/000454739)

Insulin Resistance and Diabetes Associated with Lipodystrophies

Sarah M. Leiter · Robert K. Semple

University of Cambridge Metabolic Research Laboratories, Wellcome Trust-MRC Institute of Metabolic Science, Addenbrooke's Hospital, Cambridge, UK

Abstract

Obesity is strongly associated with insulin resistance, diabetes mellitus, fatty liver disease, and dyslipidaemia. The opposite perturbation, namely absence or paucity of adipose tissue in lipodystrophy, leads to the same spectrum of disorders, often in an exaggerated form. The two states are unified by the concept of "adipose failure": when the metabolic buffering capacity of adipose tissue is exceeded, metabolic dysfunction including insulin resistance and deposition of harmful lipids in other tissues ensues. Although first described in the 1920s, it is only over the past 17 years that lipodystrophies have yielded to genetic studies. Recessive generalised lipodystrophy is rare, and is largely accounted for by mutations in *AGPAT2* or *BSCL2*. Much more common are familial partial lipodystrophies, the commonest of which are caused by dominant mutations in *LMNA* and *PPARG*. Causes of many rarer forms of lipodystrophy have been and continue to be identified; the genes thus far implicated have been involved in processes such as adipogenesis, lipid metabolism, lipid droplet function, and DNA replication or repair. Detailed study even of small groups of affected patients is improving understanding of (1) the pathophysiology of these rare, extreme conditions, and (2) the role of adipose tissue in commoner forms of metabolic disease.   © 2017 S. Karger AG, Basel

The ability to buffer widely fluctuating availability of nutrition is critical to survival of a species, and so humans, like other mammals, have evolved sophisticated mechanisms to store excess caloric intake in energy-dense triglyceride-rich adipose tissue depots at times of excess, and to mobilise it efficiently at times of privation. These dynamic processes are now known to be regulated by cues from hormones, including insulin, and substrate fluxes from key metabolically active organs [1].

Obesity, or excess adipose tissue, is a relatively recent problem related to sedentary, overnourished modern lifestyles, and has come to pose a pandemic public health threat through its attendant morbidity and mortality, accounted for by cardiovascular and metabolic sequelae and an increased risk of neoplasia [2, 3]. Obese individuals, especially when excess adipose tissue is centripetal in distribution, often develop metabolic dyslipidaemia characterised by suppressed plasma HDL cholesterol and elevated triglyceride, non-alcoholic fatty liver disease, insulin resistance, and type 2 diabetes mellitus [4].

Strikingly, individuals with a pathological paucity of adipose tissue, known as lipodystrophy, are not protected from the adverse consequences of obesity. Indeed, it has been appreciated since the 1920s that they exhibit the full spectrum of metabolic complications of obesity, including insulin resistance, diabetes, fatty liver, and dyslipidaemia, often to an extremely severe degree. This has been one key line of evidence supporting the concept of "adipose failure" as a requirement for development of the metabolic syndrome [5]. According to this notion, both patients with severe obesity and those with lipodystrophy have exceeded the energy-buffering capacity of their adipose tissue, with this failure being absolute in generalised lipodystrophy, but only relative in the case of partial lipodystrophy or obesity. The consequences of such adipose failure include remodelling of substrate fluxes to favour deposition of harmful ectopic lipids in distant, insulin-sensitive organs such as the liver and skeletal muscle, infiltration of adipose tissue with inflammatory cells, and development of insulin resistance [6].

Monogenic forms of lipodystrophy are critical to identify clinically, as intervention with nutritional measures and adjunctive therapies such as leptin may have greatly beneficial impact in addition to more conventional therapies. Moreover, they provide valuable insight into adipose tissue development and function, and the role of adipose tissue in the development of common disease in humans. In this chapter we discuss the classification and molecular basis of genetic forms of lipodystrophy, and summarise existing treatment options.

Clinical Classification of Lipodystrophies

One general definition of lipodystrophy is as a visible deficit of adipose tissue in all or part of the body. Lipodystrophies are highly heterogeneous, and many acquired forms exist. Some of these acquire forms are localised and asymmetrical, and relate to local insults such as local radiotherapy, subcutaneous drug administration or trauma, or to a localised autoimmune response [7]. Other acquired forms are symmetrical, and are caused by more systemic insults, including HIV infection and antiretroviral therapies, whole-body irradiation, some chemotherapies, or more generalised autoimmunity, usually with evidence of deranged humoral immunity and complement activation [8, 9]. Henceforth, however, this chapter will consider only genetic forms of lipodystrophy, which are invariably symmetrical, but which present to clinical attention at different stages of life (Table 1).

Congenital generalised lipodystrophies (CGL) represent the most extreme form of lipodystrophy. They are invariably autosomal recessive, and are usually easily recognisable by the mothers or health care professionals within the first few months of life due to failure of the infant to develop healthy adipose tissue and normal "plump"

Table 1. Overview of genetic causes of lipodystrophy with associated clinical features

Gene	Cell function affected	Other clinical features
Congenital generalised lipodystrophies		
Common features: SIR, T2DM, dyslipidaemia, NAFLD, PCOS, pseudoacromegaly		
AGPAT2	Triglyceride synthesis	Lytic bone lesions, preserved mechanical fat depots
BSCL2	Adipogenesis; Lipid droplet regulation	Mild mental retardation reported; sometimes cardio-myopathy
CAV1	Formation of caveolae	Short stature
PTRF	Formation of caveolae	Myopathy
Familial partial lipodystrophies		
Common features: SIR, T2DM, dyslipidaemia, NAFLD, PCOS, pseudoacromegaly		
LMNA	Nuclear lamina formation and transcriptional regulation	AD: excess facial and neck fat AR: mandibuloacral dysplasia Hutchinson-Gilford syndrome: premature aging
ZMPSTE24	Prelamin processing	Mandibuloacral dysplasia
PPARG	Adipogenesis	Preserved abdominal fat
CIDEC	Unilocular lipid droplet formation	Multilocular lipid droplets
PLIN1	Lipolysis regulation	–
PCYT1A	Phosphatidylcholine synthesis	Short stature
AKT2	Insulin signaling	
PIK3R1	Insulin signaling	Short stature, hyperextensibility, ocular depression, Rieger anomaly, delayed tooth eruption
WRN	DNA unwinding during repair	Premature aging, increased risk of cataracts, neoplasia, peripheral contractures and sarcopaenia
POLD1	DNA replication and repair	Limb sarcopaenia, sensorineural deafness, mandibular hypoplasia, male hypoganodism, scleroderma, contractures
PSMB8	Immune proteasome	Joint contractures, muscle atrophy, microcytic anaemia
FBN1	Connective tissue	Marfan syndrome, progeroid features

SIR, severe insulin resistance; T2DM, type 2 diabetes mellitus; NAFLD, non-alcoholic fatty liver disease; PCOS, polycystic ovary syndrome; AR, autosomal recessive; AD, autosomal dominant.

appearance. Affected infants are often described as "wrinkled" or "aged". Sometimes concern arises that the lack of adipose tissue is accounted for by nutritional problems or by another underlying medical disorder. Critical clues to the presence of lipodystrophy rather than another illness or malnourishment may come from observation of clinical features of insulin resistance such as acanthosis nigricans, of an unusually muscular appearance at odds with undernutrition, or of a distended abdomen due to an engorged fatty liver. Biochemical testing may also be discriminatory if hyperinsulinaemia or elevated plasma triglycerides are found, although these depend on the nutritional state at the time of testing. Patients with CGL commonly progress to develop most of the metabolic complications of lipodystrophy described below, including severe or extreme insulin resistance, severe fatty liver and sequelae, and poorly controlled diabetes. An important differential diagnosis of CGL in children is diencephalic syndrome caused by tumours in the region of the hypothalamus [10]. Such tumours may produce generalised loss of adipose tissue, without corresponding features of insulin resistance, fatty liver, and muscular hypertrophy, and this "pseudolipodystrophy" may antedate development of neurological symptoms by several years. For this reason, CNS imaging should be considered in children with atypical forms of CGL.

In partial lipodystrophies, some adipose depots are preserved, and indeed these remaining depots may show compensatory excess fat deposition, leading to considerable cosmetic distress. Familial partial lipodystrophies (FPLD) are far more common than CGL and most commonly show autosomal dominant inheritance, although rare recessive forms are also known as described below. Involvement of femorogluteal subcutaneous adipose tissue is the norm, although different molecular subtypes show differences in the extent of subcutaneous fat loss beyond those depots. Clinical presentation is usually delayed until the peripubertal period, as pathological deficits in adipose tissue are extremely difficult to discriminate in lean prepubertal children. Peripubertally, however, failure of a normal accretion of adipose tissue in girls is frequently noticed, often with attendant features of severe insulin resistance including oligomenorrhoea or amenorrhoea despite well advanced puberty, or clinical hyperandrogenism. Lean boys do not exhibit these "sentinel" clinical features, and so are commonly undiagnosed or identified only in midlife when diabetes has developed. Some genetic forms of lipodystrophy feature additional subtype-specific clinical problems as discussed later.

Complications of Lipodystrophy

Loss of energy-buffering capacity coupled to chronic positive energy balance, as seen throughout the industrialised world, leads to accumulations of triglyceride and other toxic forms of lipid in liver, muscle, pancreatic β-cells, and elsewhere. This phenomenon is often called lipotoxicity [11]. As a consequence of this systemic insulin resistance, dyslipidaemia and diabetes develop, each of which may be severe and/or refractory to the usual treatment. The important clinical consequences of this may be grouped into those which are generic to all forms of insulin resistance, and which were discussed in the context of primary insulin signalling disorders in the previous chapter [Leiter and Semple, this vol., pp. 104–118], and those which are specific to lipotoxicity.

Generic features of severe insulin resistance include ovulatory dysfunction and ovarian hyperandrogenism in women, as well as acanthosis nigricans and sometimes pseudoacromegaloid soft tissue overgrowth, the appearance of which is accentuated by lack of adipose tissue. Insulin-resistant diabetes appears when β-cell decompensation occurs, and poor glycaemic control frequently leads to severe microvascular complications.

"Lipotoxic" complications of lipodystrophy include severe dyslipidaemia, featuring hypertriglyceridaemia that is exquisitely sensitive to dietary fat intake and that may be extreme. This is commonly sufficient to cause recurrent attacks of acute pancreatitis and/or eruptive xanthomata. Fatty liver disease is also a major component of lipodystrophic syndromes, and is often severe from an early age. Steatohepatitis progressing to bridging fibrosis is common, and hepatocellular carcinoma is a significant risk. Indeed, advanced liver disease and its complications are among the major causes of mortality in lipodystrophy. Premature atherosclerosis is also highly prevalent in lipodystrophy, and is likely to be driven by both dysglycaemia and lipotoxicity.

Interestingly, mutations in proximal insulin signalling genes *INSR* and *PIK3R1* cause severe or extreme insulin resistance, and also often feature reduced adipose tissue. However, these disorders appear almost never to feature dyslipidaemia or fatty liver, which can serve as a quick and simple biochemical triage tool before genetic testing. This can be enhanced by measuring plasma adiponectin, SHBG, and IGFBP1, which are usually suppressed in lipodystrophic insulin resistance, but which are preserved and sometimes frankly elevated in insulin receptoropathies and in SHORT syndrome [12]. Plasma leptin is severely reduced or absent in CGL, but is more variable in FPLD and proximal insulin signalling disorders, depending on the overall size of whole-body adipose depots. Thus, it does not serve as a reliable marker of lipodystrophy or as a discriminator between lipodystrophic and other forms of monogenic insulin resistance. In those with lipodystrophy who have very low plasma leptin, however, its therapeutic replacement is a valuable plank of therapy, as discussed below.

Specific Genetic Subtypes of Lipodystrophy

Congenital Generalised Lipodystrophies
CGL are often referred to as Berardinelli-Seip congenital lipodystrophies (BSCL), in deference to early clinical descriptions of the syndromes [13, 14]. They are extremely rare (probably 1 in several million), but in most cases a genetic aetiology can be established. The near total absence of adipose tissue from limbs, trunk, and face in BSCL coupled to abdominal protuberance can sometimes be mistaken for the wrinkled appearance and distended abdomen seen in Donohue syndrome (see previous chapter [Leiter and Semple, this vol., pp. 104–118]); however, quite unlike the situation in Donohue syndrome, the abdominal protuberance is largely accounted for by a severely triglyceride-engorged liver, and sometimes splenomegaly, while the increased muscle mass seen in BSCL is also unlike the reduced muscle bulk seen in Donohue syndrome. Patients with BSCL also often show accelerated linear growth, unlike the marked growth retardation of recessive insulin receptoropathy, although in BSCL, as

in many other types of severe insulin resistance, bone age may be advanced and epiphyses often fuse early [15]. Another feature shared by the 2 different forms of severe insulin resistance is an increased prevalence of hypertrophic cardiomyopathy, although this is more common in the receptoropathies, where it is frequently detected in infancy.

The early description of a series of 42 cases in 31 families by Seip [16] in 1971 suggested a genetic origin of CGL, with inheritance consistent with an autosomal recessive pattern of inheritance. The first gene implicated, which was renamed *BSCL2*, was identified using linkage analysis in 3 large families in 2001 [17], and has since been shown to harbour biallelic loss-of-function mutations (most commonly frameshift or nonsense) in many patients with BSCL. *BSCL2* encodes an endoplasmic reticulum protein named seipin. Although many questions remain about its cellular function, a growing body of evidence has implicated it in different aspects of triglyceride metabolism, lipid droplet function, and adipocyte differentiation [18, 19]. Seipin is most highly expressed in the brain and testes with lower mRNA and protein levels in adipose tissue. However, although early reports suggested an increased prevalence of mental retardation in some patients with *BSCL2* mutations, it remains unclear whether this is a significant component of the syndrome or whether it may have been accounted for by co-inherited recessive mutations reported in some patients.

Soon after identification of mutations in *BSCL2*, biallelic mutations in *AGPAT2* were reported in a further major subgroup of patients. *AGPAT2* encodes the enzyme 1-acylglycerol-3-phosphate O-acyltransferase 2 (AGPAT2), which catalyses the acylation of lysophosphatidic acid to form phosphatidic acid, an intermediate product in the biosynthesis of triacylglycerides [20]. Several lines of evidence suggest that this enzyme activity may be required not only for mass synthesis of triglyceride in otherwise normal adipocytes, but also that its deficiency impairs adipocyte differentiation, perhaps due to a failure to synthesise proadipogenic lipid intermediates required for full activation of the adipogenic transcriptional network.

BSCL may confidently be divided on genetic grounds into BSCL1, caused by mutations in *AGPAT2*, and BSCL2, caused by mutations in *BSCL2*. Often it is clinically difficult to distinguish the 2 subtypes, although several differences have been described, including some preservation of "mechanical" adipose depots (e.g., in the periarticular region, palms, and soles of the feet) and an increased prevalence of lytic bone lesions within the appendicular skeleton in BSCL1, while BSCL2 has been suggested to feature more mental retardation and cardiomyopathy, and to show surprisingly higher adiponectin levels than seen in BSCL1 [21]. In practice, however, genetic screening for both *AGPAT2* and *BSCL2* simultaneously is often appropriate in patients being investigated for CGL.

Mutations in *BSCL2* and *AGPAT2* have been reported to account for a large majority of CGL; however, rare mutations in a handful of other genes have also been described. Two of these genes, *CAV1 and PTRF* [22, 23], are required for the formation of caveolae, specialised plasma membrane invaginations that are thought to play an important role in key signalling pathways, and which are particularly abundant in adipocytes. Patients with *PTRF* mutations may usually be discriminated clinically due to the co-occurrence of myopathy with CGL.

Partial Lipodystrophies

FPLD is much more common than CGL, and its genetic basis is more complex. Moreover, a substantial minority of patients remain without a genetic diagnosis. In contrast to BSCL, which are inherited in an autosomal recessive pattern, most "simple" FPLD cases are autosomal dominant or de novo, although recessive forms have been described. The defining feature of FPLD is sparing of some regions or depots of adipose tissue, in particular the visceral and head and neck adipose tissue (Fig. 1a). This means that FPLD is only rarely diagnosed prepubertally unless sought as part of family screening. Most commonly, as discussed above, FPLD presents to clinical attention in girls around the time of puberty because of cosmetic distress arising from a failure to assume a normal female body shape with, for example, lack of adipose tissue in the femorogluteal region. This distress is often accentuated by hyperandrogenism due to the actions of high levels of insulin on the ovaries, which not only produces hirsutism, but may also worsen muscular hypertrophy. Several different genes, described below, have now been implicated in FPLD.

LMNA

Heterozygous mutations in *LMNA,* encoding lamins A and C, are the most common cause of FPLD. The resulting condition is often referred to as familial partial lipodystrophy type 2 (FPLD2) or Dunnigan-type familial partial lipodystrophy, and the genetic aetiology was established in 2000 [24, 25]. Patients with lamin A/C-associated lipodystrophy have a characteristic preservation of fat in the neck, chin, face, viscera, and labia majora (fig. 1b). Failure of normal subcutaneous adipose accretion on the limbs and trunk is seen at puberty and may gradually become more pronounced. Residual fat depots in the head and neck and intra-abdominally commonly increase in size leading to a somewhat "Cushingoid" adipose topography, and also give the erroneous impression of normal or increased adipose tissue in patients still wearing clothes.

Mutations in *LMNA* are associated with a wide number of other clinical syndromes including Emery-Dreifuss muscular dystrophy, Charcot-Marie-Tooth sensorimotor neuropathy, various progeroid syndromes, and cardiomyopathy and cardiac conduction disorders [26]. Ninety per cent of "isolated" Dunnigan-type lipodystrophies are caused by a hot-spot missense mutation at arginine 482; however, some phenotypic overlap among syndromes is well recognised, especially for the minor FPLD mutations, and so vigilance is needed for clinical evidence of cardiomyopathy or skeletal myopathy in FPLD.

Lamins A and C are intermediate filaments which are a key component of the nuclear lamina, a mesh-like structure lining the inside of the nuclear membrane and

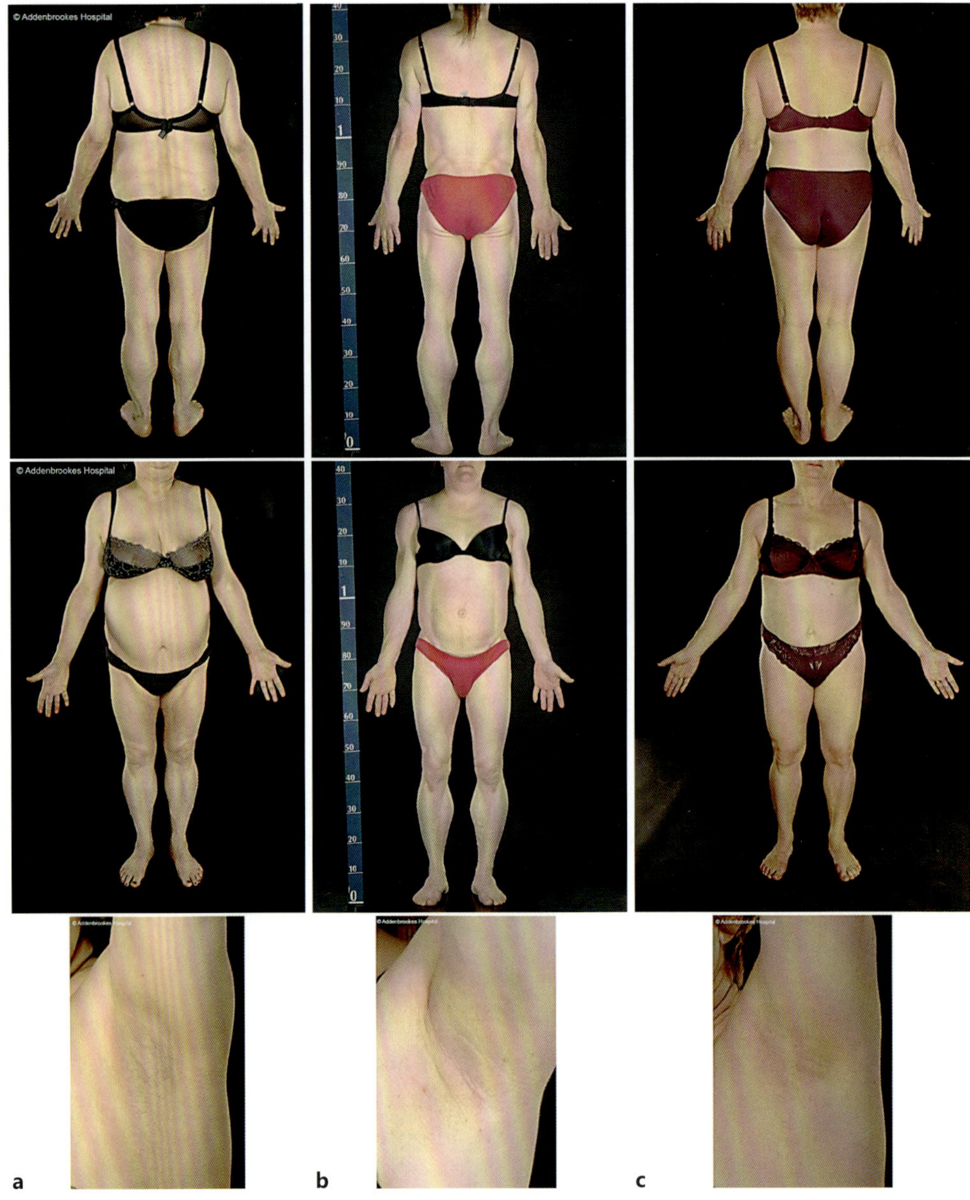

Fig. 1. Female patients with different subtypes of familial partial lipodystrophy (FPLD), demonstrating the typical phenotypes of FPLD type 1, genetic cause unknown (**a**), FPLD type 2, secondary to a mutation in *LMNA* (**b**), and FPLD type 3, secondary to a mutation in *PPARG* (**c**). All 3 patients have axillary acanthosis nigricans as shown in the bottom panel. Reproduced with permission from [48].

linked to the nuclear membrane via anchor proteins [27]. In addition to its role in organisation of the nuclear membrane and cytoskeleton, lamin A/C has also been shown to bind chromatin and regular transcription factors such as sterol regulatory element-binding protein 1c, which is suggested to play a key role in adipogenesis as well as in sterol and fatty acid synthesis [28, 29]. However, the mechanism behind the preservation of some adipose depots has not been explained, and the mechanisms explaining the very striking genotype-phenotype correlation for the wider range of *LMNA* mutations have not been fully established.

FPLD Associated with *PPARG* Mutations

Heterozygous mutations in *PPARG*, which encodes peroxisome proliferator-activated receptor-γ, the cognate receptor for the thiazolidinedione class of insulin-sensitising drugs, were first identified to cause severe insulin resistance in 1999 [30], and as further patients were identified it became clear that this was associated with a pattern of FPLD. This subgroup is now sometimes labelled FPLD3. Patients with mutations in *PPARG* show preserved visceral fat and usually also have some preserved subcutaneous abdominal adipose tissue (Fig. 1c). Indeed, it is not uncommon for patients with FPLD3 to have some degree of centripetal obesity, although relative limb lipodystrophy appears invariable. Similar to other types of FPLD, FPLD3 is often discerned at the onset of puberty. Although the appearance may be subtler than in FPLD2, unusually severe dyslipidaemia, fatty liver, insulin resistance, or early-onset hypertension should prompt genetic evaluation of *PPARG*.

Mutations in Lipid Droplet-Related Genes

Driven by growing scientific appreciation of the critical and dynamic role played by lipid droplets in adipocytes and other tissues, candidate-gene studies have focused on lipid droplet proteins in undiagnosed forms of FPLD. This has led to identification of mutations in 2 genes known to have key roles in lipid droplet formation and function. A single case of a homozygous early truncation mutation in *CIDEC* has been reported [31]. *CIDEC* encodes the highly conserved cell death-inducing Dffa-like effector C, also known as Fsp27. CIDEC is induced during adipocyte differentiation and the lipid coat protein it encodes is required for regulation of triglyceride accumulation and hydrolysis [32]. In cellular models, in the affected patient the truncation mutation identified was shown to lead to formation of multiple small droplets instead of the normal large single lipid droplet in human adipocytes.

Mutations in another lipid droplet protein, perilipin 1 (*PLIN1*), were also recently identified following a candidate screen [33]. Subcutaneous fat loss has been more uniform than in FPLD2 in patients described to date and is accompanied by generic clinical features of lipodystrophic severe insulin resistance including early adult-onset diabetes mellitus, acanthosis nigricans, and hyperandrogenism. PLIN1 has a crucial role in adipocytes where it is situated on the outer membrane of the lipid droplet, inhibiting basal lipolysis of triacylglycerol as well as attenuating stimulated lipolysis

[34]. The observed disease-related mutations are frameshift mutations that have a long aberrant C terminal tail, and this may be required to interrupt normal PLIN1 function [35].

Insulin Signalling Genes

Some mutations in genes encoding proximal components of the insulin signalling pathway have also been shown to cause severe insulin resistance associated with lipodystrophy. Mutations in *PIK3R1*, encoding the p85α catalytic subunit of PI3 kinase, in SHORT syndrome and activating mutations in *AKT2* are described in more detail in the previous chapter [Leiter and Semple, this vol., pp. 104–118]. Strikingly, SHORT syndrome, although frequently featuring femorogluteal lipodystrophy, does not feature fatty liver or dyslipidaemia in most cases, while lipodystrophy due to an *AKT2* mutation resembles other types of FPLD metabolically with severe dyslipidaemia and fatty liver.

Phospholipid Metabolism

Partial lipodystrophy has also recently been attributed in rare cases to biallelic mutations in *PCYT1A* [36], which encodes phosphate cytidylyltransferase 1α, which plays a critical role in the synthesis of phosphatidylcholine, an essential cellular phospholipid. Interruption of the normal metabolism of phosphatidylcholine underlies FPLD associated with mutations in *PCYT1A*. This gene encodes the rate-limiting enzyme phosphate cytidylyltransferase 1α of the Kennedy pathway. The pathway produces phosphatidylcholine, an essential component of the cell membrane. The 2 reported cases show short stature, severe childhood insulin resistance, very low HDL, and significant steatohepatitis.

Complex Syndromes Associated with Lipodystrophy

Lipodystrophy and severe insulin resistance is also seen as a feature of several rare complex syndromes. The first group of such syndromes are caused by perturbation of LMNA function or processing. These include "type A" mandibuloacral dysplasia, featuring small mandibles and clavicles, acro-osteolysis, delayed closure of cranial sutures, joint contractures, early aging, and a mottled pigmentation [37]. This is due to biallelic mutations in *LMNA* that are distinct from those causing FPLD2. Another rare pleiotropic laminopathy is Hutchinson-Gilford syndrome, in which de novo point mutations in exon 11 of *LMNA* produce lipodystrophy also with mandibuloacral dysplasia, and also markedly premature aging and early death [38]. The lipodystrophic phenotype is one of childhood loss of fat throughout the body with no sparing of the face and neck, unlike FPLD2. The causative *LMNA* mutation results in a cryptic splice site leading to the deletion of 50 amino acids in the C-terminus of the protein. Finally, a mechanistically related disorder caused by mutations in a different gene,

ZMPSTE24, is "type B" mandibuloacral dysplasia [39]. During protein maturation, prelamin A is cleaved by the zinc metalloproteinase STE24 (encoded by *ZMPSTE24*), removing its farnesyl anchor. Fat loss in these patients includes the face, leading to a progeroid appearance.

Other syndromes that feature dyslipidaemic severe insulin resistance with impaired adipose tissue development or maintenance are caused by defects in different aspects of DNA replication or damage repair. The associated lipodystrophy is most clearly described for Werner syndrome [40], a premature ageing syndrome caused by biallelic mutation of a DNA helicase involved in many pathways of DNA repair, and in the "MDP" syndrome, denoting "mandibular hypoplasia, deafness, and progeria syndrome" [41]. Patients with MDP syndrome have a normal birth weight and appearance, but progressive fat loss starts in early childhood and is accompanied by increased visceral adipose tissue and marked insulin resistance. Additional features seen in some cases include atrophy of limb muscles, sensorineural deafness, mandibular hypoplasia, hypoganodism, scleroderma, and ligament contractures. In contrast to lipodystrophy associated with mandibuloacral dysplasia, MDP patients are of normal height. MDP syndrome is caused by heterozygous mutation of the polymerase active site of DNA polymerase delta *(POLD1)*, which encodes the dominant lagging strand DNA polymerase in mammalian cells [42]. How such fundamental defects in DNA replication and repair produce relative tissue-selective dysfunction remains the subject of continuing study.

Several other genes have been shown to cause rare syndromic forms of lipodystrophy, including *PSMB8*, which causes a progressive and striking autoinflammatory form of lipodystrophy [43], and *FBN1*, which causes some cases of neonatal progeroid lipodystrophy [44], or Wiedemann-Rautenstrauch syndrome, but these are beyond the scope of this chapter.

Management of Lipodystrophy

The significant morbidity and early mortality associated with lipodystrophies are due to poorly controlled diabetes mellitus and dyslipidaemia as well as to acute pancreatitis and advanced liver disease related to non-alcoholic steatohepatitis. These metabolic derangements are thought to be caused by a lack of buffering capacity for dietary caloric excess, compounded in some patients with lipodystrophy by deficiency of leptin, which erroneously indicates to the brain that energy stores are critically low and thus drives hyperphagia. This leads to a pernicious interaction between pathologically reduced energy storage capacity and pathologically increased energy intake. Understanding these issues is necessary for a rational approach to management of lipodystrophy. In many respects, patients with metabolic disease-related lipodystrophy should be treated along similar lines to those with metabolic disease due to morbid obesity, which, as discussed above, may be viewed as a different form of adipose tissue failure.

To address the underlying defect in patients with lipodystrophy, it is critical to counter chronic positive energy balance. This requires dietary advice and support in following a low-fat, hypocaloric, or eucaloric diet, and promotion of exercise. In patients with CGL who have absolute leptin deficiency, and in those patients with FPLD who have relative leptin deficiency, subcutaneous leptin may exert marked metabolic improvements by reducing appetite and facilitating achievement of neutral energy balance [45, 46]. Although there is evidence in mice that leptin may exert directly beneficial effects on insulin-sensitive tissues [47], evidence for this in humans is minimal at present. Where these measures are ineffective, use of treatments commonly regarded as "obesity therapies" is rational, though guided only by clinical experience and case reports at present. Thus, GLP-1 agonists may be beneficial in part by reducing appetite, while bariatric surgery has been shown to yield major benefits in FPLD2 [48].

Despite the best efforts to achieve neutral or negative energy balance, metabolic control is frequently not achieved with these measures alone. In these cases, the use of agents that effectively addresses the consequences of the underlying lipodystrophy rather than the cause is of use. Insulin sensitivity can be improved through the use of metformin, while thiazolidinediones may have a more limited role, although their utility is limited by the expansion of residual adipose depots which they produce, often exacerbating cosmetic distress. SGLT2 inhibitors are worthy of further study. Severe hypertriglyceridaemia may be treated with conventional therapies if needed, including fibrates and dietary supplementation with n–3 polyunsaturated fatty acids [49]. Use of statins to reduce hypertriglyceridaemia is a common practice.

Glycaemic control following decompensation of pancreatic β-cell activity can be difficult to achieve in some patients with very high requirements for exogenous insulin. The use of high concentration (U-500) insulin can be beneficial both to prevent injection-site reactions and to increase glycaemic control [50].

Conclusion

Mendelian lipodystrophies are rare disorders of adipose development and function associated with a variable spectrum of clinical disorders, but nearly universally characterised by severe insulin resistance, fatty liver, and dyslipidaemia. CGL are easy to recognise and most affected patients should receive a precise genetic diagnosis. FPLD are clinically and genetically more heterogeneous, and many cases are likely to remain unrecognised, particularly men as the redistribution of fat is less easy to discern than in affected women. Diagnosis of lipodystrophy is important in the management of affected patients, who, despite having low amounts of adipose tissue and being "healthy" by criteria such as the body mass index, ideally should be viewed therapeutically as similar to those with morbid obesity and attendant metabolic complications. Dietary and pharmacological measures to "offload" limited fat reserves are critical to management.

Acknowledgement

R.K.S. is supported by a Senior Research Fellowship from the Wellcome Trust (Grant WT098498). S.M.L. is supported by the Rosetrees Trust.

Disclosure Statement

R.K.S. has received speaker fees from Novo Nordisk and Sandoz.

References

1 Frayn K: Adipose tissue as a buffer for daily lipid flux. Diabetologia 2002;45:1201–1210.
2 Grundy SM: Obesity, metabolic syndrome, and cardiovascular disease. J Clin Endocrinol Metab 2004; 89:2595–2600.
3 Pischon T, Nöthlings U, Boeing H: Obesity and cancer. Proc Nutr Soc 2008;67:128–145.
4 Carr MC, Brunzell JD: Abdominal obesity and dyslipidemia in the metabolic syndrome: importance of type 2 diabetes and familial combined hyperlipidemia in coronary artery disease risk. J Clin Endocrinol Metab 2004;89:2601–2607.
5 Danforth E: Failure of adipocyte differentiation causes type II diabetes mellitus? Nat Genet 2000;26:13.
6 Virtue S, Vidal-Puig A: It's not how fat you are, it's what you do with it that counts. PLoS Biol 2008;6: 1819–1823.
7 Misra A, Peethambaram A, Garg A: Clinical features and metabolic and autoimmune derangements in acquired partial lipodystrophy: report of 35 cases and review of the literature. Medicine (Baltimore) 2004;83:18–34.
8 Tershakovec AM, Frank I, Rader D: HIV-related lipodystrophy and related factors. Atherosclerosis 2004;174:1–10.
9 Misra A, Garg A: Clinical features and metabolic derangements in acquired generalized lipodystrophy: case reports and review of the literature. Medicine (Baltimore) 2003;82:129–146.
10 Fleischman A: Diencephalic syndrome: a cause of failure to thrive and a model of partial growth hormone resistance. Pediatrics 2005;115:e742–e748.
11 Virtue S, Vidal-Puig A: Adipose tissue expandability, lipotoxicity and the metabolic syndrome – an allostatic perspective. Biochim Biophys Acta 2010;1801: 338–349.
12 Semple RK, Cochran EK, Soos MA, Burling KA, Savage DB, Gorden P, O'Rahilly S: Plasma adiponectin as a marker of insulin receptor dysfunction: clinical utility in severe insulin resistance. Diabetes Care 2008;31:977–979.
13 Berardinelli W: An undiagnosed endocrinometabolic syndrome: report of 2 cases. J Clin Endocrinol Metab 1954;14:193–204.
14 Seip M: Lipodystrophy and gigantism with associated endocrine manifestations. A new diencephalic syndrome? Acta Paediatr 1959;48:555–574.
15 Christensen JD, Lungu AO, Cochran E, Collins MT, Gafni RI, Reynolds JC, Rother KI, Gorden P, Brown RJ: Bone mineral content in patients with congenital generalized lipodystrophy is unaffected by metreleptin replacement therapy. J Clin Endocrinol Metab 2014;99:1493–1500.
16 Seip M: Generalized Lipodystrophy; in: Ergebnisse der inneren Medizin und Kinderheilkunde. Berlin, Springer, 1971, pp 59–95.
17 Magré J, Delépine M, Khallouf E, Gedde-Dahl T, Van Maldergem L, Sobel E, et al: Identification of the gene altered in Berardinelli-Seip congenital lipodystrophy on chromosome 11q13. Nat Genet 2001;28: 365–370.
18 Boutet E, El Mourabit H, Prot M, Nemani M, Khallouf E, Colard O, Maurice M, Durand-Schneider AM, Chrétien Y, Grès S, Wolf C, Saulnier-Blache JS, Capeau J, Magré J: Seipin deficiency alters fatty acid Δ9 desaturation and lipid droplet formation in Berardinelli-Seip congenital lipodystrophy. Biochimie 2009;91:796–803.
19 Szymanski KM, Binns D, Bartz R, Grishin N V, Li W-P, Agarwal AK, Garg A, Anderson RGW, Goodman JM: The lipodystrophy protein seipin is found at endoplasmic reticulum lipid droplet junctions and is important for droplet morphology. Proc Natl Acad Sci U S A 2007;104:20890–20895.
20 Agarwal AK, Arioglu E, De Almeida S, Akkoc N, Taylor SI, Bowcock AM, Barnes RI, Garg A: AGPAT2 is mutated in congenital generalized lipodystrophy linked to chromosome 9q34. Nat Genet 2002; 31:21–23.

21 Van Maldergem L, Magré J, Khallouf TE, Gedde-Dahl T, Delépine M, Trygstad O, Seemanova E, Stephenson T, Albott CS, Bonnici F, Panz VR, Medina JL, Bogalho P, Huet F, Savasta S, Verloes A, Robert JJ, Loret H, De Kerdanet M, Tubiana-Rufi N, Mégarbané A, Maassen J, Polak M, Lacombe D, Kahn CR, Silveira EL, D'Abronzo FH, Grigorescu F, Lathrop M, Capeau J, O'Rahilly S: Genotype-phenotype relationships in Berardinelli-Seip congenital lipodystrophy. J Med Genet 2002;39:722–733.

22 Garg A, Kircher M, del Campo M, Amato RS, Agarwal AK: Whole exome sequencing identifies de novo heterozygous CAV1 mutations associated with a novel neonatal onset lipodystrophy syndrome. Am J Med Genet Part A 2015;167:1796–1806.

23 Hayashi YK, Matsuda C, Ogawa M, Goto K, Tominaga K, Mitsuhashi S, Park YE, Nonaka I, Hino-Fukuyo N, Haginoya K, Sugano H, Nishino I: Human PTRF mutations cause secondary deficiency of caveolins resulting in muscular dystrophy with generalized lipodystrophy. J Clin Invest 2009;119:2623–2633.

24 Speckman RA, Garg A, Du F, Bennett L, Veile R, Arioglu E, Taylor SI, Lovett M, Bowcock AM: Mutational and haplotype analyses of families with familial partial lipodystrophy (Dunnigan variety) reveal recurrent missense mutations in the globular C-terminal domain of lamin A/C. Am J Hum Genet 2000;66:1192–1198.

25 Shackleton S, Lloyd DJ, Jackson SN, Evans R, Niermeijer MF, Singh BM, Schmidt H, Brabant G, Kumar S, Durrington PN, Gregory S, O'Rahilly S, Trembath RC: LMNA, encoding lamin A/C, is mutated in partial lipodystrophy. Nat Genet 2000;24:153–156.

26 Scharner J, Gnocchi VF, Ellis JA, Zammit PS: Genotype-phenotype correlations in laminopathies: how does fate translate? Biochem Soc Trans 2010;38:257–262.

27 Dechat T, Pfleghaar K, Sengupta K, Shimi T, Shumaker DK, Solimando L, Goldman RD: Nuclear lamins: major factors in the structural organization and function of the nucleus and chromatin. Genes Dev 2008;22:832–853.

28 Kim JB, Spiegelman BM: ADD 1/SREBP1 promotes adipocyte differentiation and gene expression linked to fatty acid metabolism. Genes Dev 1996;10:1096–1107.

29 Lloyd DJ, Trembath RC, Shackleton S: A novel interaction between lamin A and SREBP1: implications for partial lipodystrophy and other laminopathies. Hum Mol Genet 2002;11:769–777.

30 Barroso I, Gurnell M, Crowley VE, Agostini M, Schwabe JW, Soos MA, Maslen GL, Williams TD, Lewis H, Schafer AJ, Chatterjee VK, O'Rahilly S: Dominant negative mutations in human PPARgamma associated with severe insulin resistance, diabetes mellitus and hypertension. Nature 1999;402:880–883.

31 Rubio-Cabezas O, Puri V, Murano I, Saudek V, Semple RK, Dash S, Hyden CSS, Bottomley W, Vigouroux C, Magré J, Raymond-Barker P, Murgatroyd PR, Chawla A, Skepper JN, Chatterjee VK, Suliman S, Consortium LS, Patch AM, Agarwal AK, Garg A, Barroso I, Cinti S, Czech MP, Argente J, O'Rahilly S, Savage DB: Partial lipodystrophy and insulin resistant diabetes in a patient with a homozygous nonsense mutation in CIDEC. EMBO Mol Med 2009;1:280–287.

32 Puri V, Konda S, Ranjit S, Aouadi M, Chawla A, Chouinard M, Chakladar A, Czech MP: Fat-specific protein 27, a novel lipid droplet protein that enhances triglyceride storage. J Biol Chem 2007;282:34213–34218.

33 Gandotra S, Le Dour C, Bottomley W, Cervera P, Giral P, Reznik Y, Charpentier G, Auclair M, Delépine M, Barroso I, Semple RK, Lathrop M, Lascols O, Capeau J, O'Rahilly S, Magré J, Savage DB, Vigouroux C: Perilipin deficiency and autosomal dominant partial lipodystrophy. N Engl J Med 2011;364:740–748.

34 Garcia A, Subramanian V, Sekowski A, Bhattacharyya S, Love MW, Brasaemle DL: The amino and carboxyl termini of perilipin a facilitate the storage of triacylglycerols. J Biol Chem 2004;279:8409–8416.

35 Kozusko K, Tsang VHM, Bottomley W, Cho Y-H, Gandotra S, Mimmack M, Lim K, Isaac I, Patel S, Saudek V, O'Rahilly S, Srinivasan S, Greenfield JR, Barroso I, Campbell LV, Savage DB: Clinical and molecular characterization of a novel PLIN1 frameshift mutation identified in patients with familial partial lipodystrophy. Diabetes 2015;64:299–310.

36 Payne F, Lim K, Girousse A, Brown RJ, Kory N, Robbins A, Xue Y, Sleigh A, Cochran E, Adams C, Dev Borman A, Russel-Jones D, Gorden P, Semple RK, Saudek V, O'Rahilly S, Walther TC, Barroso I, Savage DB: Mutations disrupting the Kennedy phosphatidylcholine pathway in humans with congenital lipodystrophy and fatty liver disease. Proc Natl Acad Sci U S A 2014;111:8901–8906.

37 Novelli G, Muchir A, Sangiuolo F, Helbling-leclerc A, Apice MRD, Massart C, Capon F, Sbraccia P, Federici M, Lauro R, Tudisco C, Pallotta R, Scarano G, Dallapiccola B, Merlini L: Mandibuloacral dysplasia is caused by a mutation in LMNA-encoding lamin A/C. Am J Hum Genet 2002;71:426–431.

38 Eriksson M, Brown WT, Gordon LB, Glynn MW, Singer J, Scott L, Erdos MR, Robbins CM, Moses TY, Berglund P, Dutra A, Pak E, Durkin S, Csoka AB, Boehnke M, Glover TW, Collins FS: Recurrent de novo point mutations in lamin A cause Hutchinson-Gilford progeria syndrome. Nature 2003;423:293–298.

39 Agarwal AK, Fryns JP, Auchus RJ, Garg A: Zinc metalloproteinase ZMPSTE24, is mutated in mandibuloacral dysplasia. Hum Mol Genet 2003;12:1995–2001.

40 Muftuoglu M, Oshima J, Kobbe C, Cheng WH, Leistritz DF, Bohr VA: The clinical characteristics of Werner syndrome: molecular and biochemical diagnosis. Hum Genet 2008;124:369–377.

41 Shastry S, Simha V, Godbole K, Sbraccia P, Melancon S, Yajnik CS, Novelli G, Kroiss M, Garg A: A novel syndrome of mandibular hypoplasia, deafness, and progeroid features associated with lipodystrophy, undescended testes, and male hypogonadism. J Clin Endocrinol Metab 2010;95:192–197.

42 Weedon MN, Ellard S, Prindle MJ, Caswell R, Lango Allen H, Oram R, Godbole K, Yajnik CS, Sbraccia P, Novelli G, Turnpenny P, McCann E, Goh KJ, Wang Y, Fulford J, McCulloch LJ, Savage DB, O'Rahilly S, Kos K, Loeb LA, Semple RK, Hattersley AT: An in-frame deletion at the polymerase active site of POLD1 causes a multisystem disorder with lipodystrophy. Nat Genet 2013;45:947–950.

43 Kitamura A, Maekawa Y, Uehara H, Izumi K, Kawachi I, Nishizawa M, Toyoshima Y, Takahashi H, Standley DM, Tanaka K, Hamazaki J, Murata S, Obara K, Toyoshima I, Yasutomo K: A mutation in the immunoproteasome subunit PSMB8 causes autoinflammation and lipodystrophy in humans. J Clin Invest 2011;121:4150–4160.

44 Graul-Neumann LM, Kienitz T, Robinson PN, Baasanjav S, Karow B, Gillessen-Kaesbach G, Fahsold R, Schmidt H, Hoffmann K, Passarge E: Marfan syndrome with neonatal progeroid syndrome-like lipodystrophy associated with a novel frameshift mutation at the 3′ terminus of the FBN1-gene. Am J Med Genet Part A 2010;152:2749–2755.

45 Tsoukas MA, Farr OM, Mantzoros CS: Leptin in congenital and HIV-associated lipodystrophy. Metabolism 2015;64:47–59.

46 Safar Zadeh E, Lungu AO, Cochran EK, Brown RJ, Ghany MG, Heller T, Kleiner DE, Gorden P: The liver diseases of lipodystrophy: the long-term effect of leptin treatment. J Hepatol 2013;59:131–137.

47 Shimomura I, Hammer RE, Ikemoto S, Brown MS, Goldstein JL: Leptin reverses insulin resistance and diabetes mellitus in mice with congenital lipodystrophy. Nature 1999;401:73–76.

48 Stears A, Hames C: Diagnosis and management of lipodystrophy: a practical update. Clin Lipidol 2014;9:235–259.

49 The ORIGIN Trial Investigators: n–3 fatty acids and cardiovascular outcomes in patients with dysglycemia. N Engl J Med 2012;367:309–318.

50 Cochran E, Musso C, Gorden P: The of use of U-500 in patients with extreme insulin resistance. Diabetes Care 2005;28:1240–1244.

Dr. Robert K. Semple
University of Cambridge Metabolic Research Laboratories, Level 4
Wellcome Trust-MRC Institute of Metabolic Science, Box 289, Addenbrooke's Hospital
Hills Road, Cambridge CB2 0QQ (UK)
E-Mail rks16@cam.ac.uk

Barbetti F, Ghizzoni L, Guaraldi F (eds): Diabetes Associated with Single Gene Defects and Chromosomal Abnormalities. Front Diabetes. Basel, Karger, 2017, vol 25, pp 134–144 (DOI: 10.1159/000454740)

Alström Syndrome

Pietro Maffei[a] · Francesca Favaretto[a] · Gabriella Milan[a] · Jan D. Marshall[b, c]

[a] Dipartimento di Medicina (DIMED), Padua University, Padua, Italy; [b] The Jackson Laboratory, Bar Harbor, ME, and [c] Alström Syndrome International, Mount Desert, ME, USA

Abstract

Alström syndrome is a recessively inherited disorder characterized by symptoms of cone-rod dystrophy and, in some, sudden and severe mitogenic cardiomyopathy. In early childhood, sensorineural hearing loss and truncal obesity develop. As the patients progress through the first decade of life, insulin resistance and hyperinsulinemia, type 2 diabetes, hyperlipidemia, hepatic steatosis, and progressive pulmonary fibrosis frequently develop. Typically, adults present with short adult stature and cardiac, hepatic, and renal dysfunction. Fibrosis is observed in nearly all organs and progressive development of multiorgan pathology leads to a reduced life expectancy. There is considerable variability in age of onset and severity of clinical symptoms, even within families, which is likely due to environmental or genetic modifiers. The wide range of observed phenotypes and their similarity to those of other ciliopathies such as Bardet-Biedl syndrome poses diagnostic challenges. The gene responsible for Alström syndrome, *ALMS1*, is comprised of 23 exons and codes for a protein of 4,169 amino acids. Alternate splice variants exist that may give rise to additional isoforms with specific functions. *ALMS1* mutations include insertions, deletions, and nonsense mutations leading to premature protein truncations with a clustering of disease-causing variants in exons 8, 10, and 16. The ALMS1 protein localizes to the cytosol, to the centrosomes of dividing cells, and the basal bodies of ciliated cells. ALMS1 is expressed in all tissues affected by the disease, which may explain the broad phenotypic spectrum of Alström syndrome.
© 2017 S. Karger AG, Basel

Alström syndrome (AS) (OMIM 203800) is an extremely rare disease, with a prevalence of less than 1 per million in the general population [1, 2]. It was described for the first time in 1959 by the Swedish psychiatrist C.H. Alström [3]. AS occurs in all races and ethnicities, although geographic or cultural isolation can increase the frequency of disease transmission [4–6]. The syndrome has a chronic and progressive course that severely impacts the quality of life and survival of patients. The gene responsible for AS, *ALMS1* located on chromosome 2p13, was identified in 2002 and is transmitted in an autosomal recessive manner with equal frequency in both sexes

Jan D. Marshall deceased on September 6, 2016.

[7–9]. *ALMS1* appears to play a role in protein trafficking at the base of the cilium, a cellular organelle that functions as an 'antenna' for cellular detection and management of external signals present in all the cells of the body [10]. The syndrome typically presents during the first weeks of life with nystagmus, photodysphoria, and retinopathy due to the progressive damage of the cones and subsequently of rods. Most AS patients are legally blind before the age of 20 years. Sudden congestive heart failure can present in the first weeks or months of life, which is also the leading cause of death in children. As the child grows, liver steatosis and (in some) cirrhosis, kidney failure, or recurrence of cardiac problems can occur. Other typical manifestations of the syndrome are sensorineural hearing loss, childhood obesity, insulin resistance and diabetes, short adult stature, hypertriglyceridemia, and hypogonadism [2, 11, 12]. Additional derangements involve the brain, pulmonary function, the skin, and the bones. Postmortem investigations have shown extensive systemic organ fibrosis [12]. Currently there is no cure for AS, but its early detection and prevention of complications are a valuable approach to improve the quality of life of patients and their survival.

Genetic and Molecular Mechanisms

ALMS1, a ubiquitously expressed gene composed of 23 exons, varying in length from 64 to 6,108 bp, codes for ALMS1, a protein of 4,169 amino acids whose function is only partly known. Excluding the region encoding exon 8, the deduced amino-acid sequence of mouse *Alms1* is 63.7% identical to the protein sequence of human ALMS1. The ALMS1 protein contains a predicted leucine zipper motif, a serine-rich region, and a large tandem-repeat domain comprising 34 imperfect repetitions of 47 amino acids. In addition, potential nuclear localization signals as well as a histidine-rich region in the mouse sequence have been identified [7, 8]. To date, 239 different mutations in *ALMS1* have been identified in individuals with AS and the majority are nonsense and frameshift (insertions or deletions) that result in premature termination codons [2, 9]. There is a strong clustering of disease-causing variants in exon 8 (49%), exon 10 (17%), and exon 16 (19%) [9]. Subjects harboring mutations only in exon 8 may have delayed and milder renal complications, perhaps due to tissue-specific expression of different splice isoforms [13]. So far, no disease-causing mutations have been identified in exons 1–2, 6, 7, 13, and 22–23 [9; unpublished results]. An open access, comprehensive mutation database stored and catalogued using the Leiden Open Source Variation Database (LOVD) (https://lovd.euro-wabb.org/home.php?select_db = ALMS1) listing all known AS pathogenic mutations is available online as a part of the EURO-WABB project [14]. EURO-WABB is an international multicenter large-scale observational study capturing longitudinal clinical and outcome data for patients with Wolfram, Alström, and Bardet-Biedl (WABB) syndromes [14].

The ALMS1 protein localizes to the cytosol, centrosomes of dividing cells, and basal bodies of ciliated cells, and is one of more than 100 proteins associated with the cilium present in all cells [15]. It has been observed that ALMS1 remains at the centrosome throughout mitosis, and roles in microtubule organization, intracellular transport, and the assembly and function of basal bodies and cilia have been suggested [15]. In particular, ALMS1 associates with the proximal ends of centrioles and basal bodies and is implicated in C-Nap1 and PCM1-related functions. Involvement of the ALMS motif-containing proteins C10orf90 and KIAA1731 in primary cilium assembly and centriole formation/stability have also been proposed [16]. Purvis et al. [17] suggested that the ubiquitous factor Sp1 regulates ALMS1 transcription and that the regulatory factor X proteins activate ALMS1 transcription during serum starvation-induced growth arrest. ALMS1 also interacts with the components of the CART complex including members of the actinin family. The cellular phenotype observed in patient fibroblasts during transferrin receptor recycling underscores an important role for ALMS1 in the endocytic recycling pathway of the cytoplasm [18]. In addition, fibroblasts from AS patients upregulate collagen expression and secretion, display a longer cell cycle, and are more resistant to apoptotic stimuli [19]. Butler et al. [20] observed that in adult AS subjects, members of the metallothionein gene family had a decreased expression. Furthermore, involvement of multiple snoRNAs and miRNAs impacting the cell cycle cascade, DNA replication, and repair occur [20].

Mouse Models

Several mouse models of AS which recapitulate the features observed in patients have been well characterized. Collin et al. [21] generated the first mouse model using an *Alms1* gene-trapped ES cell line, Alms1$^{\text{GT(pGT1Lxf)/Pjn}}$. The *Alms1$^{-/-}$* mice developed similar features to patients with AS including obesity, hypogonadism, hyperinsulinemia, and late-onset hearing loss. Electron microscopy revealed accumulation of intracellular vesicles in the inner segments of photoreceptors while rhodopsin transport through the connecting cilium in photoreceptor cells was impaired and mislocalization of rhodopsin to the outer nuclear layer was seen in immunohistochemical studies [21]. The fat Aussie mouse (*Alms1$^{\text{foz/foz}}$*), another mouse model of AS, is caused by a spontaneous mutation in *Alms1* [22]. *Alms1$^{\text{foz/foz}}$* mice become obese and hyperinsulinemic, and diabetes accompanied by pancreatic islet hyperplasia and cysts eventually develops. The *foz/foz* mice develop hepatomegaly and steatohepatitis with failure to upregulate PPARα, hypoadiponectinemia, and upregulation of mitochondrial UCP2 [22]. The male *foz/foz* mice are sterile due to a progressive germ cell loss followed by an almost complete block of development at the round-to-elongating spermatid stage of spermatogenesis [22]. The third mouse model, the ENU-induced *Alms1$^{L2131X/L2131X}$* mice, is characterized by impaired retinal rhodopsin transport, obesity onset at 7–10 weeks, hyperinsulinemia, hypercholesterolemia and elevated triglycerides, and defective sperm formation [23].

Although the mechanisms remain unknown, children with AS experience varying degrees of hyperphagia and food obsession with a marked increase of body weight beginning in the first 18 months of life. The rapid weight gain continues through puberty [24]. AS patients seem to be characterized by fat accumulation in subcutaneous instead of visceral regions [25]. Overweight or obesity in childhood partially normalizes as they reach adulthood, with weight and BMI trends differing by gender as reported in a group of Italian patients with AS [26]. In a study of 12 AS patients in the UK, waist circumference and fat mass were negatively correlated with age [27], contrary to the general population.

AS and Bardet-Biedl syndrome (BBS), both characterized by obesity, are genetic disorders caused by mutations resulting in ciliary dysfunction. Loss of cilia on hypothalamic POMC neurons in conditional mouse mutants resulted in hyperphagia and obesity [28]. Further studies confirmed that mutations in genes that directly influence the expression of signaling or structural proteins of the primary cilia induce disturbances in energy homeostasis in both humans and mice [29–31]. Recently, in a mouse model with obese phenotype (Ankrd26$^{-/-}$), profound regional changes and defects in the distribution of primary cilia in regions of the central nervous system that control appetite and energy homeostasis have been found [32]. When mutated or deleted, cilia-targeted proteins such as AC3, Mchr1, or Sstr3 cannot be incorporated into the primary cilia of hypothalamic circuits that control food intake [32]. In addition, neuronal cilia lengths are selectively reduced in the hypothalamus of obese mice with leptin deficiency and leptin resistance [33]. However, Berbari et al. [34] suggested that the leptin signaling axis is not the initiating event leading to hyperphagia and obesity in mice with cilia dysfunction.

In *foz/foz* mice, hyperphagia was observed prior to weight gain [22]. Recently, in the same model, there is a reduction of Alms1 at the base of the cilia in hypothalamic neurons, leading to a failure to maintain the structure and function of the cilia after birth [35]. These data suggest that ALMS1 can act on hypothalamic circuits that control the sense of hunger or satiety. Cellular studies indicate that ALMS1 mRNA levels are upregulated in response to serum starvation [36] and downregulated during adipogenesis [37]. Peripherally, in adipose tissue, changes in fat cell insulin sensitivity do not result in any effect on Alms1 expression in 3T3L1 cells [37]. In contrast, Huang-Doran and Semple [38] showed that the silencing of *Alms1* causes impaired adipogenesis in the 3T3-L1 cell line. Favaretto et al. [39] suggested that mutations in *Alms1* do not directly affect adipocyte maturation and that the adipose tissue expansion is secondary to multiple in vivo interactions.

Reduced insulin-stimulated glucose disposal and hyperinsulinemia have been observed in AS patients as young as 1 year of age and can appear before obesity begins in children, often evolving to type 2 diabetes mellitus during childhood, with a variable age of onset [2, 12, 40]. Favaretto et al. [39] showed that the

Alms1$^{GT(pGT1Lxf)/Pjn}$ mice have aberrant insulin signaling either downstream or independent of AKT signaling, before the increase of body weight and circulating insulin levels. In adipose tissue, several defects of glucose transporter 4 (GLUT4) have been demonstrated, including the reduction of total protein content, mislocalization, and impairment in insulin-induced translocation [39]. Reduced insulin receptor expression has been reported in fibroblasts derived from BBS patients, a disease which shares many clinical features with AS [41]. Recently, it has been observed in zebrafish that Alms1 and BBS genes have opposite effects on β-cell mass [42]. Alms1 is necessary for continued β-cell expansion in response to glucose, is required for β-cell regenerative capacity, and Alms1 depletion resulted in β-cell death. On the contrary, a deficiency of BBS genes (bbs1 or bbs4) showed an increased β-cell production accompanied by a decrease in α-cells and δ-cells during early developmental stages [42].

AS is characterized by severe insulin resistance, with cutaneous signs of acanthosis nigricans in many young patients. Type 2 diabetes mellitus is typically diagnosed in the second to third decade in approximately 70% of patients, with hyperinsulinemia often preceding the diabetes [2, 11, 12]. It is possible that the severe postreceptor insulin resistance in the syndrome results from impairment of intracellular trafficking along microtubules and externalization of functional glucose transporter 4 receptors also in skeletal muscle. For unknown reasons, there is a striking lack of peripheral neuropathy and preservation of protective foot sensation in AS [43]. Bettini et al. [26] demonstrated that mechanisms and time course of insulin resistance and β-cell failure in AS are distinct from that observed in control subjects, independent of body weight. β-Cell function was reduced in patients older than 18 years while those under 18 years had a significantly higher β-cell secretion; therefore, the development of type 2 diabetes mellitus could result from the metabolic effect of "β-cell exhaustion" [26]. In the wider population, preliminary data do not support a contribution for polymorphisms in *ALMS1* in type 2 diabetes [44].

Although the mechanism is not known, hypertriglyceridemia is a common clinical feature in AS. In many AS patients, hypertriglyceridemia is intractable and could result in multiple episodes of pancreatitis [45]. Paisey et al. [46] reported an overlap between hypertriglyceridemia and hyperinsulinemia in AS, but no direct correlation between the two, or with insulin resistance. Additionally, in the same study, triglyceride levels were unrelated to glycemia and hepatic or renal dysfunction.

A range of endocrinological problems have also been reported in AS, including hypothyroidism, growth hormone (GH) deficiency, primary hypogonadism in males, and irregular cycles or amenorrhea with hyperandrogenism in females. Alter and Moshang [47] described for the first time normal growth early in life with advanced bone age in 2 siblings with clinical features of AS. A low average height in adolescence and low GH concentrations were observed. Zumsteg et al. [48] observed blunted GH concentrations following an arginine stimulation test in 3 affected siblings. Tai et al. [49] described a 15-year-old Taiwanese boy whose height was below the 3rd

Table 1. Main clinical features of Alström syndrome

Organ system	Typical age onset	Clinical problem
Vision	1st month	nystagmus, photophobia, cone-rod dystrophy, cataract, blindness
Cardiac	1st month, adulthood	heart failure, dilated cardiomyopathy, restrictive cardiomyopathy, pulmonary hypertension, mitogenic cardiomyopathy
Hearing	5–10 years	sensorineural hearing loss, otitis media
Renal	variable, early adolescence	glomerulofibrosis, interstitial fibrosis, end-stage renal failure
Gastrointestinal	variable, early adolescence	liver steatosis, hepatic inflammation and fibrosis, cirrhosis, portal hypertension

percentile, and low GH secretion was documented. Recently, 3 subjects presenting with short stature have been described by Catrinoiu et al. [50]. Maffei et al. [51] reported a reduction of ALS and IGFBP-1 concentrations in AS in the presence of increased levels of IGFBP-2. However, concentrations of IGFs (-I and -II) and IGFBP-3 did not differ from controls [51]. Recently, in a large population of AS patients, Romano et al. [52] demonstrated that approximately 50% of nonobese patients have an inadequate GH reserve to the GHRH-arginine test and may be functionally GH deficient. Additionally, longitudinal auxological assessment of AS subjects established, after a period of normal or slightly increased growth, a reduced final height that is associated with an impaired GH reserve [26]. Elevated body weight, as well as elevated insulin levels, likely supports the normal or accelerated growth in the first years of life in AS. Subsequently, this mechanism cannot compensate for the failure of the pituitary to produce GH or other unknown genetic factors, which could affect final height. Histopathological alterations have been reported in the pituitary gland consisting of marked and diffuse fibrosis of the adenohypophysis [52]. Empty sella has been sporadically observed [50, 53].

General Clinical Aspects and Miscellaneous

The main clinical features of AS and their time course are summarized in Table 1. IQ is normal in the majority of AS subjects, although developmental delay and learning difficulties have been documented [2, 12, 13]. Some patients with AS have received a diagnosis of autism or autistic-spectrum disorder. Tonic-clonic seizures have been observed in a subset of AS patients. Very few studies have systematically investigated the neurological and psychological aspects of the syndrome. In a recent study using conventional brain MRI sequences, AS patients presented with mild brain atrophy and vascular-like lesions at a very young age. The white and grey matter volume decrease was more evident in the posterior regions. In addition, diffusion tensor imaging revealed a supratentorial dysmyelination which also entailed the white matter that appears normal on conventional MRI sequences [53].

Other variable conditions with a different age range of appearance have been described. Recurrent pulmonary infection and otitis have been reported in the early years of life. Some AS patients develop increasingly severe lung dysfunction, including COPD and ARDS with extensive pulmonary fibrosis. In the pediatric age until puberty, scoliosis, flat wide feet, and recurrent urinary tract infections are common. Difficulty in bladder voiding could be a disturbing problem in a subset of AS patients, and some of them will require a urinary catheter or bladder surgical procedures. Alopecia usually develops after puberty, although it has been reported very early in some cases [54].

Diagnosis

Diagnostic delay is common in AS, probably because it is still an unfamiliar disease [55]. AS patients frequently receive multiple misdiagnoses, including BBS (rod-cone dystrophy) [56], Cohen syndrome (rod-cone dystrophy), Usher syndrome, Refsum disease, congenital achromatopsia (cone dystrophy), Leber congenital amaurosis (cone dystrophy) [57, 58], Wolfram syndrome (optic atrophy), Biemond 2 syndrome (coloboma, aniridia, cataract, microphthalmia), sporadic infantile DCM, and mitochondrial disorders. The most common differential diagnosis is BBS, which is characterized by childhood obesity, developmental and intellectual delay, polydactyly, and vision loss. Notably, AS patients generally have normal digits, although polydactyly or syndactyly has been observed in 2% [11].

The diagnosis of AS is based on genetic mutations in *ALMS1* in combination with clinical criteria that are age dependent [11]. A screening strategy that first targets exons 8, 10, and 16 has been successfully used [1, 2], although *ALMS1* mutations are now being identified in other exons. The proof of AS syndrome is based on the presence of 2 *ALMS1* mutations (homozygosis or compound heterozygous). Marshall et al. [11], set forth diagnostic criteria based upon the age of the patient, when only one heterozygous *ALMS1* mutation is found.

Recently, Casey et al. [59] suggested that the current clinical diagnostic criteria and genetic testing strategy could miss some atypical cases or milder phenotypes which present with the absence of a number of key clinical features such as obesity, nystagmus, photophobia, short stature, and hearing loss. Other atypical phenotypes, without obesity, have also been reported in the literature [60]. With improvements in the availability of genetic sequencing and advances in sequencing techniques, it is becoming clear that the current diagnostic criteria for AS will need to be broadened to include patients with an isolated eye and/or heart phenotype.

Therapy

There is no definite cure or targeted treatment for AS – we can only try to prevent or delay its systemic complications. At present, complications associated with AS are treated symptomatically as in the general population [1, 2, 11, 12]. Patients have to be assessed for visual and/or hearing aids. Early intervention planning, including enrolment in specialty schools for the blind and hearing impaired or specific support for inevitable dual sensory loss is crucial for school progression. Informed family planning including the prenatal diagnosis is a feasible option when the mutation is known.

Dietary counselling beginning in early childhood to mitigate obesity and its complications remains a mainstay of therapy. Paisey et al. [61] have demonstrated that diabetes control could also be improved in AS by aerobic exercise and that all features of the metabolic syndrome are responsive to lifestyle modifications. Hyperinsulinemia and type 2 diabetes can be treated with caloric restriction, reduced carbohydrate diet, metformin, incretins, and insulin [62–64]. Lipid-lowering strategies include diet, statin, fibrates, and fish oil [63]. Severe hypertriglyceridemia with a risk of pancreatitis has been treated in some cases with fasting and insulin [63]. When cardiac dysfunction is present, medications such as ACE inhibitors, β-blockers, diuretics, or spironolactone can be given to improve heart function. Heart-lung transplantation could be a viable therapeutic option in some patients [65]. Endocrine deficiencies should be treated with replacement therapies such as L-thyroxine, testosterone, and rGH.

Future perspectives might come from new or previously established therapies that reduce systemic fibrosis such as spironolactone or AT-II inhibitors and stem cell or gene therapies for retinal disorders or the artificial retina.

Organizations such as Alström Syndrome International (ASI, www.alstrom.org), Alström Syndrome UK (AS-UK, http://www.alstrom.org.uk/), Alström Syndrome Canada, and the Associazione Sindrome di Alström Italia Onlus (ASS.A.I Onlus http://www.alstrom.it/) offer invaluable information and emotional support for patients and their families.

Acknowledgement

J.D.M. received the following grant: NIH HD036878.

References

1 Marshall JD, Maffei P, Beck S, Barrett TG, Paisey R, Naggert JK: Clinical utility gene card for: Alström Syndrome – update 2013. Eur J Hum Genet 2013, DOI: 10.10358/ejhg.2013.61.

2 Marshall JD, Maffei P, Collin GB, Naggert JK: Alström syndrome: genetics and clinical overview. Curr Genomics 2011;12:225–235.

3 Alström CH, Hallgren B, Nilsson LB, Asander H: Retinal degeneration combined with obesity, diabetes mellitus and neurogenous deafness: a specific syndrome (not hitherto described) distinct from the Laurence-Moon-Bardet-Biedl syndrome: a clinical, endocrinological and genetic examination based on a large pedigree. Acta Psychiatr Neurol Scand Suppl 1959;129:1–35.

4 Aldahmesh MA, Abu-Safieh L, Khan AO, Al-Hassnan ZN, Shaheen R, Rajab M, Monies D, Meyer BF, Alkuraya FS: Allelic heterogeneity in inbred populations: the Saudi experience with Alström syndrome as an illustrative example. Am J Med Genet A 2009; 149A:662–665.

5 Marshall JD, Ludman MD, Shea SE, Salisbury SR, Willi SM, LaRoche RG, Nishina PM: Genealogy, natural history, and phenotype of Alstrom syndrome in a large Acadian kindred and three additional families. Am J Med Genet 1997;73:150–161.

6 Ozanturk A, Marshall JD, Collin GB, Duzenli S, Marshall RP, Candan S, Tos T, Esen I, Taskesen M, Cayir A, Ozturk S, Ustun I, Ataman E, Karaca E, Ozdemir TR, Erol I, Eroglu FK, Torun D, Pariltay E, Yilmaz-Gulec E, Karaca E, Atabek ME, Elcioglu N, Satman I, Moller C, Muller J, Naggert JK, Ozgul RK: The phenotypic and molecular genetic spectrum of Alstrom syndrome in 44 Turkish kindreds and a literature review of Alstrom syndrome in Turkey. J Hum Genet 2015;60:1–9.

7 Collin GB, Marshall JD, Ikeda A, So WV, Russell-Eggitt I, Maffei P, Beck S, Boerkoel CF, Sicolo N, Martin M, Nishina PM, Naggert JK: Mutations in ALMS1 cause obesity, type 2 diabetes and neurosensory degeneration in Alström syndrome. Nat Genet 2002;31:74–78.

8 Hearn T, Renforth GL, Spalluto C, Hanley NA, Piper K, Brickwood S, White C, Connolly V, Taylor JF, Russell-Eggitt I, Bonneau D, Walker M, Wilson DI: Mutation of ALMS1, a large gene with a tandem repeat encoding 47 amino acids, causes Alström syndrome. Nat Genet 2002;31:79–83.

9 Marshall JD, Muller J, Collin GB, Milan G, Kingsmore SF, Dinwiddie D, Farrow EG, Miller NA, Favaretto F, Maffei P, Dollfus H, Vettor R, Naggert JK: Alström syndrome: mutation spectrum of ALMS1. Hum Mutat 2015;36:660–668.

10 Hildebrandt F, Benzing T, Katsanis N: Ciliopathies. N Engl J Med 2011;364:1533–1543.

11 Marshall JD, Beck S, Maffei P, Naggert JK: Alström syndrome. Eur J Hum Genet 2007;15:1193–1202.

12 Marshall JD, Bronson RT, Collin GB, Nordstrom AD, Maffei P, Paisey RB, Carey C, Macdermott S, Russell-Eggitt I, Shea SE, Davis J, Beck S, Shatirishvili G, Mihai CM, Hoeltzenbein M, Pozzan GB, Hopkinson I, Sicolo N, Naggert JK, Nishina PM: New Alström syndrome phenotypes based on the evaluation of 182 cases. Arch Intern Med 2005;165:675–683.

13 Marshall JD, Hinman EG, Collin GB, Beck S, Cerqueira R, Maffei P, Milan G, Zhang W, Wilson DI, Hearn T, Tavares P, Vettor R, Veronese C, Martin M, So WV, Nishina PM, Naggert JK: Spectrum of ALMS1 variants and evaluation of genotype-phenotype correlations in Alström syndrome. Hum Mutat 2007;28:1114–1123.

14 Farmer A, Ayme S, de Heredia ML, Maffei P, McCafferty S, Mlynarski W, Nunes V, Parkinson K, Paquis-Flucklinger V, Rohayem J, Sinnott R, Tillmann V, Tranebjaerg L, Barrett TG: EURO-WABB: an EU rare diseases registry for Wolfram syndrome, Alström syndrome and Bardet-Biedl syndrome. BMC Pediatr 2013;13:130.

15 Hearn T, Spalluto C, Phillips VJ, Renforth GL, Copin N, Hanley NA, Wilson DI: Subcellular localization of ALMS1 supports involvement of centrosome and basal body dysfunction in the pathogenesis of obesity, insulin resistance, and type 2 diabetes. Diabetes 2005;54:1581–1587.

16 Knorz VJ, Spalluto C, Lessard M, Purvis TL, Adigun FF, Collin GB, Hanley NA, Wilson DI, Hearn T: Centriolar association of ALMS1 and likely centrosomal functions of the ALMS motif-containing proteins C10orf90 and KIAA1731. Mol Biol Cell 2010; 21:3617–3629.

17 Purvis TL, Hearn T, Spalluto C, Knorz VJ, Hanley KP, Sanchez-Elsner T, Hanley NA, Wilson DI: Transcriptional regulation of the Alström syndrome gene ALMS1 by members of the RFX family and Sp1. Gene 2010;460:20–29.

18 Collin GB, Marshall JD, King BL, Milan G, Maffei P, Jagger DJ, Naggert JK: The Alström syndrome protein, ALMS1, interacts with α-actinin and components of the endosome recycling pathway. PLoS One 2012;7:e37925.

19 Zulato E, Favaretto F, Veronese C, Campanaro S, Marshall JD, Romano S, Cabrelle A, Collin GB, Zavan B, Belloni AS, Rampazzo E, Naggert JK, Abatangelo G, Sicolo N, Maffei P, Milan G, Vettor R: ALMS1-deficient fibroblasts over-express extra-cellular matrix components, display cell cycle delay and are resistant to apoptosis. PLoS One 2011;6:e19081.

20 Butler MG, Wang K, Marshall JD, Naggert JK, Rethmeyer JA, Gunewardena SS, Manzardo AM: Coding and noncoding expression patterns associated with rare obesity-related disorders: Prader-Willi and Alström syndromes. Adv Genomics Genet 2015;2015: 53–75.

21 Collin GB, Cyr E, Bronson R, Marshall JD, Gifford EJ, Hicks W, Murray SA, Zheng QY, Smith RS, Nishina PM, Naggert JK: Alms1-disrupted mice recapitulate human Alström syndrome. Hum Mol Genet 2005;14:2323–2333.

22 Arsov T, Silva DG, O'Bryan MK, Sainsbury A, Lee NJ, Kennedy C, Manji SS, Nelms K, Liu C, Vinuesa CG, de Kretser DM, Goodnow CC, Petrovsky N: Fat aussie – a new Alström syndrome mouse showing a critical role for ALMS1 in obesity, diabetes, and spermatogenesis. Mol Endocrinol 2006;20:1610–1622.

23 Li G, Vega R, Nelms K, Gekakis N, Goodnow C, Mc-Namara P, Wu H, Hong NA, Glynne R: A role for Alström syndrome protein, alms1, in kidney ciliogenesis and cellular quiescence. PLoS Genet 2007;3:e8.

24 Milani D, Cerutti M, Pezzani L, Maffei P, Milan G, Esposito S: Syndromic obesity: clinical implications of a correct diagnosis. Ital J Pediatr 2014;40:33.

25 Paisey RB, Hodge D, Williams K: Body fat distribution, serum glucose, lipid and insulin response to meals in Alström syndrome. J Hum Nutr Diet 2008; 21:268–274.

26 Bettini V, Maffei P, Pagano C, Romano S, Milan G, Favaretto F, Marshall JD, Paisey R, Scolari F, Greggio NA, Tosetto I, Naggert JK, Sicolo N, Vettor R: The progression from obesity to type 2 diabetes in Alström syndrome. Pediatr Diabetes 2012;13:59–67.

27 Minton JA, Owen KR, Ricketts CJ, Crabtree N, Shaikh G, Ehtisham S, Porter JR, Carey C, Hodge D, Paisey R, Walker M, Barrett TG: Syndromic obesity and diabetes: changes in body composition with age and mutation analysis of ALMS1 in 12 United Kingdom kindreds with Alström syndrome. J Clin Endocrinol Metab 2006;91:3110–3116.

28 Davenport JR, Watts AJ, Roper VC, Croyle MJ, van Groen T, Wyss JM, Nagy TR, Kesterson RA, Yoder BK: Disruption of intraflagellar transport in adult mice leads to obesity and slow-onset cystic kidney disease. Curr Biol 2007;17:1586–1594.

29 Girard D, Petrovsky N: Alström syndrome: insights into the pathogenesis of metabolic disorders. Nat Rev Endocrinol 2011;7:77–88.

30 Sen Gupta P, Prodromou NV, Chapple JP: Can faulty antennae increase adiposity? The link between cilia proteins and obesity. J Endocrinol 2009;203:327–336.

31 Shalata A, Ramirez MC, Desnick RJ, Priedigkeit N, Buettner C, Lindtner C, Mahroum M, Abdul-Ghani M, Dong F, Arar N, Camacho-Vanegas O, Zhang R, Camacho SC, Chen Y, Ibdah M, DeFronzo R, Gillespie V, Kelley K, Dynlacht BD, Kim S, Glucksman MJ, Borochowitz ZU, Martignetti JA: Morbid obesity resulting from inactivation of the ciliary protein CEP19 in humans and mice. Am J Hum Genet 2013; 93:1061–1071.

32 Acs P, Bauer PO, Mayer B, Bera T, Macallister R, Mezey E, Pastan I: A novel form of ciliopathy underlies hyperphagia and obesity in Ankrd26 knockout mice. Brain Struct Funct 2015;220:1511–1528.

33 Han YM, Kang GM, Byun K, Ko HW, Kim J, Shin MS, Kim HK, Gil SY, Yu JH, Lee B, Kim MS: Leptin-promoted cilia assembly is critical for normal energy balance. J Clin Invest 2014;124:2193–2197.

34 Berbari NF, Pasek RC, Malarkey EB, Yazdi SM, McNair AD, Lewis WR, Nagy TR, Kesterson RA, Yoder BK: Leptin resistance is a secondary consequence of the obesity in ciliopathy mutant mice. Proc Natl Acad Sci U S A 2013;110:7796–7801.

35 Heydet D, Chen LX, Larter CZ, Inglis C, Silverman MA, Farrell GC, Leroux MR: A truncating mutation of Alms1 reduces the number of hypothalamic neuronal cilia in obese mice. Dev Neurobiol 2013;73:1–13.

36 Yabuta N, Onda H, Watanabe M, Yoshioka N, Nagamori I, Funatsu T, Toji S, Tamai K, Nojima H: Isolation and characterization of the TIGA genes, whose transcripts are induced by growth arrest. Nucleic Acids Res 2006;34:4878–4892.

37 Romano S, Milan G, Veronese C, Collin GB, Marshall JD, Centobene C, Favaretto F, Dal Pra C, Scarda A, Leandri S, Naggert JK, Maffei P, Vettor R: Regulation of Alström syndrome gene expression during adipogenesis and its relationship with fat cell insulin sensitivity. Int J Mol Med 2008;21:731–736.

38 Huang-Doran I, Semple RK: Knockdown of the Alström syndrome-associated gene Alms1 in 3T3-L1 preadipocytes impairs adipogenesis but has no effect on cell-autonomous insulin action. Int J Obes (Lond) 2010;34:1554–1558.

39 Favaretto F, Milan G, Collin GB, Marshall JD, Stasi F, Maffei P, Vettor R, Naggert JK: GLUT4 defects in adipose tissue are early signs of metabolic alterations in Alms1GT/GT, a mouse model for obesity and insulin resistance. PLoS One 2014;9:e109540.

40 Satman I, Yilmaz MT, Gursoy N, Karsidag K, Dinccag N, Ovali T, Karadeniz S, Uysal V, Bugra Z, Okten A, Devrim S: Evaluation of insulin resistant diabetes mellitus in Alström syndrome: a long-term prospective follow-up of three siblings. Diabetes Res Clin Pract 2002;56:189–196.

41 Starks RD, Beyer AM, Guo DF, Boland L, Zhang Q, Sheffield VC, Rahmouni K: Regulation of insulin receptor trafficking by Bardet Biedl syndrome proteins. PLoS Genet 2015;11:e1005311.

42 Lodh S, Hostelley TL, Leitch CC, O'Hare EA, Zaghloul NA: Differential effects on β-cell mass by disruption of Bardet-Biedl syndrome or Alstrom syndrome genes. Hum Mol Genet 2016;25:57–68.

43 Paisey RB, Paisey RM, Thomson MP, Bower L, Maffei P, Shield JP, Barnett S, Marshall JD: Protection from clinical peripheral sensory neuropathy in Alström syndrome in contrast to early-onset type 2 diabetes. Diabetes Care 2009;32:462–464.

44 Patel S, Minton JA, Weedon MN, Frayling TM, Ricketts C, Hitman GA, McCarthy MI, Hattersley AT, Walker M, Barrett TG: Common variations in the ALMS1 gene do not contribute to susceptibility to type 2 diabetes in a large white UK population. Diabetologia 2006;49:1209–1213.

45 Wu WC, Chen SC, Dia CY, Yu ML, Hsieh MY, Lin ZY, Wang LY, Tsai JF, Chang WY, Chuang WL: Alström syndrome with acute pancreatitis: a case report. Kaohsiung J Med Sci 2003;19:358–361.

46 Paisey RB, Carey CM, Bower L, Marshall J, Taylor P, Maffei P, Mansell P: Hypertriglyceridaemia in Alström's syndrome: causes and associations in 37 cases. Clin Endocrinol (Oxf) 2004;60:228–231.

47 Alter CA, Moshang T Jr: Growth hormone deficiency in two siblings with Alström syndrome. Am J Dis Child 1993;147:97–99.

48 Zumsteg U, Muller PY, Miserez AR: Alstrom syndrome: confirmation of linkage to chromosome 2p12–13 and phenotypic heterogeneity in three affected sibs. J Med Genet 2000;37:E8.

49 Tai TS, Lin SY, Sheu WH: Metabolic effects of growth hormone therapy in an Alström syndrome patient. Horm Res 2003;60:297–301.

50 Catrinoiu D, Mihai CM, Tuta L, Stoicescu R, Simpetru A: Rare case of Alstrom syndrome with empty sella and interfamilial presence of Bardet-Biedl phenotype. J Med Life 2009;2:98–103.

51 Maffei P, Boschetti M, Marshall JD, Paisey RB, Beck S, Resmini E, Collin GB, Naggert JK, Milan G, Vettor R, Minuto F, Sicolo N, Barreca A: Characterization of the IGF system in 15 patients with Alström syndrome. Clin Endocrinol (Oxf) 2007;66:269–275.

52 Romano S, Maffei P, Bettini V, Milan G, Favaretto F, Gardiman M, Marshall JD, Greggio NA, Pozzan GB, Collin GB, Naggert JK, Bronson R, Vettor R: Alström syndrome is associated with short stature and reduced GH reserve. Clin Endocrinol (Oxf) 2013;79: 529–536.

53 Citton V, Favaro A, Bettini V, Gabrieli J, Milan G, Greggio NA, Marshall JD, Naggert JK, Manara R, Maffei P: Brain involvement in Alström syndrome. Orphanet J Rare Dis 2013;8:24.

54 Kocova M, Sukarova-Angelovska E, Kacarska R, Maffei P, Milan G, Marshall JD: The unique combination of dermatological and ocular phenotypes in Alström syndrome: severe presentation, early onset and two novel ALMS1 mutations. Br J Dermatol 2011;164:878–880.

55 Maffei P, Munno V, Marshall JD, Scandellari C, Sicolo N: The Alström syndrome: is it a rare or unknown disease? Ann Ital Med Int 2002;17:221–228.

56 Dyer DS, Wilson ME, Small KW, Pai GS: Alström syndrome: a case misdiagnosed as Bardet-Biedl syndrome. J Pediatr Ophthalmol Strabismus 1994;31: 272–274.

57 Wang X, Wang H, Cao M, Li Z, Chen X, Patenia C, Gore A, Abboud EB, Al-Rajhi AA, Lewis RA, Lupski JR, Mardon G, Zhang K, Muzny D, Gibbs RA, Chen R: Whole-exome sequencing identifies ALMS1, IQCB1, CNGA3, and MYO7A mutations in patients with Leber congenital amaurosis. Hum Mutat 2011; 32:1450–1459.

58 Xu Y, Guan L, Xiao X, Zhang J, Li S, Jiang H, Jia X, Yin Y, Guo X, Wang J, Zhang Q: ALMS1 null mutations: a common cause of Leber congenital amaurosis and early-onset severe cone-rod dystrophy. Clin Genet 2015, DOI: 10.1111/cge.12617.

59 Casey J, McGettigan P, Brosnahan D, Curtis E, Treacy E, Ennis S, Lynch SA: Atypical Alstrom syndrome with novel ALMS1 mutations precluded by current diagnostic criteria. Eur J Med Genet 2014;57: 55–59.

60 Koc E, Bayrak G, Suher M, Ensari C, Aktas D, Ensari A: Rare case of Alstrom syndrome without obesity and with short stature, diagnosed in adulthood. Nephrology (Carlton) 2006;11:81–84.

61 Paisey RB, Geberhiwot T, Waterson M, Cramb R, Steeds R, Williams K, White A, Hardy C: Modification of severe insulin resistant diabetes in response to lifestyle changes in Alström syndrome. Eur J Med Genet 2014;57:71–75.

62 Lee NC, Marshall JD, Collin GB, Naggert JK, Chien YH, Tsai WY, Hwu WL: Caloric restriction in Alström syndrome prevents hyperinsulinemia. Am J Med Genet A 2009;149A:666–668.

63 Paisey RB: New insights and therapies for the metabolic consequences of Alström syndrome. Curr Opin Lipidol 2009;20:315–320.

64 Sinha SK, Bhangoo A, Anhalt H, Maclaren N, Marshall JD, Collin GB, Naggert JK, Ten S: Effect of metformin and rosiglitazone in a prepubertal boy with Alström syndrome. J Pediatr Endocrinol Metab 2007;20:1045–1052.

65 Goerler H, Warnecke G, Winterhalter M, Muller C, Ballmann M, Wessel A, Haverich A, Struber M, Simon A: Heart-lung transplantation in a 14-year-old boy with Alström syndrome. J Heart Lung Transplant 2007;26:1217–1218.

Pietro Maffei, MD, PhD
Dipartimento di Medicina (DIMED), Padua University
Via Giustiniani 2, IT–35128 Padua (Italy)
E-Mail pietromaffei@libero.it, pietro.maffei@aopd.veneto.it

Barbetti F, Ghizzoni L, Guaraldi F (eds): Diabetes Associated with Single Gene Defects and Chromosomal Abnormalities. Front Diabetes. Basel, Karger, 2017, vol 25, pp 145–150 (DOI: 10.1159/000454741)

Prader-Willi Syndrome

Graziano Grugni

Division of Auxology, S. Giuseppe Hospital Research Institute, Italian Auxological Institute, Verbania, Italy

Abstract

Prader-Willi syndrome (PWS) is due to genetic alterations on chromosome 15q11-q13, and represents the most common genetic cause of obesity. Weight excess associated with PWS is often massive, and its complications are the major causes of morbidity and mortality, including diabetes mellitus. Type 2 diabetes mellitus (T2DM) accounts for the vast majority of cases of PWS patients with diabetes. The relationship between the obese condition and the development of diabetes, however, is not clear and may be different than that seen in individuals with simple obesity. The bulk of evidence has demonstrated that PWS subjects exhibit a state of relative hypoinsulinemia, with higher insulin sensitivity, despite severe obesity. Data about differences in insulin secretion in PWS, however, are still conflicting. Other reports have shown that PWS subjects and BMI-matched controls have similar insulin levels and are similarly insulin resistant. T2DM may be present with the classic symptoms, but most PWS subjects are asymptomatic and diabetes-related complications are infrequent. In spite of this, periodic surveillance for T2DM should be undertaken, and evaluation of diabetes risk is recommended prior and during growth hormone (GH) therapy. Apart from diet and increased exercise, management of T2DM needs similar pharmacological agents as with nonsyndromic obesity-related diabetes.

Prader-Willi syndrome (PWS) is a rare chromosomal disorder caused by the absent expression of paternally inherited genes in the PWS critical region on chromosome 15 [1]. In approximately 55–60% of affected individuals there is a microdeletion of the long arm of paternal chromosome 15 (15q11-q13), whereas up to the 45% of subjects have a maternal uniparental disomy for the same chromosome (UPD15) [2]. Abnormalities of the imprinting center controlling the activity of imprinted genes or translocations involving chromosome 15 have been found in few cases. PWS represents the single most common known genetic cause of obesity, with a population prevalence of no less than 1:52,000 [3]. A complex hypothalamic-pituitary dysregulation is currently thought to be partly responsible for the PWS phenotype. The syndrome affects multiple organ systems and its most consistent characteristics include muscular hypotonia, characteristic appearance, neuropsychomotor developmental delay, behavioral and psychiatric disturbances, hypogonadism, restricted longitudinal growth, growth hormone (GH) insufficiency, and hyperphagia [4]. Combined with a low metabolic rate and decreased activity level, hyperphagia leads most patients to develop morbid obesity. In this respect, patients with PWS go through 5 major nutritional phases, and excessive weight gain typically begins between 2 and 4 years of age [5]. In absence of appropriate intervention, the frequency of obesity and overweight progressively increase with age. Obesity associated with PWS is often massive, and its complications are the major causes of morbidity and mortality, including cardiovascular disease, respiratory insufficiency, and diabetes mellitus. Type 2 diabetes mellitus (T2DM) accounts for the vast majority of cases of PWS patients with diabetes, while both type 1 diabetes mellitus [6, 7] and monogenic diabetes [8] occur very rarely.

T2DM has been found in 7–24% of adults with PWS [9], and affects 50% of patients after the 5th decade, with a mean age at the time of diagnosis ranging from 20 to 41.6 years [10]. Altered glucose tolerance seems to be less frequent in the pediatric age range. T2DM was detected in 1/50 (2%) PWS patients under 18 years of age [11], while the prevalence of impaired glucose tolerance is reported to be 4.3–17%. A study performed in children with PWS has observed only 3 patients with impaired glucose tolerance by an oral glucose tolerance test and none of the 118 patients with filled data with T2DM [12]. On the other hand, an earlier onset of T2DM was observed in Japanese PWS patients, but this occurrence may be due to the higher rate of T2DM in Asian children than in Caucasians [13]. Nevertheless, early onset of T2DM in PWS may be related to the duration of weight problems, as has been suggested in non-PWS populations. In this light, nonobese PWS children have shown a lower frequency of glucose homeostasis alterations in comparison to obese PWS subjects [14].

The relationship between the obese condition and the development of diabetes, however, is not clear and may be different than that seen in individuals with simple obesity. A large number of studies have demonstrated that PWS subjects exhibit a state of relative hypoinsulinemia in spite of severe obesity. Low fasting insulin concentrations and greater insulin sensitivity, compared with BMI-matched controls, have been reported both in children and in adults with PWS [15, 16]. Despite a similar degree of body weight excess and glucose response, the insulin response to both a mixed meal and an oral glucose tolerance test was significantly lower in children with PWS in respect to obese controls [17]. In addition, a reduced first- and second-phase insulin and C-peptide secretion response to intravenous glucose was found in PWS adults when compared to obese subjects [18]. Proposed reasons for the reduced insulin resistance in people with PWS include a selective reduction of visceral fat in PWS after adjustment for total adiposity [19], the presence of GH/IGF-I axis dysfunction, and higher ghrelin levels for the degree of obesity [20]. Another possible reason for β-cell dysfunction in PWS is a decreased vagal parasympathetic efferent tone to the pancreas, as demonstrated by the blunted pancreatic polypeptide secretion in PWS children [21]. Furthermore, increased concentrations of adiponectin, a protein secreted by adipocytes that exerts a dominant role in modulation of insulin sensitivity, might contribute to the heightened insulin sensitivity of PWS subjects [15].

Data about differences in insulin secretion and body composition in PWS, however, are still conflicting. Other reports have shown that PWS subjects and BMI-matched controls have similar insulin levels and are similarly insulin resistant, both in children [14] and in adults [22]. Moreover, a similar amount of abdominal subcutaneous and visceral fat has been detected in PWS in comparison to obese controls [23, 24]. In addition, it has been found that a clear relationship between obesity status and insulin levels was still detectable in PWS children, as obese subjects showed higher insulin levels and HOMA-index than nonobese patients [14]. These discrepancies might be due to the different clinical characteristics of the study groups, including age, degree of weight excess, variable percentage of fat body mass, and number of patients undergoing GH therapy. Furthermore, a familial component in insulin resistance, as in the general population, may also be present in PWS patients.

The clinical impact of T2DM is quite variable, and most PWS subjects are asymptomatic. In some cases, however, T2DM may be present with the classic symptoms, including polyuria, polydipsia, and, rarely, unexpected weight loss despite hyperphagia. Consequently, periodic surveillance for signs and symptoms of T2DM should be undertaken, mainly in obese individuals, as recommended for obesity in the general population. Similarly, evaluation of diabetes risk is recommended prior to initiation of GH therapy, with periodic surveillance for those on GH treatment [25]. In fact, doubts on whether GH administration can impair glucose homeostasis in subjects prone to develop diabetes have risen in recent years. In this context, it has been reported that GH therapy could contribute to increase insulin resistance and to develop hyperinsulinemia in PWS children, especially in obese subjects [26], as well as in adults [27]. On the other hand, several studies have recently demonstrated that long-term GH treatment does not adversely affect glucose homeostasis in all age groups [8, 28].

Physical activity and nutritional management remains the mainstay of treatment of altered glucose metabolism (AGM) in obese PWS. A caloric restriction of 6–8 calories/cm of height is requested to allow for weight loss, while a target of 10–12 calories/cm of height usually maintains weight in children with PWS [29]. Adult patients generally need no more than 1,000–1,200 kcal/day. Apart from caloric restriction and increased exercise, management of T2DM in PWS requires similar pharmacological agents as with nonsyndromic obesity-related diabetes, e.g., initially insulin-sensitizing agents, such as metformin or thiazolidinediones, with the introduction of insulin as required [30]. In addition, the use of glucagon-like peptide 1 receptor agonists seems to induce an improvement/stabilization of AGM [31].

With appropriate therapy, few diabetic complications are reported in PWS subjects, but this may simply be due to the reduced life expectancy of these individuals since diabetic retinopathy and nephropathy are generally observed after early adulthood. In this regard, the average age of patients with PWS has increased substantially in recent years. Thus, it is presumable that the increased risk of T2DM and associated comorbidities will become more important with the aging of PWS population, particularly because the frequency of obesity is significantly higher in older patients [32]. Consequently, additional surveillance protocols concerning this issue are needed in the future. Moreover, further research in large population cohorts is warranted in order to better understand the role of adipose tissue distribution and other possible confounders, such as ethnicity, concomitant therapy, diet, and physical activity, which may affect insulin sensitivity and the prevalence of T2DM in PWS. In this respect, a national collaborative study from the Italian Network for PWS has recently demonstrated a positive correlation of AGM with age and BMI, whereas gender, genotypes, and GH therapy did not seem to influence AGM development [33].

In conclusion, PWS subjects show a high prevalence of AGM that appears more common in obese and in adult subjects. The negative influence of weight excess on the individual metabolic risk clustering in the PWS population supports the view that an early intervention to prevent obesity remains the most important goal of any PWS treatment program. The challenge is to demonstrate that appropriate weight management throughout one's life will lead to an improvement of glucose homeostasis in PWS individuals and more generally to an amelioration of morbidity and mortality in these subjects.

References

1 Butler MG: Prader-Willi syndrome: obesity due to genomic imprinting. Curr Genomics 2011;12:204–215.

2 Lionti T, Reid SM, White SM, Rowell MM: A population-based profile of 160 Australians with Prader-Willi syndrome: trends in diagnosis, birth prevalence and birth characteristics. Am J Med Genet Part A 2015;67:371–378.

3 Whittington JE, Holland AJ, Webb T, Butler JV, Clarke DJ, Boer H: Population prevalence and estimated birth incidence and mortality rate for people with Prader-Willi syndrome in one UK health region. J Med Genet 2001;38:792–798.

4 Cassidy SB, Schwartz S, Miller JL, Driscoll DJ: Prader-Willi syndrome. Genet Med 2012;14:10–26.

5 Miller JL, Lynn CH, Driscoll DC, Goldstone AP, Gold JA, Kimonis V, Dykens E, Butler MG, Shuster JJ, Driscoll DJ: Nutritional phases in Prader-Willi syndrome. Am J Med Genet A 2011;155A:1040–1049.

6 Anhalt H, Eckert KH, Hintz RL, Neely EK: Type I diabetes mellitus, ketoacidosis and thromboembolism in an adolescent with Prader-Willi syndrome. Acta Paediatr 1996;85:516.

7 Bakker NE, Kuppens RJ, Siemensma EP, Tummers-de Lind van Wijngaarden RF, Festen DA, Bindels-de Heus GC, Bocca G, Haring DA, Hoorweg-Nijman JJ, Houdijk EC, Jira PE, Lunshof L, Odink RJ, Oostdijk W, Rotteveel J, Schroor EJ, Van Alfen AA, Van Leeuwen M, Van Pinxteren-Nagler E, Van Wieringen H, Vreuls RC, Zwaveling-Soonawala N, de Ridder MA, Hokken-Koelega AC: Eight years of growth hormone treatment in children with Prader-Willi syndrome: maintaining the positive effects. J Clin Endocrinol Metab 2013;98:4013–4022.

8 Mariani B, Cammarata B, Grechi E, Di Candia S, Chiumello G: Maturity onset diabetes of the young in a child with Prader-Willi syndrome. Horm Res 2012;78(suppl 1):162.

9 Sinnema M, Maaskant MA, van Schrojenstein Lantman-de Valk HMJ, Caroline van Nieuwpoort I, Drent ML, Curfs LMG, Schrander-Stumpel CTRM: Physical health problems in adults with Prader-Willi syndrome. Am J Med Genet Part A 2011;155:2112–2124.

10 Sinnema M, Schrander-Stumpel CT, Maaskant MA, Boer H, Curfs LM: Aging in Prader-Willi syndrome: twelve persons over the age of 50 years. Am J Med Genet A 2012;158A:1326–1336.

11 Butler JV, Whittington JE, Holland AJ, Boer H, Clarke D, Webb T: Prevalence of, and risk factors for, physical ill-health in people with Prader-Willi syndrome: a population-based study. Dev Med Child Neurol 2002;44:248–255.

12 Diene G, Mimoun E, Feigerlova E, Caula S, Molinas C, Grandjean H, Tauber M: Endocrine disorders in children with Prader-Willi syndrome – data from 142 children of the French database. Horm Res Paediatr 2010;74:121–128.

13 Tsuchiya T, Oto Y, Ayabe T, Obata K, Murakami N, Nagai T: Characterization of diabetes mellitus in Japanese Prader-Willi syndrome. Clin Pediatr Endocrinol 2011;20:33–38.

14 Brambilla P, Crinò A, Bedogni G, Bosio L, Cappa M, Corrias A, Delvecchio M, Di Candia S, Gargantini L, Grechi E, Iughetti L, Mussa A, Ragusa L, Sacco M, Salvatoni A, Chiumello G, Grugni G; Genetic Obesity Study Group of the Italian Society of Pediatric Endocrinology and Diabetology (ISPED): Metabolic syndrome in children with Prader-Willi syndrome: the effect of obesity. Nutr Metab Cardiovasc Dis 2011;21:269–276.

15 Haqq AM, Muehlbauer M, Newgard CB, Grambow SC, Freemark MS: The metabolic phenotype of Prader-Willi syndrome (PWS) in childhood: heightened insulin sensitivity relative to body mass index. J Clin Endocrinol Metab 2011;96:E225–E232.

16 Hoybye C, Hilding A, Jacobsson H, Thoren M: Metabolic profile and body composition in adults with Prader-Willi syndrome. J Clin Endocrinol Metab 2002;87:3590–3597.

17 Zipf WB, Schuster D, Osei K: Glucose homeostasis in Prader-Willi syndrome; in Eiholzer U, l'Allemand D, Zipf WB (eds): Prader-Willi Syndrome as a Model for Obesity. Basel, Karger, 2003, pp 102–118.

18 Schuster D, Osei K, Zipf WB: Characterization of alterations in glucose and insulin metabolism in Prader-Willi subjects. Metabolism 1996;45:1514–1520.

19 Goldstone AP, Thomas EL, Brynes AE, Bell JD, Frost G, Saeed N, Hajnal JV, Howard JK, Holland A, Bloom SR: Visceral adipose tissue and metabolic complications of obesity are reduced in Prader-Willi syndrome female adults: evidence for novel influences on body fat distribution. J Clin Endocrinol Metab 2001;86:4330–4338.

20 Emerick JE, Vogt KS: Endocrine manifestations and management of Prader-Willi syndrome. Int J Pediatr Endocrinol 2013;21:14.

21 Zipf WB, Odorisio TM, Cataland S, Dixon K: Pancreatic polypeptide responses to protein meal challenges in obese but otherwise normal children and obese children with Prader-Willi syndrome. J Clin Endocrinol Metab 1983;57:1074–1080.

22 Purtell S, Sze L, Loughnan G, Smith E, Herzog H, Sainsbury A, Steinbeck K, Campbell LV, Viardot A: In adults with Prader-Willi syndrome, elevated ghrelin levels are more consistent with hyperphagia than high PYY and GLP-1 levels. Neuropeptides 2011;45:301–307.

23 Talebizadeh Z, Butler MG: Insulin resistance and obesity-related factors in Prader-Willi syndrome: comparison with obese subjects. Clin Genet 2005;67:230–239.

24 Marzullo P, Marcassa C, Minocci A, Campini R, Eleuteri E, Gondoni LA, Aimaretti G, Sartorio A, Scacchi M, Grugni G: Long-term echocardiographic and cardioscintigraphic effects of growth hormone treatment in adults with Prader-Willi syndrome. J Clin Endocrinol Metab 2015;100:2106–2114.

25 Deal CL, Tony M, Höybye C, Allen DB, Tauber M, Christiansen JS; 2011 Growth Hormone in Prader-Willi Syndrome Clinical Care Guidelines Workshop Participants: Growth Hormone Research Society workshop summary: consensus guidelines for recombinant human growth hormone therapy in Prader-Willi syndrome. J Clin Endocrinol Metab 2013;98:E1072–E1087.

26 Crinò A, Di Giorgio G, Manco M, Grugni G, Maggioni A: Effects of growth hormone therapy on glucose metabolism and insulin sensitivity indices in prepubertal children with Prader-Willi syndrome. Horm Res 2007;68:83–90.

27 Sanchez-Ortiga R, Klibanski A, Tritos NA: Effects of recombinant human growth hormone therapy in adults with Prader-Willi syndrome: a meta-analysis. Clin Endocrinol 2012;77:86–93.

28 Höybye C: Growth hormone treatment of Prader-Willi syndrome has long-term, positive effects on body composition. Acta Paediatr 2015;104:422–427.

29 Butler MG, Hanchett JM, Thompson T: Clinical findings and natural history of Prader-Willi syndrome; in Butler MG, Lee PDK, Whitman BY (eds): Management of Prader-Willi Syndrome. New York, Springer, 2006, pp 3–48.

30 Goldstone AP, Holland AJ, Hauffa BP, Hokken-Koelega AC, Tauber M; speakers contributors at the Second Expert Meeting of the Comprehensive Care of Patients with PWS: Recommendations for the diagnosis and management of Prader-Willi syndrome. J Clin Endocrinol Metab 2008;93:4183–4197.

31 Fintini D, Grugni G, Brufani C, Bocchini S, Cappa M, Crinò A: Use of GLP-1 receptor agonists in Prader-Willi Syndrome: report of six cases. Diabetes Care 2014;37:e76–e77.

32 Grugni G, Crinò A, Bosio L, Corrias A, Cuttini M, De Toni T, Di Battista E, Franzese A, Gargantini L, Greggio N, Iughetti L, Livieri C, Naselli A, Pagano C, Pozzan G, Ragusa L, Salvatoni A, Trifirò G, Beccaria L, Bellizzi M, Bellone J, Brunani A, Cappa M, Caselli G, Cerioni V, Delvecchio M, Giardino D, Iannì F, Memo L, Pilotta A, Pomara C, Radetti G, Sacco M, Sanzari A, Sartorio A, Tonini G, Vettor R, Zaglia F, Chiumello G: The Italian National Survey for Prader-Willi syndrome: an epidemiologic study. Am J Med Genet A 2008;146A:861–872.

33 Fintini D, Grugni G, Bocchini S, Brufani C, Di Candia S, Corrias A, Delvecchio M, Salvatoni A, Ragusa L, Greggio N, Franzese A, Scarano E, Trifirò G, Mazzanti L, Chiumello G, Cappa M, Crinò A; Genetic Obesity Study Group of the Italian Society of Pediatric Endocrinology and Diabetology (ISPED): Disorders of glucose metabolism in Prader-Willi syndrome: results of a multicenter Italian cohort study. Nutr Metab Cardiovasc Dis 2016;26:842–847.

Graziano Grugni, MD
Division of Auxology
S. Giuseppe Hospital Research Institute
Italian Auxological Institute
Corso Mameli 199
IT–28921 Verbania (Italy)
E-Mail g.grugni@auxologico.it

Barbetti F, Ghizzoni L, Guaraldi F (eds): Diabetes Associated with Single Gene Defects and Chromosomal Abnormalities. Front Diabetes. Basel, Karger, 2017, vol 25, pp 151–159 (DOI: 10.1159/000454742)

47,XXY Klinefelter Syndrome Is Associated with an Increased Risk of Insulin Resistance: The Impact of Hypogonadism and Visceral Obesity

Francesca Panimolle · Antonio F. Radicioni

Center of Rare Diseases, Section of Medical Pathophysiology, Department of Experimental Medicine, Sapienza University of Rome, Rome, Italy

Abstract

Klinefelter syndrome (KS) is the most common male sex chromosome disorder, affecting 1/660 men. It is caused by the presence of extra X chromosomes. The KS phenotype is traditionally described as a tall, slim, narrow-shouldered, broad-hipped man with hypergonadotropic hypogonadism and small testes. An association between KS and type 2 diabetes has long been recognized, but the pathogenesis is still unknown. If both hypogonadism and visceral obesity play a role in the development of insulin resistance in men, KS offers an interesting window into this relationship. Indeed, in addition to hypergonadotropic hypogonadism, with variable degrees of androgen deficiency, most 47,XXY KS patients present an unfavorable change in body composition, with increased truncal fat. In KS, both hypotestosteronemia and visceral obesity not only play an important and independent role in determining impaired insulin sensitivity, but may also be reciprocally influenced in a self-perpetuating vicious circle. Other possible mechanisms that may lead to insulin resistance in KS involve the extra copies of X chromosomes. This chapter discusses the main evidence linking KS and impaired insulin sensitivity, leading to insulin resistance and type 2 diabetes.

© 2017 S. Karger AG, Basel

Klinefelter Syndrome and Insulin Resistance

Klinefelter syndrome (KS) was first described in 1942 as a male endocrine disorder characterized by small firm testes, gynecomastia, hypogonadism, and a higher than normal concentration of follicle-stimulating hormone [1]. The genetic background for the KS phenotype is based on the presence of 1 or more extra X chromosomes compared to the normal 46,XY male karyotype. About 80% of cases are due to the congenital numerical chromosome aberration 47,XXY; the remaining 20% have higher-grade chromosome aneuploidies (48,XXXY; 48,XXYY; 49,XXXXY), 46,XY/47,XXY mosaicism, or

Small testes (<4–6 mL)
Cryptorchidism
Gynecomastia
Infertility
Azoospermia
Decreased facial and pubic hair
Varicose veins
Decreased libido and potency
Decreased muscle strength

structurally abnormal X chromosomes [2]. The prototypical adult KS patient phenotype is traditionally described as tall, with narrow shoulders, broad hips, sparse body hair, gynecomastia, small testicles, learning disabilities, and psychiatric disorders (Table 1).

Looking at the function of the hypothalamic-pituitary-testicular axis, adult KS patients show hypergonadotropic hypogonadism characterized by high serum concentrations of luteinizing hormone and follicle-stimulating hormone, estradiol, and sex-hormone-binding globulin; undetectable serum levels of inhibin B; low serum concentrations of insulin-like factor 3; and normal or low serum testosterone concentrations (androgen deficiency) [2]. With an estimated prevalence of about 1 in 660 men, KS is the most common sex chromosome abnormality [1]. Diagnosis is based on the presence of suggestive clinical findings and is confirmed by cytogenetic determination of supernumerary X chromosomes. This syndrome is often underdiagnosed during the postnatal period because pituitary-gonadal function is relatively normal during puberty, childhood, and adolescence, and is characterized by physiological low androgen levels and the absence of specific clinical features [3]. Even in adults, diagnosis may be severely delayed or missed because of a highly variable phenotype associated with hypergonadotropism with a varying degree of androgen deficiency [4, 5]. In Denmark, for example, only 25% of the expected numbers are diagnosed, and barely 10% of these are diagnosed before puberty [5].

Epidemiological studies have shown increased morbidity and mortality in KS due to a variety of diseases and conditions, with an estimated life expectancy reduction of 11.5 years compared to the healthy male population [5]. The main disorders associated with KS are varicose veins, diabetes, thrombosis, embolism, bone fractures, epilepsy, and neurological and mental disorders [6, 7]. All the clinical findings and long-term consequences of the syndrome may be caused directly by supernumerary X chromosomes, or by the hormonal imbalances secondary to hypogonadism.

Hypogonadism and Insulin Sensitivity
Sex steroid hormones are secreted mainly by the ovaries and testis and regulate diverse physiological processes in target tissues. There is extensive experimental evidence that sex steroids and insulin interact in their actions on tissues [8]. At

physiological levels, androgens and estrogens are thought to be involved in maintaining normal insulin sensitivity. However, outside this physiological window these steroids may promote insulin resistance. The molecular basis of such resistance has been reported to involve various phases of the insulin pathway, reducing insulin receptor autophosphorylation, reducing expression or translocation of insulin-responsive glucose transporters, and increasing insulin signaling defects [8].

An important role in determining insulin sensitivity has been described for testosterone. Among its various actions, testosterone has a major action on biochemical pathways of metabolism of lipids and cholesterol and inflammation in men. The cumulative effects of testosterone could account for its overall benefits on insulin sensitivity observed in clinical trials [9]. In the literature, Rancho Bernardo and the Massachusetts Male Aging Study stated that low levels of testosterone predict insulin resistance. Furthermore, the NHANES III study found a higher incidence of type 2 diabetes mellitus (T2DM) even in men who had low testosterone levels but were not obese at the beginning of the study. Similarly, the Health in Men Study showed that low levels of total testosterone are associated with insulin resistance, independently of measures of central obesity in elderly men (>70 years) [10].

The mechanisms linking testosterone with insulin sensitivity/resistance are still not fully understood. There is, however, increasing biochemical evidence from animal, cell, and clinical studies that testosterone may influence the molecular expression of important regulatory proteins involved in glucose uptake, glycolysis, and mitochondrial oxidative phosphorylation, suggesting a complex regulatory role of testosterone on metabolism [9]. Testosterone affects the main target tissues responding to insulin, including skeletal muscle, adipose tissue, and liver. In detail, testosterone has an anabolic effect on skeletal muscle, with a deficiency associated with a decrease in lean body mass, while relative muscle mass is inversely associated with insulin resistance and prediabetes [10]. Another potential mechanism for the beneficial effect of testosterone may be the increase of the metabolic rate in skeletal muscle, promoting the acquisition of energy from adipose tissue and thus reducing fat mass with increasing insulin sensitivity. Furthermore, fat is oxidized in the liver and in extrahepatic tissue such as skeletal muscle, and this component of lipid metabolism may be influenced by testosterone. In this light, male hypogonadism, which is the clinical syndrome caused by a lack of androgens or their action, impairs glucose tolerance and, as reported in the literature, reduces insulin sensitivity. Several prospective and cross-sectional studies have in fact shown that T2DM is common in hypogonadal patients [7]; vice versa, a higher prevalence of hypogonadism (up to 50%) has been found in men with T2DM than in age-matched controls [11, 12].

Visceral Adiposity and Insulin Sensitivity
Adipose tissue influences glucose homoeostasis and insulin sensitivity through the regulation of lipid and glucose metabolism [9]. There is strong evidence in the literature showing adipose tissue dysfunction plays a crucial role in the development of

insulin resistance, and thus T2DM. To better underline this link, the term "diabesity" has recently been adopted, and several studies have shown that 60–90% of patients with T2DM are or have been obese [13]. However, rather than obesity per se, it is fat distribution, and above all visceral obesity, that is strongly linked with the development of impaired glucose tolerance and subsequent insulin resistance. Several mechanisms mediating the interaction between insulin resistance and visceral fatness have been identified. Adipose tissue can modulate whole-body glucose metabolism by regulating levels of circulating nonesterified fatty acids and also by acting as secretory tissue, producing adipokines that can modulate insulin signaling [14].

The increased mass of adipocytes, especially in visceral or deep subcutaneous depots, is in fact resistant to the ability of insulin to suppress lipolysis. This results in increased release and circulating levels of nonesterified fatty acids that, via portal circulation into the liver, can induce/aggravate peripheral insulin resistance in muscle, liver, and pancreatic β-cells [14].

As previously mentioned, adipose tissue is not only specialized in the storage and mobilization of lipids, but it is also a remarkable endocrine organ. Adipose tissue releases numerous proinflammatory adipocytokines such as IL-1 and IL-6, TNF-α, and adipokines, such as leptin and resistin, which are consequently found at higher levels in obese subjects [14]. Adiponectin levels are reduced in obese individuals, particularly among patients with excess visceral adiposity. This is because visceral adiposity enhances inhibition of hepatic glucose output as well as of glucose uptake and use in fat and muscle. Insulin resistance is induced both directly and indirectly by the overproduction of proinflammatory cytokines and of adipokines with insulin-antagonist effects and the reduction of adiponectin levels resulting from excess adipose tissue.

Hypogonadism, Change in Body Composition, and Insulin Resistance in KS
Given that hypogonadism and visceral obesity both have a role in the development of insulin resistance in men, KS offers an interesting window into this relationship. As reported above, 47,XXY KS patients are characterized by hypergonadotropic hypogonadism, with various degrees of androgen deficiency. Bojesen and colleagues [1] measured the body composition of 70 KS patients and 70 age-matched controls, finding dramatic changes in body composition. Although there was no significant difference in BMI, KS men presented significantly increased levels of truncal fat and decreased lean body mass (Fig. 1). This clinical evidence is so important that some authors suggested the diagnosis of KS may be confounded by obesity.

Furthermore, low testosterone levels and visceral obesity not only play an important and role in determining impaired insulin sensitivity, but they are also reciprocally influenced in a self-perpetuating vicious circle (Fig. 2). Specifically, as testosterone has an anabolic effect on skeletal muscle and reduces fat mass [9], hypogonadal men exhibit reduced lean body mass and increased abdominal or central obesity. Therefore, increased visceral obesity is a well-known clinical feature of hypogonadism [12]. Vice versa, testicular function declines with obesity [15]. The pathogenesis of reduced androgen levels

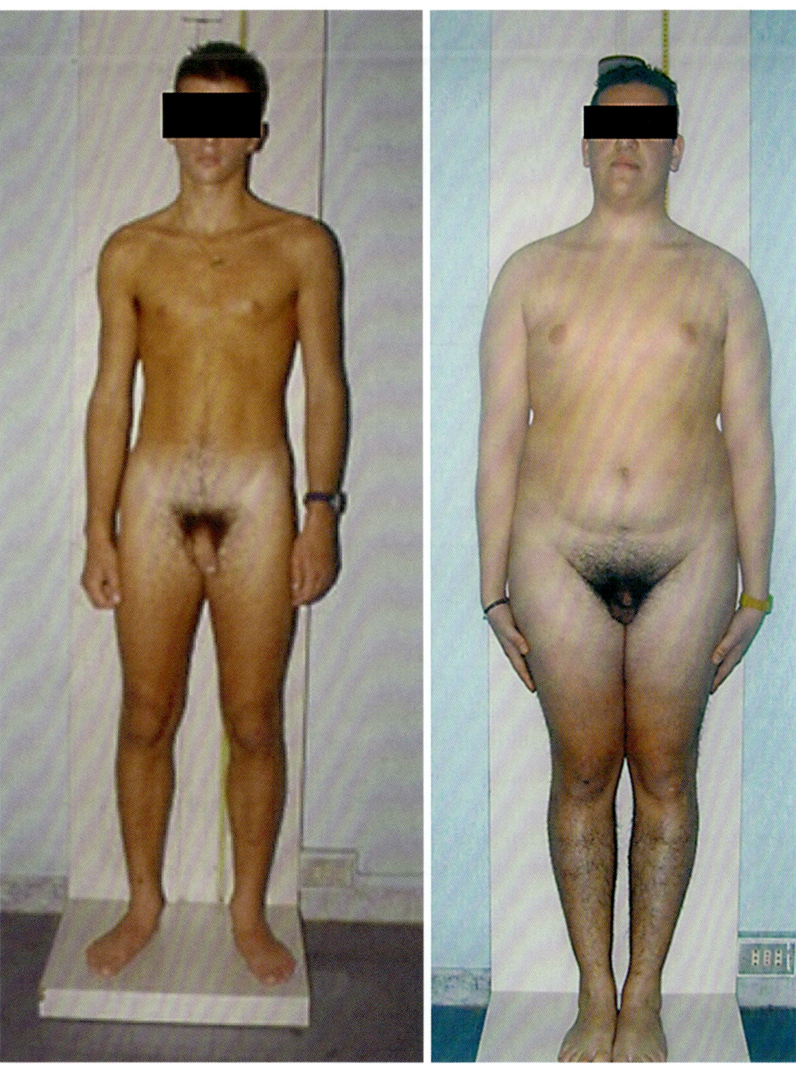

Fig. 1. 47,XXY adult KS patients with different visceral adiposity distribution.

in obese men is multifactorial, involving both central and peripheral mechanisms, such as increased levels in estrogens, which feed back at the hypothalamic axis to suppress gonadotropin secretion, and a direct inhibitory effect of leptin on the testes [13].

The temporal sequence of events is still unknown and both scenarios may be present. The 'hypogonadal-obesity cycle hypothesis' suggested by Cohen and colleagues in 1999 considers low testosterone levels as a promoter of increased visceral adiposity and obesity as an enhancer of hypogonadism [9]. In detail, testosterone production is regulated by the hypothalamic-pituitary-testicular axis. Pulsatile release of gonadotropin-releasing hormone from the hypothalamus stimulates the release of luteinizing hormone and follicle-stimulating hormone from the pituitary gland, which then

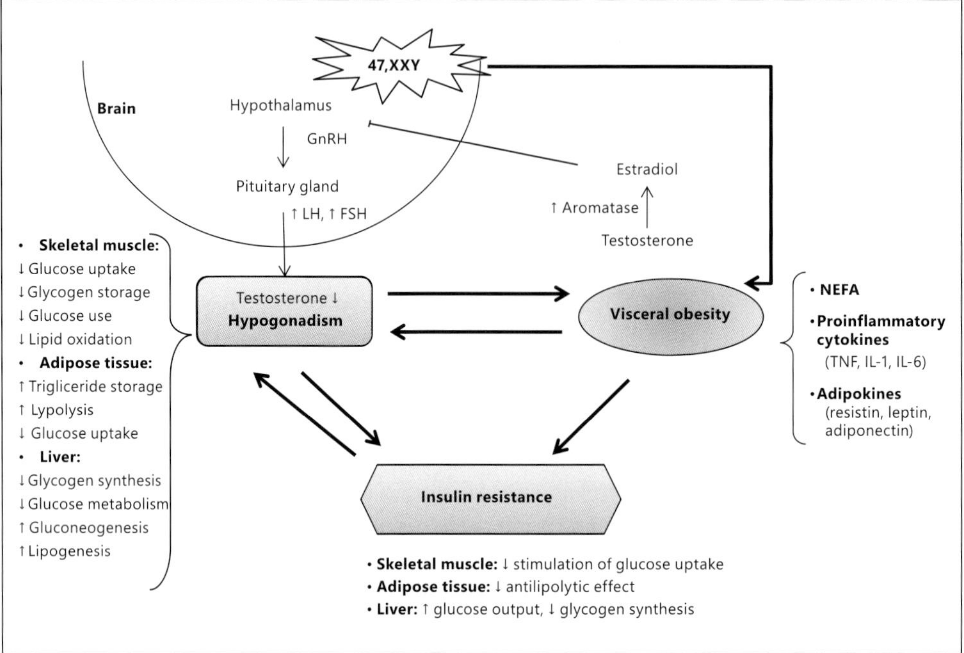

Fig. 2. The proposed vicious circle of hypogonadism, visceral adipose tissue, and insulin resistance in Klinefelter syndrome: insulin action normally reduces glucose output and stimulation of glycogen synthesis by the liver, enhances glucose uptake by skeletal muscle, and suppresses fatty acid release from adipose tissue. In Klinefelter syndrome, the major risk factors for impairment of insulin sensitivity, namely obesity-induced androgen deficiency and hypogonadism-induced obesity, coexist and both contribute to a bidirectional effect on insulin resistance. Furthermore, an X chromosome dosage effect seems to induce abdominal adiposity, thus determining insulin resistance and leading to the development of type 2 diabetes. FSH, follicle-stimulating hormone; LH, luteinizing hormone; NEFA, nonesterified fatty acids.

stimulate the testes to synthesize and secrete testosterone. The axis is regulated by the direct negative feedback of testosterone on the hypothalamus. In adipose tissue, testosterone is metabolized to estradiol by aromatase, which has an increased activity in visceral fat. Estradiol directly feeds back and inhibits the hypothalamic-pituitary-testicular axis. Furthermore, adipocytokines, including the proinflammatory cytokines TNF, IL-6, and IL-1β, secreted by visceral adipose tissue, inhibit both hypothalamic-pituitary and testicular secretion of testosterone.

Leptin usually stimulates the release of gonadotropin-releasing hormone. However, in obesity, where excess leptin is produced by adipocytes, the hypothalamic-pituitary axis becomes resistant to leptin. In addition, leptin inhibits the stimulatory action of gonadotropin on the testes, thereby further reducing testosterone production [13]. In this light, the pathophysiological interaction between chronic hypogonadism, truncal fat, and proinflammatory cytokines helps explain why the body cannot respond to low testosterone levels by normal compensatory homoeostatic production of androgens to stimulate the testis to secrete testosterone. This vicious circle extends Cohen's theory to the "hypogonadal-obesity-adipocytokine hypothesis" [9].

In KS, the causality of the relationship between low testosterone levels, visceral obesity, and insulin resistance is even more intriguing, with obesity-induced androgen deficiency and hypogonadism-induced obesity both probably contributing to a bidirectional effect on impairment of insulin sensitivity [9]. As reported by Yesilova et al., [16] testosterone is an independent determinant of whole-body glucose levels, irrespective of BMI. It is still unknown whether the change in body composition with increased body fat in KS is a consequence of the specific genotype, the hormonal milieu, or their combination. In these patients, it is reasonable to assume that gonadal dysfunction precedes visceral obesity and that both characteristics then enhance insulin resistance. However, in 2008 Aksglaede et al. [17] analyzed 24 boys with KS, finding an increase in body fat mass before puberty, when pituitary-gonadal function is relatively normal and androgen levels are physiologically low [13, 18]. This suggests a possible genetic influence of body fat in KS hypogonadism.

Other possible mechanisms for the increased risk of diabetes in KS may involve the extra copies of X chromosomes. In 2012, Jiang-Feng et al. [19] described a close relationship between karyotypes and diabetes. They evaluated the prevalence and risk factors of diabetes in 39 KS patients and 40 idiopathic hypogonadotropic hypogonadal patients. The prevalence of diabetes was higher in KS than in idiopathic hypogonadotropic hypogonadal patients, possibly due to the abnormal karyotype. They speculated that a gene-dosage effect, similar to that observed for seminiferous tubule hyaline degeneration in men with KS, might cause insulin secretion deficiency and/or increased insulin resistance, contributing to T2DM.

Klinefelter Syndrome and Diabetes Mellitus

An association between KS and diabetes was first reported in 1966 [20], followed by numerous studies. In 1998, Pei et al. [21] reported a higher percentage of insulin resistance in 7 patients with KS. Insulin resistance was evaluated by 2 methods: the incremental area under the curve of serum insulin concentrations in response to a 75-g oral glucose load, and the insulin suppression test. In 2005, Yesilova et al. [16] evaluated insulin sensitivity by the hyperinsulinemic-euglycemic clamp technique, the gold standard for this evaluation. They found decreased insulin sensitivity and elevated fasting insulin levels in 13 patients with KS. Similar findings were described by Bojesen et al. [18], who assessed insulin sensitivity and pancreatic β-cell function by homeostasis model assessment (HOMA) in 70 adult patients with KS and a healthy age-matched control group.

Recent epidemiological studies have demonstrated an increased risk of dying due to diabetes-related causes in KS subjects (standardized mortality rate 5.8 and HR 1.6) and of hospital admissions due to diagnosis of diabetes (HR 2.21 for T1DM and 3.71 for T2DM) [18]. It is worth noting that the classification and diagnosis of diabetes have been revised and improved over the years, and possible misclassification of the different types of diabetes in KS patients in past literature should be considered.

There is only sporadic information, coming essentially from a few case reports [22], on the prevalence of T1DM in KS patients, whereas an increasing number of studies have focused on the association between KS and T2DM. The mechanisms leading to an increased prevalence of T2DM in KS patients are still largely unknown. Recent findings have considered the role of *hypogonadism* and *change in body composition* in the molecular basis of insulin resistance in this condition [2, 11, 18].

Conclusions

The genomic imbalance caused by the overexpression of noninactivated genes on the supernumerary X chromosome(s) is the fundamental reason for KS phenotype, but many comorbidities (e.g., diabetes, obesity, anemia, osteoporosis, and osteoporotic fractures) may be directly or indirectly linked to hormonal imbalances caused by gonadal dysfunction, or by a combination of these factors. Furthermore, other clinical implications may be considered as an expression of poor general health, possibly combined with unfavorable lifestyle factors. It is important to underline that many KS-related diagnoses pertain to preventable diseases, such as T2DM. The development of insulin resistance involves multiple organs including the liver, muscle, and adipose tissue, which suggests a diversity of mechanisms, with possible implications for intervention strategies. In this light, clinical management of KS should consider careful monitoring of the preclinical and clinical phases of T2DM, improving the management of overnutrition, physical inactivity, and overweight/obesity, and evaluating the effects of testosterone replacement therapy (TRT). TRT could reduce the negative consequences of tissue-specific insulin insensitivity and improve metabolic function. The beneficial effects of testosterone on insulin resistance might be attributable to a complex regulatory influence on insulin signaling and glucose homeostasis in the major insulin-responsive target tissues, such as skeletal muscle, liver, and adipose tissue [12]. Early interventional studies suggest that TRT has beneficial effects on lipids, adiposity, and parameters of insulin sensitivity and glucose control. In a double-blind placebo-controlled crossover study analyzing 24 hypogonadal men with type 2 diabetes, TRT reduced the HOMA index, indicating improved fasting insulin sensitivity. Glycated hemoglobin was also reduced. TRT also produced a reduction in visceral adiposity, as assessed by waist circumference [23]. These effects may be both short- and long-term in the liver and adipose and muscle tissue, with a rapid improvement in insulin sensitivity. However, TRT should be preceded by a careful assessment of both the benefits and the risks of potential adverse effects. National guidelines and recommendations are still needed to improve the treatment of patients with KS.

This chapter is part of a research project (MRAR08Q009) on rare diseases funded by the Italian Ministry of Health and the Italian Medicines Agency (AIFA).

Disclosure Statement

No potential conflicts of interest relevant to this article were reported.

References

1 Groth KA, Skakkebæk A, Høst C, Gravholt CH, Bojesen A: Klinefelter syndrome – a clinical update. J Clin Endocrinol Metab 2013;98:20–30.
2 Lanfranco F, Kamischke A, Zitzmann M, Nieschlag E: Klinefelter's syndrome. Lancet 2004;364:273–283.
3 Radicioni AF, De Marco E, Gianfrilli D, Granato S, Gandini L, Isidori AM, Lenzi A: Strategies and advantages of early diagnosis in Klinefelter's syndrome. Mol Hum Reprod 2010;16:434–440.
4 Kamischke A, Baumgardt A, Horst J, Nieschlag E: Clinical and diagnostic features of patients with suspected Klinefelter syndrome. J Androl 2003;24:41–48.
5 Bojesen A, Stochholm K, Juul S, Gravholt CH: Socioeconomic trajectories affect mortality in Klinefelter syndrome. J Clin Endocrinol Metab 2011;96:2098–2104.
6 Swerdlow AJ, Higgins CD, Schoemaker MJ, Wright AF, Jacobs PA: Mortality in patients with Klinefelter syndrome in Britain: a cohort study. J Clin Endocrinol Metab 2005;90:6516–6522.
7 Bojesen A, Juul S, Birkebaek NH, Gravholt CH: Morbidity in Klinefelter syndrome: a Danish register study based on hospital discharge diagnoses. J Clin Endocrinol Metab 2006;91:1254–1260.
8 Livingstone C, Collison M: Sex steroids and insulin resistance. Clin Sci 2002;102:151–166.
9 Kelly DM, Jones TH: Testosterone: a metabolic hormone in health and disease 2013;217:25–45.
10 Wild S, Roglic G, Green A, Sicree R, King H: Global prevalence of diabetes: estimates for the year 2000 and projections for 2030. Diabetes Care 2004;27:1047–1053.
11 Høst C, Skakkebæk A, Groth KA, Bojesen A: The role of hypogonadism in Klinefelter syndrome. Asian J Androl 2014;16:185–191.
12 Rao PM, Kelly DM, Jones TH: Testosterone and insulin resistance in the metabolic syndrome and T2DM in men. Nat Rev Endocrinol 2013;9:479–493.
13 Golay A, Ybarra J: Link between obesity and type 2 diabetes. Best Pract Res Clin Endocrinol Metab 2005;19:649–663.
14 Schinner S, Scherbaum WA, Bornstein SR, Barthel A: Molecular mechanisms of insulin resistance. Diabet Med 2005;22:674–682.
15 Pasquali R: Obesity and androgens: facts and perspectives. Fertil Steril 2006;85:1319–1340.
16 Yesilova Z, Oktenli C, Sanisoglu SY, Musubak U, Cakir E, Ozata M, Dagalp K: Evaluation of insulin sensitivity in patients with Klinefelter's syndrome. Endocrine 2005;27:11–15.
17 Aksglaede L, Molgaard C, Skakkebaek NE, Juul A: Normal bone mineral content but unfavourable muscle/fat ratio in Klinefelter syndrome. Arch Dis Child 2008;93:30–34.
18 Bojesen A, Høst C, Gravholt CH: Klinefelter's syndrome, type 2 diabetes and the metabolic syndrome: the impact of body composition. Mol Hum Reprod 2010;16:396–401.
19 Jiang-Feng M, Hong-Li X, Xue-Yan W, Min N, Shuang-Yu L, Hong-Ding X, Liang-Ming L: Prevalence and risk factors of diabetes in patients with Klinefelter syndrome: a longitudinal observational study. Fertil Steril 2012;98:1331–1135.
20 Jackson IM, Buchanan KD, McKiddie MT, Prentice CR: Carbohydrate metabolism in Klinefelter's syndrome. J Endocrinol 1966;35:169–172.
21 Pei D, Sheu WH, Jeng CY, Liao WK, Fuh MM: Insulin resistance in patients with Klinefelter's syndrome and idiopathic gonadotropin deficiency. J Formos Med Assoc 1998;97:534–540.
22 Kota S, Lalit KM, Jammula S, Kota SK, Kirtikumar DM: Clinical profile of coexisting conditions in type 1 diabetes mellitus patients. Diabetes Metab Syndr 2012;6:70–76.
23 Kapoor D, Goodwin E, Channer KS, Jones TH: Testosterone replacement therapy improves insulin resistance, glycaemic control, visceral adiposity and hypercholesterolaemia in hypogonadal men with type 2 diabetes. Eur J Endocrinol 2006;154:899–906.

Antonio F. Radicioni, MD
Center of Rare Diseases, Section of Medical Pathophysiology
Department of Experimental Medicine, Sapienza University of Rome
Viale del Policlinico 155
IT–00161 Rome (Italy)
E-Mail antonio.radicioni@uniroma1.it

Barbetti F, Ghizzoni L, Guaraldi F (eds): Diabetes Associated with Single Gene Defects and Chromosomal Abnormalities. Front Diabetes. Basel, Karger, 2017, vol 25, pp 160–165 (DOI: 10.1159/000454743)

Down Syndrome (Trisomy 21) and Diabetes

Carla Bizzarri · Marco Cappa

Endocrinology and Diabetes Unit, Bambino Gesù Children's Hospital, IRCCS, Rome, Italy

Abstract

An increased prevalence of diabetes mellitus in Down syndrome (DS) was reported in studies published more than 30 years ago, but these studies did not distinguish between type 1 diabetes mellitus (T1DM) and type 2 diabetes mellitus (T2DM). More recently, a 4-fold increased prevalence of T1DM has been reported in DS people as compared to the general population of similar age. Insulin resistance, metabolic syndrome, and early T2DM are also relatively common in DS subjects due to premature ageing, obesity, and sedentary lifestyle. For this reason, a bias may exist when simple age criteria are used to differentiate between T1DM and T2DM. The etiopathogenesis of T1DM in DS seems to be related to an autoimmune process with earlier onset but with similar mechanisms to those underlying classic T1DM. The low frequency of detection of HLA haplotypes typically associated with T1DM, the common coexistence of multiorgan autoimmunity, and the long-lasting persistence of islet autoantibodies support the hypothesis that genes located on chromosome 21 contribute to increase the penetrance of T1DM and other autoimmune disorders in DS. Understanding how autoimmunity occurs in the absence of HLA risk genotypes in children with DS could provide important insights into disease mechanisms in the general population.

Down syndrome (DS), caused by the trisomy of chromosome 21 (OMIM No. 190685), is characterized by mental retardation, well-defined dysmorphic facial appearance and body proportions, and an increased prevalence of different autoimmune disorders, i.e., autoimmune thyroiditis and celiac disease [1, 2]. Studies published more than 30 years reported an increased prevalence of diabetes mellitus in DS. However, all of these early studies showed clear limitations. Above all, they often did not distinguish between the various forms of diabetes mellitus [1, 2]. Milunsky and Neurath [1] described a 0.43% prevalence of type 1 diabetes mellitus (T1DM) in DS subjects. The study was based on data collected from questionnaires, and the reply rates were around 50%. No age distribution was defined and only a portion of the cases were on insulin treatment, suggesting that several subjects could be affected by type 2 diabetes mellitus (T2DM). A second study [2] reported a prevalence of

1.7%, but it was based on a group of DS subjects attending a training center, and glycosuria was the only test used for the diagnosis of diabetes, without any differentiation between T1DM and T2DM. A more recent Dutch study reported a 3-fold increase in the prevalence of both T1DM and T2DM in DS patients [3]. In Scotland, a study based on interviews and data collected from a clinical registry [4] provided a prevalence rate ranging between 1.4 and 10.6%. DS diagnosis was based only on clinical examination, without confirmatory karyotype analysis in all but 2 subjects. No clinical or biochemical information regarding diabetes characteristics and presentation were reported.

It is important to emphasize that insulin resistance, metabolic syndrome, and early T2DM are relatively common in DS subjects due to premature ageing, obesity, and sedentary lifestyle. As a result, a potential bias may exist when simple age criteria are used to differentiate between T1DM and T2DM.

Recently, a nationwide population-based Danish study demonstrated that T1DM prevalence among patients with DS is 4.2 times higher than in the general population [5]. Going into the specifics of this study, the number of live births in Denmark in the years 1981–2000 was 1,230,933. Based on this background population, registry-validated data about current diabetes status were obtained. A total of 2,094 subjects affected by T1DM were identified, corresponding to a T1DM prevalence in the general Danish population of 2,094/1,230,933 subjects (0.17%). From 1981 to 2000, a total of 1,151 DS individuals were registered in Denmark, corresponding to a DS prevalence of 1,151/1,230,933 (0.09%). Eight out of 2,094 T1DM cases were identified as being affected by DS. Therefore, the prevalence of DS in T1DM was 8/2,094 (0.38%), in comparison with DS prevalence in the Danish background population of 0.09%, corresponding to a 4.2-fold increased DS prevalence in T1DM individuals. Accordingly, T1DM prevalence among DS patients was equivalent to 8/1,151 (0.7%), which appears more than 4-fold higher than the T1DM prevalence described in the background population (0.7 vs. 0.17%).

Pancreatic Histopathology

The landmark study by Foulis et al. [6] examined pancreatic histopathology in a group of T1DM subjects who had died before the age of 20 years. Three cases of DS associated with T1DM were described. A diffuse lymphocytic infiltration of the pancreatic islets (insulitis) was evident in a 14-year-old boy with longstanding T1DM and in a 12-year-old boy with newly diagnosed T1DM. Insulin staining was absent in the 14-year-old boy, consistent with typical autoimmune T1DM. However, the pancreas of the third DS child, who was diagnosed with diabetes at age 18 months and examined 2 weeks after clinical presentation of T1DM, displayed normal insulin staining without morphological abnormalities of the islets, suggesting a different nonimmune-mediated pathogenesis.

Age at Onset

A study published by Burch and Milunsky in 1969 [7] reported a peak age at clinical presentation of T1DM in DS patients of around 8 years, in comparison with a mean age of 14 years in childhood diabetes in the background population. This finding supports the hypothesis of a different pathogenesis of T1DM in DS subjects, which is probably genetically determined and not related to a progressive autoimmune destruction of the pancreatic β-cells.

The aforementioned Danish study [5] described a median age of 6 years (range: 0–13) at T1DM onset in 8 DS subjects, whereas the median age at T1DM onset in the background population was 8 years (range: 0–17). Rohrer et al. [8] compared data from 159 patients with DS and T1DM, and 41,983 patients with T1DM only. Mean age at diabetes onset was similar between groups (8.2 ± 5.3 vs. 8.4 ± 4.3 years, respectively). On the other hand, age distribution significantly differed. Disease onset during the first 3 years of life occurred in 18.9% of the patients with DS and T1DM versus 6.4% of the patients with T1DM only ($p < 0.001$). Moreover, age at diabetes onset showed 2 peaks in the DS and T1DM group, whereas it was approximately Gaussian in shape in the T1DM group.

The results of an international collection of clinical, immunological, and genetic data from children with DS and T1DM (Diaploidy), established in 2010, have been recently published [9]. By June 2012, 136 individuals had been registered (80 from the United Kingdom, 30 from Austria and Germany, 7 from other European countries and Australia, and 19 from Kuwait). Twenty-six (22%) of the 118 DS patients with T1DM onset before 21 years of age were diagnosed during the first 2 years of life, a significantly higher prevalence when compared to patients with T1DM only (91/1,822 patients = 5%), matched for age. A biphasic pattern in age at T1DM presentation was evident in DS subjects, with a peak incidence at 1 year of age and another peak around the age of 10 years.

Genetic Susceptibility

An age-related association between the HLA class II haplotypes DRB1*04-DQB1*0302 (DR4-DQ8) and DRB1*03-DQB1*0201 (DR3-DQ2) and T1DM susceptibility is well established in populations of Caucasian origin. An inverse relationship between the frequency of risk haplotypes and the age at T1DM onset has been recognized [10].

In the Danish study previously quoted [5], HLA-DQB1 genotyping was performed in 6/8 individuals with DS and T1DM: 1 subject carried 2 risk alleles (0302/0201), 3 carried 1 risk allele (0302 or 0201) in combination with a neutral allele, 1 carried exclusively neutral alleles, and another subject carried 1 neutral allele and 1 allele normally considered as dominantly protective (0602).

The distribution of the specific HLA haplotypes determining T1DM risk has been investigated in DS children by Gillespie et al. [11]. The comparison of HLA class II genotypes showed a similar distribution of diabetes-associated genotypes in DS children and healthy controls. The frequency of the most strongly T1DM-associated genotypes (DR4-DQ8/DR3-DQ2) was increased in children with DS and T1DM, indicating that T1DM in DS subjects and T1DM in the general population share the same HLA associations. Children with DS and T1DM were found to be positive for DR4-DQ8/DR3-DQ2, DR4-DQ8/X, or DR3-DQ2/X in 70% of cases, compared with 44% in healthy controls. No child with DS and T1DM presented the protective HLA DRB1*02-DQB1*0602 (DR2-DQ6). The frequency of DR4-DQ8/DR3-DQ2 in patients with DS and T1DM (40 subjects) was 25%, compared with more than 43% in the age and sex-matched T1DM population (120 subjects).

In the study by Aitken et al. [9], 3% of the 621 healthy control subjects showed the highest-risk haplotype (DR4-DQ8/DR3-DQ2), 13% carried the DR4-DQ8/X haplotype, 27% had DR3-DQ2/X, and 57% had no risk haplotypes. HLA class II frequencies in the control population of patients with DS were very similar to the healthy control population. The risk haplotypes were increased in 194 individuals with T1DM (38% had DR4- DQ8/DR3-DQ2, 40% had DR4-DQ8/X, 17% had DR3-DQ2/X, and 5% had no risk haplotypes). HLA frequencies in the DS + T1DM cohort were intermediate between the T1DM and control cohorts. Specifically, 17 DS + T1DM subjects (17%) had the highest-risk diplotype (DR4-DQ8/DR3-DQ2); 23 (24%) and 31 (32%) had the moderate-risk DR4-DQ8 and DR3/DQ2 haplotypes, respectively; and 26 (27%) had no risk haplotypes. In contrast, 5% of 194 age- and sex-matched T1DM children and 64% of 222 DS individuals had no risk haplotypes.

Taken together, these findings suggest that DS-specific genetic loci could be relevant in determining the increased T1DM risk in these subjects. It is intriguing to speculate that the explanation for the increased prevalence may be related to genes located on chromosome 21.

Islet Cell Autoimmunity

DS confers susceptibility to organ- and nonorgan-specific forms of autoimmunity, although no mechanism has been definitely recognized to explain this phenomenon.

Gillespie et al. [11] tested islet autoantibodies in 106 children with DS. Autoantibodies against GAD65 (GADA) were found positive in 8 children, autoantibodies against insulinoma-associated protein 2 (IA-2A) in 5 children, and autoantibodies against insulin in 9 children. Overall, 2 or more islet autoantibodies were present in 6/106 (5.6%) children with DS, compared with 13/2,860 (0.45%) healthy school children. Titers of GADA in the samples from DS children were found to be particularly elevated.

The study by Aitken et al. [9] analyzing 136 individuals with DS and T1DM found coexisting thyroid disease in 68 subjects (74%) and celiac disease in 11 subjects (14%). Despite the relatively extended diabetes duration at the time of investigation, islet autoantibodies were found positive in 72% of the cases. All children (n = 5) with T1DM onset in the first 2 years of life were positive for GADA.

Clinical Presentation and Management

No differences have been observed in the severity of diabetic ketoacidosis at diagnosis or during disease progression. It has been reported that patients with DS and T1DM received a lower number of daily insulin injections and lower average insulin doses than T1DM patients. The use of conventional insulin therapy (i.e., 2 daily injections of mixed insulin) has been reported as the most commonly used scheme in patients with DS and T1DM. Metabolic control, expressed by HbA$_{1c}$ levels, has been reported to be better in DS subjects with T1DM than in T1DM patients, without differences in the occurrence of severe hypoglycemia. These results could be explained by the simpler lifestyle and the good acceptance of the daily routine by DS people. No significant differences have been described with regard to diabetic complications, such as nephropathy or retinopathy [8].

Conclusions and Perspectives

A 4-fold increased prevalence of T1DM has been reported in DS people as compared to the general population of similar age.

So far, no evidence that T1DM in DS children may be genetically determined has been found. Conversely, the etiopathogenesis seems to be related to an autoimmune process with earlier onset but with similar mechanisms to those underlying classic T1DM.

The low frequency of detection of HLA haplotypes typically associated with T1DM, the common coexistence of multiorgan autoimmunity, and the long-lasting persistence of islet autoantibodies support the hypothesis that genes located on chromosome 21 may contribute to increase the penetrance of T1DM and other autoimmune disorders in DS.

A recent Scandinavian genome scan for T1DM associated genes identified an area of interest on chromosome 21 [12]. Fine mapping of the region in 253 Danish families supported the existence of a gene on chromosome 21q21.11-q22.3 conferring a specific susceptibility to T1DM [13]. These data support the need for further studies to identify genetic variants on chromosome 21 contributing to increased risk of autoimmune diseases.

On the other hand, the increased penetrance of low-risk HLA haplotypes in children with DS and T1DM may simply reflect the trend, already observed in the general population, toward an increase in T1DM incidence [14–16]. Understanding how autoimmunity occurs in the absence of HLA risk genotypes in children with DS could therefore provide important insights into disease mechanisms in the general population.

References

1 Milunsky A, Neurath PW: Diabetes mellitus in Down's syndrome. Arch Environ Health 1968;17: 372–376.

2 Jeremiah DE, Leyshon GE, Rose T, Francis HW, Elliott RW: Down's syndrome and diabetes. Psychol Med 1973;3:455–457.

3 Van Goor JC, Massa GG, Hirasing R: Increased incidence and prevalence of diabetes mellitus in Down's syndrome. Arch Dis Child 1997;77:186.

4 Anwar A, Walker J, Frier B: Type 1 diabetes mellitus and Down's syndrome: prevalence, management and diabetic complications. Diabet Med 1998;15: 160–163.

5 Bergholdt R, Eising S, Nerup J, Pociot F: Increased prevalence of Down's syndrome in individuals with type 1 diabetes in Denmark: a nationwide population-based study. Diabetologia 2006;49:1179–1182.

6 Foulis AK, Liddle CN, Farquharson MA, Richmond JA, Weir RS: The histopathology of the pancreas in type 1 (insulin dependent) diabetes mellitus: a 25-year review of deaths in patients under 20 years of age in the United Kingdom. Diabetologia 1986;29: 267–274.

7 Burch PR, Milunsky A: Early-onset diabetes mellitus in the general and Down's syndrome populations. Genetics, aetiology, and pathogenesis. Lancet 1969; 1:554–558.

8 Rohrer TR, Hennes P, Thon A, Dost A, Grabert M, Rami B, Wiegand S, Holl W, DPV Initiative: Down's syndrome in diabetic patients aged, 20 years: an analysis of metabolic status, glycaemic control and autoimmunità in comparison with type 1 diabetes. Diabetologia 2010;53:1070–1075.

9 Aitken RJ, Mehers KL, Williams AJ, Brown J, Bingley PJ, Holl RW, Rohrer TR, Schober E, Abdul-Rasoul MM, Shield JP, Jillespied KM: Early-onset, coexisting autoimmunity and decreased HLA-mediated susceptibility are the characteristics of diabetes in Down syndrome. Diabetes Care 2013;36:1181–1185.

10 Gillespie KM, Gale EA, Bingley PJ: High familial risk and genetic susceptibility in early onset childhood diabetes. Diabetes 2002;51:210–214.

11 Gillespie KM, Dix RJ, Williams AJ, Newton R, Robinson ZF, Bingley PJ, Gale EA, Shield JP: Islet autoimmunity in children with Down's syndrome. Diabetes 2006;55:3185–3188.

12 Nerup J, Pociot F; European Consortium for IDDM Studies: A genomewide scan for type 1-diabetes susceptibility in Scandinavian families: identification of new loci with evidence of interactions. Am J Hum Genet 2001;69:1301–1313.

13 Bergholdt R, Nerup J, Pociot F: Fine mapping of a region on chromosome 21q21.11-q22.3 showing linkage to type 1 diabetes. J Med Genet 2005;42:17–25.

14 Fourlanos S, Varney MD, Tait BD, Morahan G, Honeyman MC, Colman PG, Harrison LC: The rising incidence of type 1 diabetes is accounted for by cases with lower-risk human leukocyte antigen genotypes. Diabetes Care 2008;31:1546–1549.

15 Steck AK, Armstrong TK, Babu SR, Eisenbarth GS: Stepwise or linear decrease in penetrance of type 1 diabetes with lower-risk HLA genotypes over the past 40 years. Diabetes 2011;60:1045–1049.

16 Gillespie KM, Bain SC, Barnett AH, Bingley PJ, Christie MR, Gill GV, Gale EA: The rising incidence of childhood type 1 diabetes and reduced contribution of high-risk HLA haplotypes. Lancet 2004;364: 1699–1700.

Prof. Marco Cappa, MD, PhD
Endocrinology and Diabetes Unit
Bambino Gesù Children's Hospital, IRCCS
Piazza S. Onofrio 4
IT–00165 Rome (Italy)
E-Mail marco.cappa@opbg.net

Barbetti F, Ghizzoni L, Guaraldi F (eds): Diabetes Associated with Single Gene Defects and Chromosomal Abnormalities. Front Diabetes. Basel, Karger, 2017, vol 25, pp 166–171 (DOI: 10.1159/000454744)

Turner Syndrome and Diabetes

Armando Grossi · Marco Cappa

Endocrinology and Diabetes Unit, Bambino Gesù Children's Hospital, IRCCS, Rome, Italy

Abstract

Turner syndrome (TS) is associated with a significant risk of developing autoimmune diseases, including type 1 diabetes. Suggested etiopathogenic mechanisms include inactivation and transcriptional silencing of genes in the X chromosome during early embryonic development, leading to abnormal thymic deletion of autoreactive T-lymphocytes, with impaired immune recognition and tolerance; deletion of genes (i.e., FOWP3) playing a crucial role for the function of natural regulatory T-cells; and upregulation of proinflammatory cytokines. On the other hand, abnormal gametogenesis and nondysjunctional events could be secondary to abnormal autoimmune responsiveness. Starting in childhood, TS patients also present an increased rate of insulin resistance and type 2 diabetes in comparison with age-matched controls. The negative role of the haploinsufficiency of the genes on the Xp chromosome on the transcription factors involved in pancreatic islet and β-cell function, as well as hormonal and metabolic factors, have been suggested. The role of growth hormone treatment and timing of pubertal induction on metabolic profile is still a subject of debate.

Turner syndrome (TS) is one of the most common chromosomal abnormalities in live births [1, 2], with a prevalence of 1:2,500–1:3,000 live-born girls [1, 3]; the 45,X karyotype is found in approximately 10% of spontaneous abortions [2]. Approximately 50% of the affected individuals have the 45,X karyotype, while 20–30% have mosaicisms; less common structural abnormalities include deletions of the short and long arm of the X chromosome, duplications, ring chromosomes, and presence of Y-positive material [4]. TS should be suspected in girls with unexplained short stature or pubertal delay, and short women with incomplete sexual development and/or inability to conceive. Other suggestive clinical features include edema of the hands or feet, nuchal folds, cardiac defects, low posterior hairline, low-set ears, cubitus valgus, short fourth metacarpal, triangular facies, high-arched palate, multiple pigmented nevi, nail abnormalities, chronic otitis media, and unexplained markedly elevated follicle-stimulating hormone levels [5, 6]. Cardiovascular defects, atherosclerosis, osteoporosis and fractures, endocrine and metabolic disorders, hearing loss, and specific cognitive deficits contribute to the increased morbidity and mortality as well as decreased life expectancy in these patients [6–8].

Autoimmunity in Turner Syndrome

Several studies reported an increased frequency of autoimmunity in TS patients [1, 9, 10], likely secondary to a complex interplay between genetic and environmental factors [9, 11, 12].

Sexual dimorphism 45,X has been hypothesized to be associated with gene inactivation and transcriptional silencing in the X chromosome of paternal (XPat) or maternal (XMat) origin during early embryonic development, leading to abnormal thymic deletion of autoreactive T-lymphocytes with impaired immune recognition and tolerance, as an autoimmune process would be enhanced if autoreactive T-lymphocytes encounter specific XPat- rather than XMat-specific antigens in tissues [13].

In addition, several genes located on the X chromosome have been demonstrated to have possible immune regulatory functions [14]. Of note, FOXP3 (Xp11.23, http://omim.org/entry/300292) plays a crucial role for the function of natural regulatory T-cells; deletions in this gene cause X-linked (IPEX) syndrome characterized by immune dysregulation, polyendocrinopathy, and enteropathy [14].

Moreover, the proinflammatory cytokines IL-6, IL-8, and TNF seem to be upregulated in women with TS [15]; autoantibody positivity is seen in a high proportion of patients [10, 16], although a clear association of cytokine levels and autoimmune diseases in TS has not been fully established [17].

It has also been hypothesized that since autoimmune disorders are frequent in relatives of TS patients, abnormal gametogenesis and nondysjunctional events are due to abnormal autoimmune responsiveness [5, 9, 18].

Hashimoto's thyroiditis is the most common autoimmune disease reported in TS, although the prevalence and incidence of antithyroid antibodies is highly variable among studies (3.9–87.5% and 4.3–40%, respectively) [19, 20]. Other autoimmune disorders commonly associated with TS are celiac disease, ulcerative colitis, Crohn's disease, psoriasis, idiopathic thrombocytopenic purpura, vitiligo, and juvenile rheumatoid arthritis [1, 3, 9]. According to a Danish registry, women with TS exhibit a 4-fold increased risk of developing type 1 diabetes as compared to nonaffected women [7], as well as other typically male-predominant autoimmune diseases (i.e., amyotrophic lateral sclerosis, ankylosing spondylitis, reactive arthritis, and Dupuytren contracture) [21].

Bakalov et al. [17] recently reported a significant increase in lymphocytic thyroiditis in both TS and karyotypically normal women with primary ovarian insufficiency, suggesting an increased risk of autoimmunity-associated factors underlying ovarian insufficiency.

In general, the rate of autoimmunity in TS is more pronounced in females with isochromosome Xq [10, 20]. Allelic variations of the other genes located on different chromosomes (i.e., the PTPN22 gene located on chromosome 1) [18, 22] also appear to contribute to the development of autoimmunity in TS. A recent study [12] found no significant association between karyotype 45,X and overall antibody prevalence, but confirmed an increased rate of antithyroperoxidase, thyroglobulin, and glutamic acid decarboxylase (isoform 65) (GADA) in IsoXq patients.

Glucose Homeostasis in Turner Syndrome

An increased prevalence of insulin resistance and impairment of nonoxidative glucose disposal has been reported in girls with TS, in comparison with age-matched controls [23, 24]. Impaired glucose tolerance and overt type 2 diabetes have been described both in children and adults with TS [25–29]. Other studies found normal insulin sensitivity [29], but relative impairment in the first-phase insulin response, considered a potential hallmark of development of type 2 diabetes [30]. Epidemiological studies on large cohorts of TS females of various ages showed type 1 and 2 diabetes to be very frequent [7, 30].

Muscle biopsies in TS showed a similar size of type I and IIx fibers in TS patients and controls, but an increased size of type IIa fibers, suggestive for a decreased substrate supply for metabolic processes, which could be indicative of prediabetes [31].

A recent cross-sectional study [32] showed higher glucose responses during an oral glucose tolerance test and intravenous glucose tolerance test, but a similar amplitude of insulin response in adults with TS in comparison with matched controls. Insulin sensitivity, response to dynamic β-cell function tests, and secretion patterns appeared similar between TS patients and controls, also when examined by deconvolution analysis, approximate entropy, spectral analysis and autocorrelation analysis. On the other hand, lower IGF-I, but higher cortisol and norepinephrine levels, and an increased waist-to-hip ratio was found in TS, suggesting that a number of hormonal and metabolic factors (i.e., prevailing levels of IGF-I, norepinephrine, and triglycerides; glucose toxicity and lipotoxicity) might play a role in the perturbed β-cell function in TS [33].

Diabetes in Turner Syndrome

In 1963, Forbes and Engel [34] reported an increased incidence of diabetes in a cohort of 41 subjects with 'gonadal dysgenesis'. More recently, prevalence of GADA was found to be higher in TS than in the general population.

In a Danish registry of TS patients, type 1 diabetes was found in 18 out of 798 subjects, instead of the expected 4.4 (standardized incidence ratios = 4.4 at 95% CI), together with a 4-fold increase of male-predominant and 1.7-fold increase in female-predominant autoimmunity. Type 1 diabetes was the most frequent male-predominant autoimmune disorder [10]. However, conflicting results on the increased prevalence of type 1 diabetes in TS have been reported in the literature. For example, Bakalov et al. [17], studying 224 patients with TS and 451 with precocious ovarian insufficiency of adult age, found a similar prevalence of type 1 diabetes as compared to the general female population.

TS patients are more prone to be overweight in childhood, which is considered a risk factor for the development of diabetes and cardiovascular disease in adult life [7, 35, 36]. According to a recent study by Reinehr et al. [37] in 887 TS subjects, weight gain was associated with an earlier start of puberty induction. However, weight increase occurred even before puberty onset, and did not differ between TS girls with induced and spontaneous puberty, indicating the involvement of other factors.

Moreover, an increased prevalence of abnormalities in glucose metabolism (i.e., insulin resistance and type 2 diabetes) has been observed in X-monosomy as compared to mosaic TS [38], suggesting a negative role of the haploinsufficiency of the genes on the Xp chromosome on the transcription factors involved in pancreatic islet and β-cell function.

A Japanese survey performed on 492 adult TS women demonstrated a mean diabetes prevalence of 5.5% (6.3% in the age 20–39 years) versus 0.8% in the general female population, with a significantly smaller proportion of mosaicism and isochromosome karyotype in affected cases. Rates of obesity, dyslipidemia, hypertension, and liver dysfunction were also increased in TS. Interestingly, low birth weight was associated with hypertension, dyslipidemia, and liver dysfunction, but not diabetes. Although BMI in TS patients was overall much higher than in the general population, no significant increase with age was observed, indicating a tendency toward obesity from young age [39].

The impact of growth hormone (GH) treatment on glucose metabolism in TS has been widely investigated with conflicting results. Treatment appears to worsen insulin sensitivity which, however, normalizes after GH discontinuation. On the other hand, GH has a positive effect on body composition by increasing lean body mass and reducing fat mass [40], and it improves the metabolic profile by decreasing total and LDL cholesterol, while increasing HDL cholesterol and triglycerides [41]. At the same time, GH does not affect age-related BMI increase [42].

Conclusions

A complex interplay between genetic and immunological factors has been suggested in women with TS. Indeed, haploinsufficiency of some genes expressed on the X chromosome appear to play a primary role in the pathogenesis of both autoimmune diseases and metabolic alterations, including type 1 and 2 diabetes, highly prevalent in these patients. On the other hand, abnormal gametogenesis and nondysjunctional events could be secondary to abnormal autoimmune responsiveness. The exact underlying mechanisms, as well as real disease prevalence and effects of GH and gonadal replacement therapy (timing and doses) remain to be elucidated, and thus deserving of in vitro studies and the creation of national and international registries.

References

1 McCarthy K, Bondy CA: Turner syndrome in childhood and adolescence. Expert Rev Endocrinol Metab 2008;3:771–775.
2 Rapaport R: Disorders of the gonads; in Kliegman RM, Behrman RE, Jenson HB, et al (eds): Nelson Text Book of Pediatrics, ed 18. Philadelphia, Saunders Elsevier, 2007, pp 2374–2384.
3 Dias Mdo C, Castro LC, Gandolfi L, Almeida RC, Córdoba MS, Pratesi R: Screening for celiac disease among patients with Turner syndrome in Brasília, DF, midwest region of Brazil. Arq Gastroenterol 2010;47:246–249.
4 Davenport ML: Approach to the patient with Turner syndrome. J Clin Endocrinol Metab 2010;95:1487–1495.
5 Larizza D, Calcaterra V, Martinetti M: Autoimmune stigmata in Turner syndrome: when lacks an X chromosome. J Autoimmun 2009;33:25–30.
6 Bondy CA: Care of girls and women with Turner syndrome: a guideline of the Turner Syndrome Study Group. J Clin Endocrinol Metab 2007;92:10–25.
7 Gravholt CH, Juul S, Naeraa RW, Hansen J: Morbidity in Turner syndrome. J Clin Epidemiol 1998;51:147–158.
8 Schoemaker MJ, Swerdlow AJ, Higgins CD, Wright AF, Jacobs PA: Mortality in women with turner syndrome in Great Britain: a national cohort study. J Clin Endocrinol Metab 2008;93:4735–4742.
9 Bianchi I, lleo A, Gershwin ME, Invernizzi P: The X chromosome and immune associated genes. J Autoimmun 2012;38:J187–J192.
10 Jørgensen KT, Rostgaard K, Bache I, Biggar RJ, Nielsen NM, Tommerup N, Frisch M: Autoimmune diseases in women with Turner's syndrome. Arthritis Rheum 2010;62:658–666.
11 Menasha J, Levy B, Hirschhorn K, Kardon NB: Incidence and spectrum of chromosome abnormalities in spontaneous abortions: new insights from a 12-year study. Genet Med 2005;7:251–263.
12 Fierabracci A: Unravelling the role of infectious agents in the pathogenesis of human autoimmunity: the hypothesis of the retroviral involvement revisited. Curr Mol Med 2009;9:1024–1033.
13 Chitnis S, Monteiro J, Glass D, et al: The role of X-chromosome inactivation in female predisposition to autoimmunity. Arthritis Res 2000;2:399–406.
14 Pessach IM, Notarangelo LD: X-linked primary immunodeficiencies as a bridge to better understanding X-chromosome related autoimmunity. J Autoimmun 2009;33:17–24.
15 Gravholt CH, Hjerrild BE, Mosekilde L, Hansen TK, Rasmussen LM, Frystyk J, et al: Body composition is distinctly altered in Turner syndrome: relations to glucose metabolism, circulating adipokines, and endothelial adhesion molecules. Eur J Endocrinol 2006;155:583–592.
16 Mortensen KH, Cleemann L, Hjerrild BE, Nexo E, Locht H, Jeppesen EM, et al: Increased prevalence of autoimmunity in Turner syndrome: influence of age. Clin Exp Immunol 2009;156:205–210.
17 Bakalov VK, Gutin L, Cheng CM, Zhou J, Sheth P, Shah K, Arepalli S, Vanderhoof V, Nelson LM, Bondy CA: Autoimmune disorders in women with Turner syndrome and women with karyotypically normal primary ovarian insufficiency. J Autoimmun 2012;38:315–321.
18 Grossi A, Palma A, Zanni G, Novelli A, Loddo S, Cappa M, Fierabracci A: Multiorgan autoimmunity in a Turner syndrome patient with partial monosomy 2q and trisomy 10p. Gene 2013;515:439–443.
19 Germain EL, Plotnick LP: Age-related anti-thyroid antibodies and thyroid abnormalities in Turner syndrome. Acta Paediatr Scand 1986;75:750–755.
20 Grossi A, Crinò A, Luciano R, Lombardo A, Cappa M, Fierabracci A: Endocrine autoimmunity in Turner syndrome. Ital J Pediatr 2013;39:79.
21 Ferrera F, Rizzi M, Sprecacenere B, Balestra P, Sessarego M, Di Carlo A, Filaci G, Gabrielli A, Ravazzolo R, Indiveri F: AIRE gene polymorphisms in systemic sclerosis associated with autoimmune thyroiditis. Clin Immunol 2007;122:13–17.
22 Bianco B, Verreschi IT, Oliveira KC, Guedes AD, Galera BB, Galera MF, Barbosa CP, Lipay MV: PTPN22 polymorphism is related to autoimmune disease risk in patients with Turner syndrome. Scand J Immunol 2010;72:256–259.

23 Caprio S, Boulware S, Diamond M, Sherwin RS, Carpenter TO, Rubin K, Amiel S, Press M, Tamborlane WV: Insulin resistance: an early metabolic defect of Turner's syndrome. J Clin Endocrinol Metab 1991; 72:832–836.

24 Cicognani A, Mazzanti L, Tassinari D, Pellacani A, Forabosco A, Landi L, Pifferi C, Cacciari E: Differences in carbohydrate tolerance in Turner syndrome depending on age and karyotype. Eur J Pediatr 1988; 14:864–868.

25 Wilson DM, Frane JW, Sherman B, Johanson AJ, Hintz RL, Rosenfeld RG: Carbohydrate and lipid metabolism in Turner syndrome: effect of therapy with growth hormone, oxandrolone, and a combination of both. J Pediatr 1988;112:210–221.

26 Nielsen J, Johansen K, Yde H: The frequency of diabetes mellitus in patients with Turner's syndrome and pure gonadal dysgenesis. Blood glucose, plasma insulin and growth hormone level during an oral glucose tolerance test. Acta Endocrinol (Copenh) 1969;62:251–269.

27 Rasio E, Antaki A, Van Campenhout J: Diabetes mellitus in gonadal dysgenesis: studies of insulin and growth hormone secretion. Eur J Clin Invest 1976;6: 59–66.

28 Holl RW, Kunze D, Etzrodt H, Teller W, Heinze E: Turner syndrome: final height, glucose tolerance, bone density and psychosocial status in 25 adult patients. Eur J Pediatr 1994;15:311–316.

29 Gravholt CH, Naeraa RW, Nyholm B, Gerdes U, Christiansen E, Schmitz O, Christiansen JS: Glucose metabolism, lipid metabolism, and cardiovascular risk factors in adult Turner syndrome: the impact of sex hormone replacement. Diabetes Care 1998;21: 1062–1070.

30 Gravholt CH: Epidemiological, endocrine and metabolic features in Turner syndrome. Eur J Endocrinol 2004;151:657–687.

31 Gravholt CH, Nyholm B, Saltin B, Schmitz O, Christiansen JS: Muscle fiber composition and capillary density in Turner syndrome: evidence of increased muscle fiber size related to insulin resistance. Diabetes Care 2001;24:1668–1673.

32 Hjerrild BE, Holst JJ, Juhl CB, Christiansen JS, Schmitz O, Gravholt CH: Delayed β-cell response and glucose intolerance in young women with Turner syndrome. BMC Endocr Disord 2011;11:6.

33 Gravholt CH, Chen JW, Oxvig C, Overgaard MT, Christiansen JS, Frystyk J, Flyvbjerg A: The GH-IGF-IGFBP axis is changed in Turner syndrome: partial normalization by HRT. Growth Horm IGF Res 2006; 16:332–339.

34 Forbes AP, Engel E: The high incidence of diabetes mellitus in 41 patients with gonadal dysgenesis, and their close relatives. Metabolism 1963;12:428–439.

35 Franks PW, Hanson RL, Knowler WC, et al: Childhood obesity, other cardiovascular risk factors, and premature death. N Engl J Med 2010;362:485–493.

36 Hanaki K, Ohzeki T, Ishitani N, et al: Fat distribution in overweight patients with Ullrich-Turner syndrome. Am J Med Genet 1992;42:428–430.

37 Reinehr T, Lindberg A, Toschke C, Cara J, Chrysis D, Camacho-Hubner C: Weight gain in Turner Syndrome: association to puberty induction? – longitudinal analysis of KIGS data. Clin Endocrinol (Oxf) 2016;85:85–91.

38 Cicognani A, Mazzanti L, Tassinari D, et al: Differences in carbohydrate metabolism in Turner syndrome dependence on age and karyotype. Pediatrics 1988;12:1072–1080.

39 Hanew K, Tanaka T, Horikawa R, Hasegawa T, Fujita K, Yokoya S: Women with Turner syndrome are at high risk of lifestyle related disease – from questionnaire surveys by the Foundation for Growth Science in Japan. Endocr J 2016;63:449–456.

40 Gravholt CH: Clinical practice in Turner syndrome. Nat Clin Pract Endocrinol Metab 2005;1:41–52.

41 Mavinkurve M, O'Gorman CS: Cardiometabolic and vascular risks in young and adolescent girls with Turner syndrome. BBA Clin 2015;3:304–309.

42 Blackett PR, Rundle AC, Frane J, Blethen SL: Body mass index (BMI) in Turner syndrome before and during growth hormone (GH) therapy. Int J Obes Relat Metab Disord 2000;24:232–235.

Dr. Armando Grossi
Endocrinology and Diabetes Unit
Bambino Gesù Children's Hospital, IRCCS
Piazza S. Onofrio 4
IT–00165 Rome (Italy)
E-Mail armando.grossi@opbg.net

Barbetti F, Ghizzoni L, Guaraldi F (eds): Diabetes Associated with Single Gene Defects and Chromosomal Abnormalities. Front Diabetes. Basel, Karger, 2017, vol 25, pp 172–181 (DOI: 10.1159/000454745)

Diabetes in Friedreich Ataxia

Shaolu Ran · Rosella Abeti · Paola Giunti

Department of Molecular Neuroscience, Ataxia Centre, Institute of Neurology, University College London (UCL), London, UK

Abstract

Friedreich ataxia (FRDA) is the most common hereditary ataxia. It is a progressive autosomal recessive neurodegenerative disorder associated with an increased risk of impaired glucose tolerance and overt diabetes mellitus. FRDA is caused by a genetic mutation inserting a GAA (guanine-adenine-adenine) repeat expansion within intron 1 of the *FXN* gene, resulting in its transcriptional silencing. The *FXN* gene encodes for frataxin, a protein ubiquitously expressed and located in the inner mitochondrial membrane. Frataxin is involved in the biogenesis of iron-sulphur clusters (ISCs). The progressive lack of frataxin leads to iron accumulation and decreased activity of those proteins that contain ISCs, such as complex I, II, and III of the mitochondrial electron transport chain, and aconitase, a crucial enzyme of the Krebs cycle (TCA). As a result, FRDA has been linked to mitochondrial dysfunction due to increased reactive oxidative species generation and decreased ATP production. Mitochondria of pancreatic β-cells are central to stimulus-secretion coupling, which is responsible for triggering and amplifying insulin secretion. Furthermore, the intrinsic pathway of apoptosis occurs in the mitochondria and has also been implicated in the pathogenesis of diabetes in FRDA. This chapter focuses on what is currently known about the pathophysiology of diabetes mellitus in the context of frataxin deficiency and its clinical management.   © 2017 S. Karger AG, Basel

Friedreich ataxia (FRDA) is the most common inherited ataxia, with an estimated prevalence in Western European populations varying from 1:125,000 to 1:20,000 [1] and an estimated carrier frequency varying from 1:110 to 1:60 [2, 3]. It is characterized by gait and limb ataxia, loss of proprioception, areflexia, square wave jerks/nystagmus, dysarthria, and extra-neurological signs, such as scoliosis, pes cavus, and hypertrophic cardiomyopathy [4]. The onset of FRDA is usually in childhood or adolescence, and usually first presents with neurological symptoms. It is associated with reduced life expectancy with cardiac complications being the most common cause of death. There is an increased risk of impaired glucose metabolism with the disease. Indeed, the prevalence of diabetes is increased with respect to the normal population and ranges from 8 to 32% depending on the diagnostic criteria and tools applied [5–7].

This wide range is the result of the considerable changes in diagnostic criteria of diabetes that have occurred over time. Ultimately, diabetic patients with FRDA will require insulin therapy [5–7]. The mean time at which diabetes develops is around 15 years after the onset of neurological symptoms [8].

The following chapter will discuss the pathogenesis of FRDA, from genetic to physiology, with a specific focus on diabetes, and ultimately its possible management.

Genetics

The genetic basis of FRDA in 96% of the patients is the insertion of GAA (guanine-adenine-adenine) repeat expansions in the *FXN* gene located at chromosome region 9q13 [6]. The other 4% of the patients have a compound heterozygous genotype with a GAA expansion allele and either a frataxin point mutation or an intragenic *FXN* deletion, which leads to the loss of the protein function [6, 9]. The threshold for genomic stability is suggested to be between 26 and 44 GAA repeats [4]. In contrast, FRDA patients generally have around 500 to over 1,000 repeats of the trinucleotide [4]. These pathologically expanded repeats impair transcription of the gene, resulting in decreased expression of the mitochondrial protein frataxin [4]. The tissues primarily affected by frataxin deficiency are the dorsal root ganglia, spinal cord, cerebellum, heart, and pancreas [4]. Interestingly, linkage of type 2 diabetes mellitus to frataxin encoding locus 9q13 has been reported in at least 4 different populations worldwide, suggesting a role of the locus 9q13 in the pathogenesis of type 2 diabetes mellitus [10–12].

Frataxin Function

Frataxin mRNA is translated in the cytosol and the protein is then localized to the inner mitochondrial membrane, where it acts as an iron chaperone and storage protein [4]. Frataxin deficiency leads to a disruption of iron homeostasis and consequential iron accumulation in the mitochondria, resulting in its dysfunction [4]. Thus, there is a reduction in ATP formation and the generation of reactive oxygen species [4].

Frataxin is directly involved in the de novo formation of iron-sulphur clusters (ISCs, i.e., 2 or more iron molecules bridged by a sulphur centre) through allosteric activation of the surface donor enzyme nutrient and stress factor 1 (NSF1) and modulation and presentation of Fe^{2+} to Fe-S scaffold proteins [13]. Key enzymes in the electron transport chain (ETC) and TCA contain ISCs, such as complex I, II, and III (ETC) and aconitase (TCA). Numerous other proteins involved in a large variety of different functions also contain ISCs, including enzymes involved in iron metabolism and purine synthesis, as well as a number of enzymes essential to DNA replication and repair [14, 15]. Frataxin deficiency results in impaired function of these enzymes [4]. Impairment of key ETC enzymes leads to electron leakage from the ETC and, consequently, free radical generation and oxidative stress [4, 14, 16]. In FRDA, one key way free radicals seem to be generated is from the reaction between Fe^{2+} and H_2O_2 in Fenton's reaction:

$$(1)\ Fe^{2+} + H_2O_2 \rightarrow Fe^{3+} + HO^\cdot + OH^-$$
$$(2)\ Fe^{3+} + H_2O_2 \rightarrow Fe^{2+} + HOO^\cdot + H^+$$

Fe^{2+} is first oxidized by H_2O_2 to form Fe^{3+} and the highly reactive free radical $HO^\cdot$; then Fe^{3+} is reduced back to Fe^{2+} by reacting with H_2O_2, and generating the free radical $HOO^\cdot$.

Frataxin deficiency leads to increased intracellular levels of both substrates of Fenton's reaction, Fe^{2+} and H_2O_2, which are responsible for the increased production of the free radicals $HO^\cdot$ and $HOO^\cdot$ [17]. Fe^{2+} accumulates in the mitochondria due to defective ISC synthesis through the mechanism outlined above. H_2O_2 is also increased through a series of steps. First, defective ETC enzymes lead to electron leakage from the ETC [4, 16]. Next, the reaction between these electrons and O_2 in the cell generates the superoxide anion O_2^-. Finally, in the mitochondria, dismutation of O_2^- forms H_2O_2 through the action of the catalyst superoxide dismutase 2 (SOD2) [14, 18]. In normal physiology, antioxidant defence mechanisms, i.e., glutathione peroxidase and cellular antioxidant ascorbic acid, restrict the amount of H_2O_2 available for Fenton's reaction. An imbalance between free radical production and antioxidant mechanisms leads to oxidative stress [19].

Diabetes in Friedreich Ataxia

The occurrence of diabetes in FRDA has been known since before the genetic basis of the disease was uncovered in 1996 [20]. The association is unsurprising considering the importance of mitochondria for the essential functions of the pancreatic β-cells. In FRDA, both insulin deficiency and resistance have been reported, secondary to mitochondrial dysfunction in the pancreas and insulin-responsive tissues [13, 21, 22]. In pancreatic β-cells, mitochondria are fundamental for stimulus-secretion coupling, the process involved in sensing plasma glucose levels and generating signals that trigger and amplify insulin secretion [21]. Principally, β-cell mitochondrial metabolism is driven by the available fuel supply, which means that insulin secretion is directly coupled to plasma glucose levels, thus allowing distribution of glucose to the insulin-sensitive tissues of the body, namely skeletal muscle, liver, and adipose tissue [21, 23]. This response maintains glucose homeostasis throughout the body. Theoretically, the impairment of this system would lead to diabetes, but data regarding this topic are inconclusive. In vitro models of frataxin-deficient pancreatic β-cells have shown that frataxin deficiency leads to the impairment of the stimulus-secretion pathways, as there is a decrease in mitochondrial membrane potential, the glucose-induced

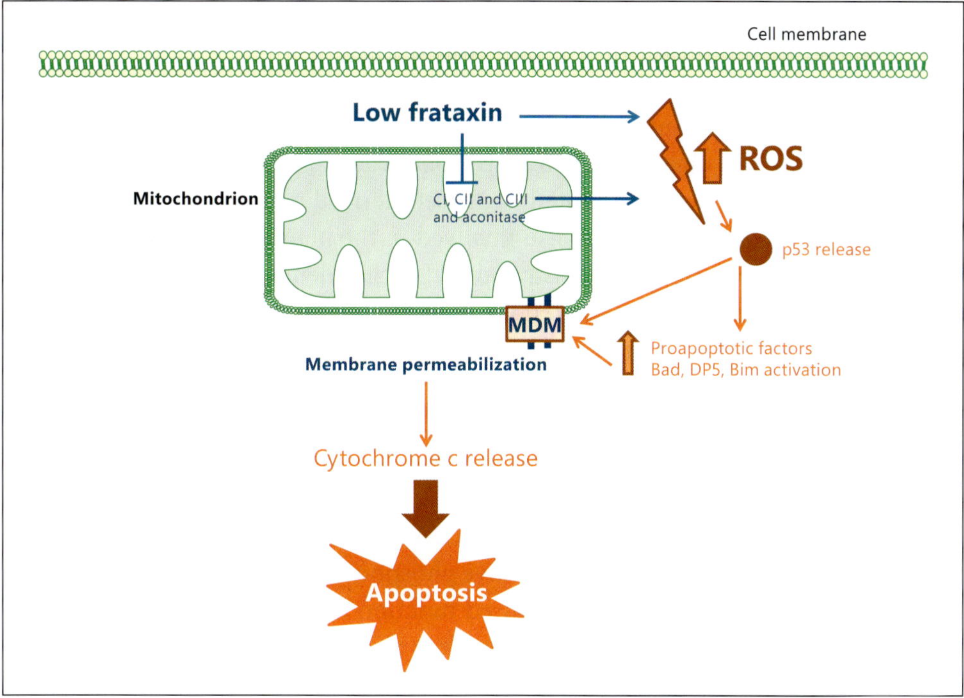

Fig. 1. Proposed pathway for pancreatic β-cell apoptosis. Frataxin deficiency leads to the impairment of ISC formation and decreases the activity of key mitochondrial enzymes, including complex I, II, and III of the mitochondrial electron transport chain (ETC), and aconitase of the Krebs cycle (TCA). The 2 processes are strictly linked and lead to the generation of oxygen free radicals (reactive oxygen species [ROS]). In turn, ROS generation triggers p53 release and activates proapoptotic factors, such as associated death promoter (Bad), death protein 5 (DP5), and Bcl-2 interacting mediator of death (Bim). Release of these factors culminates in mitochondrial membrane permeabilization and release of cytochrome c, and, finally, cell apoptosis. MDM, multidomain members.

ATP:ADP ratio, and insulin secretion [24]. On the other hand, other studies monitoring glucose-stimulated insulin secretion in isolated islets have reported unaltered insulin secretion [22].

In addition to the uncoupling of stimulus-secretion pathways, a mass reduction of pancreatic islets also contributes to insulin deficiency in FRDA. This is caused by the increased reactive oxygen species generation that triggers the activation of apoptotic pathways and results in increased apoptosis and decreased proliferation of β-cells [13, 22]. A recent study [13] has suggested β-cell death to be a consequence of oxidative stress-mediated activation of the intrinsic pathway of apoptosis (Fig. 1). The susceptibility of a cell to undergo apoptosis depends on the balance between the multidomain members (pro- and antiapoptotic proteins) of the Bcl-2 family. Evidence indicates that key mediators of frataxin deficiency-induced β-cell apoptosis are the proapoptotic Bcl-2 family members Bcl-2-associated death promoter (Bad), death protein 5 (DP5), and Bcl-2-interacting mediator of death (Bim) [13]. The activation of these members of the intrinsic pathway leads to the permeabilization of the outer mitochondrial membrane, release of cytochrome c, and activation of caspases, which ultimately results in cell death. In FRDA patients, these mechanisms lead to the non-autoimmune loss of the insulin-producing pancreatic β-cells, impaired glucose tolerance, and, eventually, diabetes. The intrinsic pathway of apoptosis was also found to be activated in the induced pluripotent stem-cell-derived neurons of FRDA patients, suggesting that this mechanism is also involved in the neuronal atrophy seen in the disease [13]. The same study demonstrated that cyclic adenosine monophosphate induction by an incretin analogue, exendin-4, and activator of adenylate cyclase, forskolin, attenuated the activation of the intrinsic pathway and was protective in both frataxin-deficient β-cells and neuronal cells, implying an important therapeutic role of these drugs [13]. These results are consistent with previous findings obtained by the same group through work on frataxin-deficient rat pancreatic β-cells and human dispersed islet cells [24].

In conjunction with insulin deficiency, FRDA is associated with insulin resistance, which is a consequence of reduced oxidative phosphorylation capacity and decreased ATP production arising from the impaired function of ISCs containing respiratory chain enzymes [21]. Insulin resistance is evident also in non-diabetic FRDA patients and has been shown to exist at the systemic level as well as the cellular level [25].

Additionally, the examination of the liver of non-diabetic mice genetically altered to exhibit a 65% decrease in frataxin showed an upregulation of the networks associated with insulin resistance and an overall shift of genetic networks towards systemically increased lipogenesis. This included upregulation of the PPAR-γ/PGC-1α pathway, which is involved in the regulation of fatty acid oxidation, mitochondrial DNA replication, and oxidative phosphorylation. Furthermore, it has been hypothesized that frataxin may be a possible target of PGC-1α, and PGC-1α expression may alter frataxin expression [25]. To investigate this hypothesis, PGC-1α was downregulated in cells from FRDA patients and controls using siRNA, and frataxin levels were recorded after 72 h. A significant frataxin decrease was observed within 72 h in transfected cells of both FRDA patients and controls, suggesting a potential positive feedback loop between PGC-1α and frataxin. Based on these premises, pharmacological activation of PGC-1α may lead to the increase of frataxin levels [25].

The PPAR-γ/PGC-1α pathway is known to be involved in the pathogenesis of diabetes. Thiazolidinediones are PPAR-γ agonists and are used in the treatment of diabetes. These work by upregulating the PPAR-γ/PGC-1α pathway [26]. Furthermore, PPAR-γ agonists may be used to treat mitochondrial disorders, such as FRDA, as they have been shown to induce mitochondrial biogenesis and synthesis of mitochondrial proteins [27]. Azelaoyl-PAF, a synthetic PPAR-γ agonist, has been demonstrated to increase frataxin levels in the fibroblasts of FRDA patients, as well as in neuroblastoma cells [28]. Pioglitazone, a thiazolidinedione, has been reported to increase fatty acid oxidation and mitochondrial function, and decrease oxidative stress and inflammation [29]. These observations led to a French proof-of-concept trial, ACTFRIE,

Table 1. Comparison of *p* values for comparing GAA1 and presence of diabetes versus absence in varies independent studies

	Dürr et al. [5], 1996 ($n = 61$)	Filla et al. [34], 1996 ($n = 63$)	Montermini et al. [33], 1997 ($n = 150$)	Delaytcki et al. [7], 1999 ($n = 51$)
Patients assessed for diabetes, *n*	61	63	150	51
p value	ns	<0.001	ns	0.08

ns, not significant.

aimed at establishing the effects of pioglitazone on neurological functions in FRDA patients. Results from the study, completed in March 2013, have not been released yet.

Ketoacidosis has been reported as the presenting symptom of diabetes in FRDA [8, 21]. However, according to several studies, impaired fasting glucose and/or impaired glucose tolerance occurs in FRDA long before a clinical diagnosis of diabetes is made [30, 31]. In one study, 49% of participants had impaired fasting glucose and/or impaired glucose tolerance, while 12% only had diabetes [24]. The current prevalence of diabetes is estimated at 6% in the UK population [32]. Furthermore, have studies demonstrated that even in non-diabetic, young, and lean FRDA patients there was increased adipose tissue content as compared to the control population. These FRDA individuals also displayed insulin resistance, which was not compensated for by increased insulin secretion, indicating β-cell failure at the cellular level prior to clinical presentation [24].

Genotype-Phenotype Correlations

The length of the smallest expansion, GAA1, inversely correlates with both age at disease onset and disease progression, measured by the time until the patients become wheelchair bound [4, 5]. Current data [5, 7, 33, 34], summarized in Table 1, are inconclusive regarding whether the GAA trinucleotide repeat length correlates with the incidence of diabetes.

As is often the case with rare genetic diseases, development of treatment and accurate genotype-phenotype correlation is constrained by limited systematic clinical information. The recent development of the European Friedreich's Ataxia Consortium for Translational Studies (EFACTS) aims to address this problem by producing a cross-sectional baseline analysis of 592 FRDA patients across 7 countries in Europe [35]. These patients will be followed and periodically evaluated to obtain longitudinal data, thus providing a powerful tool to investigate disease features [35].

A review of cases of diabetes associated with FRDA pointed out a net (>2/3 of the cases) female predominance [36]. These data were confirmed in our diabetic FRDA patients cohort ($n = 15$): females presented a 1.5-fold increased risk of developing

Table 2. Data from our FRDA patient cohort regarding gender and incidence of diabetes

	Male	Female	Total
% of total FRDA	43.6	56.4	100
% diabetic in corresponding gender	6.8	10.2	8.7

diabetes with respect to males, with an overall prevalence of 10.2 and 6.8%, respectively (Table 2). No correlation between GAA repeat length and the age at the onset of diabetes was found. This is particularly interesting as some research suggest oestrogens to be neuroprotective by attenuating Fenton's reaction, but there is not a preponderance of them in FRDA patients developing diabetes [37]. It is possible that other tissue-specific genetic and/or epigenetic factors contribute to the development of diabetes.

Recommended Management

It is currently recommended that all FRDA patients make lifestyle changes (i.e., diet control, increase of physical activity, and monitoring of weight and waist circumference) long before there is any evidence of glucose intolerance and prior to starting pharmacological treatment [38]. As FRDA patients are at risk of ketoacidosis, it is advocated to assess any hyperglycaemic derangement by oral glucose tolerance test on a yearly basis [38]. If a diagnosis of diabetes is made, therapy should be started promptly, and the importance of diet and exercise should be stressed.

A multitude of drugs have been developed to treat diabetes, each with some risks and benefits. It is common practice to prescribe metformin as the first-line agent for type 2 diabetes mellitus. At the same time, metformin inhibits complex I of the ETC and, therefore, should be used with caution in mitochondrial disorders, such as FRDA [39]. Thiazolidinediones are agonists of PPAR-γ, which is downregulated in FRDA, and they may increase frataxin levels through a positive feedback mechanism between PGC-1α and frataxin. They have also been shown to have an antioxidative effect. On the other hand, this family of drugs is associated with an increased risk of congestive heart failure due to water retention. As hypertrophic cardiomyopathy is a known manifestation of FRDA and the decompensation of heart failure is the leading cause of death in these patients, thiazolidinediones should be used with caution [40]. Pioglitazone has a safer cardiovascular profile than rosiglitazone, and therefore should be preferred [41].

Incretin analogues may have an important therapeutic role in FRDA patients as they have been shown to prevent apoptosis in both β-cells and neuronal cells. Current NICE guidelines allow prescribing the prolonged-release incretin analogue exenatide when given as triple therapy under very particular circumstances [42]. Further studies are required to determine the exact mechanisms through which incretin analogues act in FRDA patients with diabetes, and thus their efficacy. Ultimately, it is likely that insulin sensitization and lifestyle changes will not be sufficient, making it necessary to initiate insulin therapy.

Conclusion

FRDA is associated with a higher prevalence of diabetes than the general population with a rate ranging from 8 to 32% [5–7]. It has shown that both insulin resistance and insulin deficiency play a key role in the manifestation of diabetes in FRDA [13, 21, 22]. Pancreatic islet mass reduction due to increased apoptosis and decreased proliferation of β-cells also contributes to insulin deficiency in the condition [13, 22]. In terms of diabetic management, we recommend optimizing glucose control through diet and exercise before there is any evidence of glucose intolerance. From the pharmacological point of view, caution should be taken when using metformin, which inhibits complex I of the ETC, and thiazolidinediones, which are associated with water retention. Further research may build a case for incretin analogues to be used in diabetic management in FRDA.

References

1 Filla A, De Michele G, Marconi R, Bucci L, Carillo C, Castellano AE, Iorio L, Kniahynicki C, Rossi F, Campanella G: Prevalence of hereditary ataxias and spastic paraplegias in Molise, a region of Italy. J Neurol 1992;239:351–353.

2 Harding AE, Zilkha KJ: "Pseudo-dominant" inheritance in Friedreich's ataxia. J Med Genet 1981;18: 285–287.

3 Cossée M, Schmitt M, Campuzano V, Reutenauer L, Moutou C, Mandel JL, Koenig: Evolution of the Friedreich's ataxia trinucleotide repeat expansion: founder effect and premutations. Proc Natl Acad Sci U S A 1997;94:7452–7457.

4 Marmolino D: Friedreich's ataxia: past, present and future. Brain Res Rev 2011;67:311–330.

5 Dürr A, Cossee M, Agid Y, Campuzano V, Mignard C, Penet C, Mandel JL, Brice A, Koenig M, England TN: Clinical and genetic abnormalities in patients with Friedreich's ataxia. N Engl J Med 1996;335: 1169–1175.

6 Cossée M, Dürr A, Schmitt M, Dahl N, Trouillas P, Allinson P, Kostrzewa M, Nivelon-Chevallier A, Gustavson KH, Kohlschütter A, Müller U, Mandel JL, Brice A, Koenig M, Cavalcanti F, Tammaro A, De Michele G, Filla A, Cocozza S, Labuda M, Montermini L, Poirier J, Pandolfo M: Friedreich's ataxia: point mutations and clinical presentation of compound heterozygotes. Ann Neurol 1999;45:200–206.

7 Delatycki MB, Paris DB, Gardner RJ, Nicholson GA, Nassif N, Storey E, MacMillan JC, Collins V, Williamson R, Forrest SM: Clinical and genetic study of Friedreich ataxia in an Australian population. Am J Med Genet 1999;87:168–174.

8 Harding AE: Friedreich's ataxia: a clinical and genetic study of 90 families with an analysis of early diagnostic criteria and intrafamilial clustering of clinical features. Brain 1981;104:589–620.

9 Martelli A, Napierala M, Puccio H: Understanding the genetic and molecular pathogenesis of Friedreich's ataxia through animal and cellular models. Dis Model Mech 2012;5:165–176.

10 Hanis CL, Boerwinkle E, Chakraborty R, Ellsworth DL, Concannon P, Stirling B, Morrison VA, Wapelhorst B, Spielman RS, Gogolin-Ewens KJ, Shepard JM, Williams SR, Risch N, Hinds D, Iwasaki N, Ogata M, Omori Y, Petzold C, Rietzch H, Schröder HE, Schulze J, Cox NJ, Menzel S, Boriraj VV, Chen X, Lim LR, Lindner T, Mereu LE, Wang YQ, Xiang K, Yamagata K, Yang Y, Bell GI: A genome-wide search for human non-insulin-dependent (type 2) diabetes genes reveals a major susceptibility locus on chromosome 2. Nat Genet 1996;13:161–166.

11 Lindgren CM, Mahtani MM, Widén E, McCarthy MI, Daly MJ, Kirby A, Reeve MP, Kruglyak L, Parker A, Meyer J, Almgren P, Lehto M, Kanninen T, Tuomi T, Groop LC, Lander ES: Genomewide search for type 2 diabetes mellitus susceptibility loci in Finnish families: the Botnia study. Am J Hum Genet 2002;70:509–516.

12 Luo TH, Zhao Y, Li G, Yuan WT, Zhao JJ, Chen JL, Huang W, Luo M: A genome-wide search for type II diabetes susceptibility genes in Chinese Hans. Diabetologia 2001;44:501–506.

13 Igoillo-Esteve M, Gurgul-Convey E, Hu A, Romagueira Bichara Dos Santos L, Abdulkarim B, Chintawar S, Marselli L, Marchetti P, Jonas J-C, Eizirik DL, Pandolfo M, Cnop M: Unveiling a common mechanism of apoptosis in β-cells and neurons in Friedreich's ataxia. Hum Mol Genet 2015;24:2274–2286.

14 Pandolfo M, Pastore A: The pathogenesis of Friedreich ataxia and the structure and function of frataxin. J Neurol 2009;256(suppl):9–17.

15 Perdomini M, Hick A, Puccio H, Pook MA: Animal and cellular models of Friedreich ataxia. J Neurochem 2013;126(suppl):65–79.

16 Abeti R, Urzun E, Renganathan I, Honda T, Pook MA, Giunti P: Targeting lipid peroxidation and mitochondrial imbalance in Friedreich's ataxia. Pharmacol Res 2015;99:344–350.

17 Stohs S, Bagchi D: Oxidative mechanisms in the toxicity of metal ions. Free Radic Biol Med 1995;18:321–336.

18 Seznec H, Simon D, Bouton C, Reutenauer L, Hertzog A, Golik P, Procaccio V, Patel M, Drapier J-C, Koenig M, Puccio H: Friedreich ataxia: the oxidative stress paradox. Hum Mol Genet 2005;14:463–474.

19 Isaya G, O'Neill HA, Gakh O, Park S, Mantcheva R, Mooney SM: Functional studies of frataxin. Acta Paediatr Suppl 2004;93:68–71; discussion 72–73.

20 Thorén C: Diabetes mellitus in Friedreich's ataxia. Acta Paediatr 1962;51:239–247.

21 Cnop M, Mulder H, Igoillo-Esteve M: Diabetes in Friedreich ataxia. J Neurochem 2013;126:94–102.

22 Ristow M, Mulder H, Pomplun D, Schulz TJ, Müller-Schmehl K, Krause A, Fex M, Puccio H, Müller J, Isken F, Spranger J, Müller-Wieland D, Magnuson MA, Möhlig M, Koenig M, Pfeiffer AFH: Frataxin deficiency in pancreatic islets causes diabetes due to loss of beta cell mass. J Clin Invest 2003;112:527–534.

23 Szendroedi J, Phielix E, Roden M: The role of mitochondria in insulin resistance and type 2 diabetes mellitus. Nat Rev Endocrinol 2011;8:92–103.

24 Cnop M, Igoillo-Esteve M, Rai M, Begu A, Serroukh Y, Depondt C, Musuaya AE, Marhfour I, Ladrière L, Moles Lopez X, Lefkaditis D, Moore F, Brion J-P, Cooper JM, Schapira AHV, Clark A, Koeppen AH, Marchetti P, Pandolfo M, Eizirik DL, Féry F: Central role and mechanisms of β-cell dysfunction and death in Friedreich ataxia-associated diabetes. Ann Neurol 2012;72:971–982.

25 Coppola G, Marmolino D, Lu D, Wang Q, Cnop M, Rai M, Acquaviva F, Cocozza S, Pandolfo M, Geschwind DH: Functional genomic analysis of frataxin deficiency reveals tissue-specific alterations and identifies the PPARgamma pathway as a therapeutic target in Friedreich's ataxia. Hum Mol Genet 2009;18:2452–2461.

26 Cha B-S, Ciaraldi TP, Park K-S, Carter L, Mudaliar SR, Henry RR: Impaired fatty acid metabolism in type 2 diabetic skeletal muscle cells is reversed by PPARgamma agonists. Am J Physiol Endocrinol Metab 2005;289:E151–E159.

27 Wu Z, Puigserver P, Andersson U, Zhang C, Adelmant G, Mootha V, Troy A, Cinti S, Lowell B, Scarpulla RC, Spiegelman BM: Mechanisms controlling mitochondrial biogenesis and respiration through the thermogenic coactivator PGC-1. Cell 1999;98:115–124.

28 Marmolino D, Acquaviva F, Pinelli M, Monticelli A, Castaldo I, Filla A, Cocozza S: PPAR-gamma agonist azelaoyl PAF increases frataxin protein and mRNA expression: new implications for the Friedreich's ataxia therapy. Cerebellum 2009;8:98–103.

29 Babady NE, Carelle N, Wells RD, Rouault TA, Hirano M, Lynch DR, Delatycki MB, Wilson RB, Isaya G, Puccio H: Advancements in the pathophysiology of Friedreich's ataxia and new prospects for treatments. Mol Genet Metab 2007;92:23–35.

30 Khan RJ, Andermann E, Fantus IG: Glucose intolerance in Friedreich's ataxia: association with insulin resistance and decreased insulin binding. Metabolism 1986;35:1017–1023.

31 Hebinck J, Hardt C, Schöls L, Vorgerd M, Briedigkeit L, Kahn CR, Ristow M: Heterozygous expansion of the GAA tract of the X25/frataxin gene is associated with insulin resistance in humans. Diabetes 2000;49:1604–1607.

32 Prescribing and Primary Care Team and Health and Social Care Information Centre. Quality and Outcomes Framework: Achievement, Prevalence and Exceptions Data, 2012/13. Leeds, Health and Social Care Information Centre, 2013, vol 1, p 5.

33 Montermini L, Richter A, Morgan K, Justice CM, Julien D, Castellotti B, Mercier J, Poirier J, Capozzoli F, Bouchard JP, Lemieux B, Mathieu J, Vanasse M, Seni MH, Graham G, Andermann F, Andermann E, Melançon SB, Keats BJB, Di Donato S, Pandolfo M: Phenotypic variability in Friedreich ataxia: role of the associated GAA triplet repeat expansion. Ann Neurol 1997;41:675–682.

34 Filla A, De Michele G, Cavalcanti F, Pianese L, Monticelli A, Campanella G, Cocozza S: The relationship between trinucleotide (GAA) repeat length and clinical features in Friedreich ataxia. Am J Hum Genet 1996;59:554–560.

35 Reetz K, Dogan I, Costa AS, Dafotakis M, Fedosov K, Giunti P, Parkinson MH, Sweeney MG, Mariotti C, Panzeri M, Nanetti L, Arpa J, Sanz-Gallego I, Durr A, Charles P, Boesch S, Nachbauer W, Klopstock T, Karin I, Depondt C, Vom Hagen JM, Schöls L, Giordano IA, Klockgether T, Bürk K, Pandolfo M, Schulz JB: Biological and clinical characteristics of the European Friedreich's Ataxia Consortium for Translational Studies (EFACTS) cohort: a cross-sectional analysis of baseline data. Lancet Neurol 2015;14: 174–182.

36 Podolsky S, Sheremata WA: Insulin-dependent diabetes mellitus and Friedreich's ataxia in siblings. Metabolism 1970;19:555–561.

37 Richardson TE, Yu AE, Wen Y, Yang S-H, Simpkins JW: Estrogen prevents oxidative damage to the mitochondria in Friedreich's ataxia skin fibroblasts. PLoS One 2012;7:e34600.

38 Corben LA, Lynch D, Pandolfo M, Schulz JB, Delatycki MB: Consensus clinical management guidelines for Friedreich ataxia. Orphanet J Rare Dis 2014; 9:184.

39 Brunmair B, Staniek K, Gras F, Scharf N, Althaym A, Clara R, Roden M, Gnaiger E, Nohl H, Waldhäusl W, Fürnsinn C: Thiazolidinediones, like metformin, inhibit respiratory complex I: a common mechanism contributing to their antidiabetic actions? Diabetes 2004;53:1052–1059.

40 Chung SS, Kim M, Lee JS, Ahn BY, Jung HS, Lee HM, Park KS: Mechanism for antioxidative effects of thiazolidinediones in pancreatic β-cells. Am J Physiol Endocrinol Metab 2011;301:E912–E921.

41 Graham DJ, Ouellet-Hellstrom R, MaCurdy TE, Ali F, Sholley C, Worrall C, Kelman JA: Risk of acute myocardial infarction, stroke, heart failure, and death in elderly Medicare patients treated with rosiglitazone or pioglitazone. JAMA 2010;304:411–418.

42 Waugh N, Cummins E, Shyangdan DS, Court R, Mohiuddin S: Exenatide prolonged-release suspension for injection in combination with oral antidiabetic therapy for the treatment of type 2 diabetes. 2012. http://www.nice.org.uk/guidance/ta248/resources/ta248-diabetes-type-2-exenatide-prolonged-release-understanding-nice-guidance (accessed on March 22, 2015).

Paola Giunti, MD, PhD
Department of Molecular Neuroscience, Ataxia Centre
Institute of Neurology, University College London (UCL)
Queen Square
WC1N 3BG London (UK)
E-Mail p.giunti@ucl.ac.uk

Barbetti F, Ghizzoni L, Guaraldi F (eds): Diabetes Associated with Single Gene Defects and Chromosomal Abnormalities. Front Diabetes. Basel, Karger, 2017, vol 25, pp 182–187 (DOI: 10.1159/000454746)

Diabetes in Myotonic Dystrophy

Julia R. Dahlqvist · John Vissing

Copenhagen Neuromuscular Center, Department of Neurology, Rigshospitalet, University of Copenhagen, Copenhagen, Denmark

Abstract

The myotonic dystrophies are the most common muscular dystrophies worldwide. There are 2 major types of the myotonic dystrophies: type 1 (DM1) and type 2 (DM2). Both DM1 and DM2 are microsatellite expansion disorders in which a sequence of nucleotides expands to a pathogenic range. The transcripts containing repeat expansions interfere with the normal RNA metabolism resulting in disrupted regulation of alternative splicing. DM1 and DM2 are multisystem diseases, affecting skeletal muscle, the heart, the central nervous system, the eyes, and the endocrine system. Individuals with DM1 and DM2 have peripheral insulin resistance and increased proinsulin levels that can lead to glucose intolerance, hyperinsulinemia, and an increased risk of developing type 2 diabetes. In studies on individuals with DM1, impaired glucose tolerance was found in 15% compared to 10% in the background population and diabetes in 6–9 versus 3–4% in the general population.

Muscular dystrophies are inherited degenerative diseases of skeletal muscle. They cause progressive muscle weakness and atrophy in disease-specific patterns. The most common muscular dystrophies are the myotonic dystrophies. Unlike most other muscular dystrophies, myotonic dystrophies affect a great variety of other organs than muscle. Progressive wasting and weakness affects the muscles and, as the name implies, patients suffer from delayed relaxation after muscle contraction (myotonia) due to hyperexcitability of the sarcolemma. Symptoms from the brain are fatigue, cognitive impairment, and behavioral changes. There is an increased risk of cardiac arrhythmias and cardiomyopathy, hair loss, cataracts, and multiple endocrine abnormalities, including diabetes [1].

The genetic basis of the disease was discovered in 1992, almost 100 years after the first clinical description of myotonic dystrophy by Steinert. It became clear that another myotonic dystrophy type was not related to this genetic defect, and generally had a more proximal affection of muscles. This second myotonic dystrophy was referred to as proximal myotonic myopathy, or myotonic dystrophy type 2 (DM2), and the first one as Steinert disease, or myotonic dystrophy type 1 (DM1). The specific genetic mutation causing DM2 was identified in 2001. It has been suggested that there are more types of myotonic dystrophies, clinically similar to DM1 and DM2, but without the known genetic mutations [2].

Genetics and Pathogenesis

DM1 and DM2 are autosomal dominant diseases. They are microsatellite expansion disorders in which a sequence of nucleotides, typically containing a variable number of repeats within the population, expands to a pathogenic range (Fig. 1). DM1 is caused by a trinucleotide repeat expansion of cytosine-thymine-guanine (CTG) in a noncoding region of the *DMPK* (dystrophia myotonica protein kinase) gene on chromosome 19. Unaffected individuals carry 5–37 repeats, and the cutoff limit at which persons become symptomatic has been set at 50 or more repeats. The age of onset and disease severity correlates directly with the number of CTG repeats [3].

DM2 is caused by a repeat of 4 nucleotides, CCTG, on intron 1 of the *ZNF9* (zinc finger protein-9) gene on chromosome 3. The repeat expansion is larger than for DM1, ranging from 75 to over 10,000 repeats. No correlation between repeat size and disease severity has been found [3].

Different models of myotonic dystrophy pathogenesis have been proposed. The most accepted model involves toxic gain-of-function of the expanded RNAs [1]. The transcripts containing repeat expansions of CUG/CCUG fold into hairpin structures that accumulate in the nuclei and interfere with the activity of RNA-binding proteins. The interference results, for example, in elevated levels of the CUG-binding protein (CUG-BP) and inactivation of muscle-blind proteins (MBNL1). These affected proteins regulate alternative splicing and when dysfunctional lead to expression of abnormal embryonic protein isoforms in different adult tissues [4]. For example, myotonia is caused by abnormal splicing of the skeletal muscle-specific chloride channel.

Clinical Features

The prevalence of myotonic dystrophy is estimated at 1 in 8,000 worldwide, and DM1 appears to be more common than DM2, although DM2 is as common in some populations, such as in Eastern Europe and Finland [2].

Myotonic Dystrophy Type 1
DM1 can be divided into different subtypes based on the age of onset of the disease: congenital, childhood-onset, adult-onset (classical), late-onset (mild), and non-symptomatic. The great variability in phenotypes can be explained by the instable nature

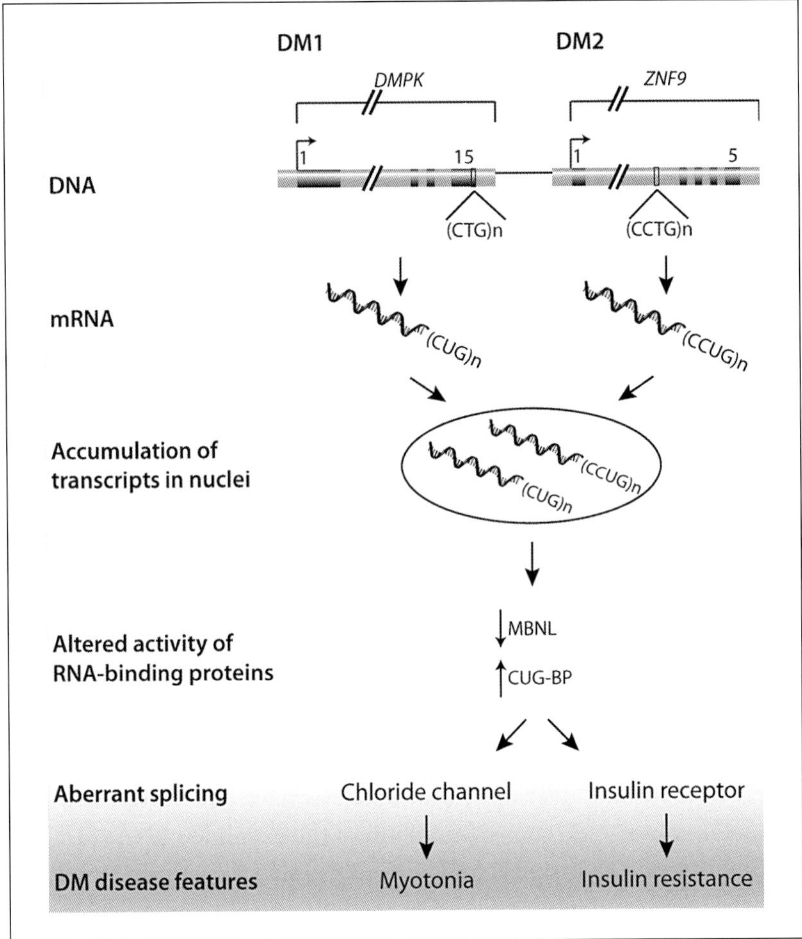

Fig. 1. Model of myotonic dystrophy pathogenesis. DM1 is caused by a repeat of 3 nucleotides, CTG, in the *DMPK* gene, and DM2 by a repeat of 4 nucleotides, CCTG, in the *ZNF9* gene. The transcripts containing the repeat expansions of CUG/CCUG accumulate in the nuclei and interfere with the activity of RNA-binding proteins such as the CUG-binding protein (CUG-BP) and muscle-blind proteins (MBNL). These affected proteins regulate alternative splicing and when dysfunctional, lead to expression of abnormal proteins causing different clinical features.

of the nucleotide expansions, which can lead to anticipation (worsening of the disease from one generation to the next) [3, 5].

The first symptoms of classical DM1 are usually myotonia and muscle weakness. Myotonia is often present in the hands as grip myotonia, but can also affect facial and pharyngeal muscles and the tongue. Muscle wasting preferentially affects facial and masticatory muscles, neck and finger flexors, and the tibialis anterior muscles first, but at later stages, diffuse and profound weakness can develop involving bulbar and respiratory muscles [5].

The extramuscular tissues involved in DM1 are the eyes, heart, brain and endocrine system. Cataract is seen in the majority of individuals. Cardiac involvement is also very frequent, and common features are conduction abnormalities and arrhythmias. Sudden death has been described in DM1, and cardiac complications have been proposed to be one of the main causes of the early mortality seen in DM1 [6, 7]. Respiratory failure, a result of the respiratory muscle weakness, is also one of the causes of early mortality [5]. Involvement of the central nervous system causes hypersomnia, altered behavior, and impaired cognitive function.

The most common endocrine dysfunctions in DM1 are hypogonadism, hyperparathyroidism, and diabetes [8–10]. Hypogonadism is seen in up to 80% of male individuals, and testicular atrophy with associated reduced fertility has been described. In women, habitual abortion and menstrual irregularities are common [3].

Myotonic Dystrophy Type 2
DM2 shares many of the multisystemic features of DM1; however, there are important differences including age of onset, the pattern of muscle weakness, and disease severity. Onset is typically in adulthood and neither anticipation nor congenital DM2 have been reported [5]. DM2 is characterized by more proximal muscle involvement, and weakness is often milder than in DM1 [2]. Cataracts, cardiac involvement, and endocrine dysfunctions are common. Hypersomnia is also commonly reported, but cognitive dysfunction is uncommon [5].

Diabetes in Myotonic Dystrophy

Individuals with DM1 and DM2 have abnormal glucose metabolism. The peripheral insulin sensitivity is decreased, which can lead to glucose intolerance, hyperinsulinemia, and an increased risk of developing type 2 diabetes [3]. This has been demonstrated with oral glucose tolerance tests (OGTT) [9, 10], insulin tolerance tests (ITT) [9], and forearm and whole-body insulin infusion tests [11, 12]. Impaired glucose tolerance was found in 15% of individuals with DM1 compared to 10% in the background population, and diabetes in 6–9 versus 3–4% in the general population [9, 10, 13].

The insulin resistance is explained by altered splicing of the *INSR* gene that encodes for the insulin receptor (IR) in skeletal muscle in DM1 and DM2. The expression of IR is physiologically regulated by alternative splicing of exon 11, generating 2 isoforms: IR-A, which lacks exon 11, and IR-B, which includes it. IR-A has a higher insulin affinity, but a lower signaling capacity than IR-B, and it has been shown that there is a positive correlation between relative IR-B expression and insulin sensitivity. IR-A generally predominates in embryonic tissues while IR-B predominates in adult skeletal muscle, liver, and adipose tissue, thus tissues that are responsive to insulin and responsible for glucose homeostasis. The expression of the IR isoforms is regulated by

RNA-binding proteins such as CUG-BP and MBNL1 proteins. CUG-BP inhibits the inclusion of exon 11, while MBNL1 proteins, which bind to CUG-BP and block its inhibitory function, are required for the exon inclusion. In skeletal muscle of patients with myotonic dystrophy, CUG-BP levels are elevated and MBNL1 function is inactivated. These alterations inhibit the inclusion of exon 11 and cause a predominant expression of the embryonic IR-A isoform, resulting in insulin resistance [4, 14].

In addition to insulin resistance, abnormal insulin secretion has been suggested to be a part of the pathogenesis of type 2 diabetes in myotonic dystrophy. A study that used OGTT and a euglycemic-hyperinsulinemic clamp to evaluate glucose metabolism found that patients with DM1 have abnormal plasma proinsulin levels in the fasting state, during clamp, and during OGTT compared to healthy controls [15].

A pathogenesis similar to that of type 1 diabetes has been rejected since patients with DM1 have normal levels of plasma C-peptide [15].

A major predisposing factor to diabetes is overweight and obesity, which has been reported in 50% of individuals with DM1 compared to 59% in the background population [16, 17]. However, it has also been reported that DM1 individuals with diabetes have a higher prevalence of overweight than DM1 individuals without diabetes, and overweight may therefore play a role in the development of diabetes [12]. Relative immobility caused by the muscle disease may also influence the prevalence of abnormal glucose metabolism.

For individuals with myotonic dystrophy that have diabetes, treatment should be similar to that of individuals without myotonic dystrophy. Low-dose metformin has been recommended in individuals with DM1 and lean diabetes [18], while thiazolidinedione or glitazone have been shown to have a good effect in overweight diabetic individuals with DM1 [19].

Conclusion

The myotonic dystrophies, DM1 and DM2, are collectively the most common muscular dystrophies worldwide. Individuals with DM1 and DM2 have abnormal glucose metabolism with an increased risk of developing type 2 diabetes. In studies on individuals with DM1, diabetes was found in 6–9% compared to 3–4% in the background population. Both insulin resistance and increased proinsulin levels have been suggested to cause the high risk of developing diabetes in these patients.

The increased incidence of diabetes suggests that glucose metabolism should be investigated regularly in patients with myotonic dystrophy. Since OGTT is inconvenient in general clinical practice for individuals with myotonic dystrophy, HbA_{1c} can possibly be used as a marker [10, 20]. Exercise should also be encouraged since it has been proved safe for DM1 patients and improves fitness and insulin sensitivity and reduces overweight [21, 22].

References

1 Lee JE, Cooper TA: Pathogenic mechanisms of myotonic dystrophy. Biochem Soc Trans 2009;37:1281–1286.

2 Ulane CM, Teed S, Sampson J: Recent advances in myotonic dystrophy type 2. Curr Neurol Neurosci Rep 2014;14:429.

3 Turner C, Hilton-Jones D: Myotonic dystrophy: diagnosis, management and new therapies. Curr Opin Neurol 2014;27:599–606.

4 Santoro M, Masciullo M, Bonvissuto D, Bianchi ML, Michetti F, Silvestri G: Alternative splicing of human insulin receptor gene (INSR) in type I and type II skeletal muscle fibers of patients with myotonic dystrophy type 1 and type 2. Mol Cell Biochem 2013;380:259–265.

5 Day JW, Ranum LP: RNA pathogenesis of the myotonic dystrophies. Neuromuscul Disord 2005;15:5–16.

6 Lund M, Diaz LJ, Ranthe MF, Petri H, Duno M, Juncker I, Eiberg H, Vissing J, Bundgaard H, Wohlfahrt J, Melbye M: Cardiac involvement in myotonic dystrophy: a nationwide cohort study. Eur Heart J 2014;35:2158–2164.

7 Petri H, Witting N, Ersboll MK, Sajadieh A, Duno M, Helweg-Larsen S, Vissing J, Kober L, Bundgaard H: High prevalence of cardiac involvement in patients with myotonic dystrophy type 1: a cross-sectional study. Int J Cardiol 2014;174:31–36.

8 Orngreen MC, Arlien-Soborg P, Duno M, Hertz JM, Vissing J: Endocrine function in 97 patients with myotonic dystrophy type 1. J Neurol 2012;259:912–920.

9 Matsumura T, Iwahashi H, Funahashi T, Takahashi MP, Saito T, Yasui K, Saito T, Iyama A, Toyooka K, Fujimura H, Shinno S: A cross-sectional study for glucose intolerance of myotonic dystrophy. J Neurol Sci 2009;276:60–65.

10 Dahlqvist JR, Orngreen MC, Witting N, Vissing J: Endocrine function over time in patients with myotonic dystrophy type 1. Eur J Neurol 2015;22:116–122.

11 Moxley RT, Griggs RC, Goldblatt D, VanGelder V, Herr BE, Thiel R: Decreased insulin sensitivity of forearm muscle in myotonic dystrophy. J Clin Invest 1978;62:857–867.

12 Moxley RT, Corbett AJ, Minaker KL, Rowe JW: Whole body insulin resistance in myotonic dystrophy. Ann Neurol 1984;15:157–162.

13 Glumer C, Jorgensen T, Borch-Johnsen K; Inter99 Study: Prevalences of diabetes and impaired glucose regulation in a Danish population: the Inter99 Study. Diabetes Care 2003;26:2335–2340.

14 Savkur RS, Philips AV, Cooper TA: Aberrant regulation of insulin receptor alternative splicing is associated with insulin resistance in myotonic dystrophy. Nat Genet 2001;29:40–47.

15 Perseghin G, Caumo A, Arcelloni C, Benedini S, Lanzi R, Pagliato E, Sereni LP, Testolin G, Battezzati A, Comi G, Comola M, Luzi L: Contribution of abnormal insulin secretion and insulin resistance to the pathogenesis of type 2 diabetes in myotonic dystrophy. Diabetes Care 2003;26:2112–2118.

16 Gagnon C, Chouinard MC, Laberge L, Brisson D, Gaudet D, Lavoie M, Leclerc N, Mathieu J: Prevalence of lifestyle risk factors in myotonic dystrophy type 1. Can J Neurol Sci 2013;40:42–47.

17 Tjepkema M: Adult obesity. Health Rep 2006;17:9–25.

18 Kouki T, Takasu N, Nakachi A, Tamanaha T, Komiya I, Tawata M: Low-dose metformin improves hyperglycaemia related to myotonic dystrophy. Diabet Med 2005;22:346–347.

19 Kashiwagi K, Nagafuchi S, Sekiguchi N, Yamagata A, Iwata I, Furuya H, Kato M, Niho Y: Troglitazone not only reduced insulin resistance but also improved myotonia in a patient with myotonic dystrophy. Eur Neurol 1999;41:171–172.

20 Jorgensen ME, Bjerregaard P, Borch-Johnsen K, Witte D: New diagnostic criteria for diabetes: is the change from glucose to HbA$_{1c}$ possible in all populations? J Clin Endocrinol Metab 2010;95:E333–E336.

21 Reyna SM, Tantiwong P, Cersosimo E, Defronzo RA, Sriwijitkamol A, Musi N: Short-term exercise training improves insulin sensitivity but does not inhibit inflammatory pathways in immune cells from insulin-resistant subjects. J Diabetes Res 2013;2013:107805.

22 Orngreen MC, Olsen DB, Vissing J: Aerobic training in patients with myotonic dystrophy type 1. Ann Neurol 2005;57:754–757.

Julia R. Dahlqvist, MD
Copenhagen Neuromuscular Center, Section 3342
Department of Neurology, Rigshospitalet, University of Copenhagen
Blegdamsvej 9
DK–2100 Copenhagen (Denmark)
E-Mail julia.rebecka.dahlqvist@regionh.dk

Author Index

Abeti, R. 172
Arvan, P. 1

Bacchetta, R. 78
Barbetti, F. IX, 1
Bizzarri, C. 160

Cappa, M. 160, 166

Dahlqvist, J.R. 182
d'Annunzio, G. 69

Fattorusso, V. 49
Favaretto, F. 134
Fierabracci, A. 91
Franzese, A. 49
Froguel, P. 26

Ghizzoni, L. IX
Giunti, P. 172
Grasso, V. 1
Grossi, A. 166
Grugni, G. 145
Guaraldi, F. IX

Leiter, S.M. 104, 119
Liu, M. 1

Maccari, M.E. 78
Maffei, P. 134
Mammì, C. 1
Marshall, J.D. 134
Milan, G. 134
Mozzillo, E. 49

Ng, Y.S. 55
Nichols, C.G. 1
Novelli, G. VII

Panimolle, F. 151

Radicioni, A.F. 151
Ran, S. 172
Remedi, M. 1
Rigoli, L.C. 69
Russo, B. 91

Schaefer, A.M. 55
Semple, R.K. 104, 119

Taylor, R.W. 55

Vaxillaire, M. 26
Vissing, J. 182

Subject Index

AADC 92, 99, 100
ABCC8
    maturity-onset diabetes of the young
        mutations 34
    neonatal diabetes mellitus mutations
        3–6
Acanthosis nigricans (AN), insulin resistance
    association 106
Adiponectin 154
AGPAT2 124
AIRE, autoimmune polyglandular syndrome
    type 1 mutations 92, 94, 96, 97
AKT2 114
ALMS1 134–136, 138, 140
Alström syndrome (AS)
    clinical features 134, 135, 139, 140
    diagnosis 140
    molecular pathogenesis 135, 136
    mouse models 138
    obesity, metabolism, and
        endocrinology 137–139
    treatment 141
AN, *see* Acanthosis nigricans
Anemia, *see* Thiamine-responsive
    megaloblastic anemia syndrome
APS1, *see* Autoimmune polyglandular
    syndrome type 1
AS, *see* Alström syndrome
Autoimmune polyglandular syndrome type 1
    (APS1)
    AIRE mutations 92, 94, 96, 97
    autoantibodies 92, 93
    clinical features 92–94
    diabetes
        genetic predisposing factors 95–97
        pancreatic autoimmunity
            markers 98–100

        presentation 94, 95
        prospects for study 100

Bardet-Biedl syndrome (BBS) 137
BBWS, *see* Bardet-Biedl syndrome
Beratdinelli-Seip congenital lipodystrophies
    (BSCL) 123, 124
BLK, maturity-onset diabetes of the young
    mutations 33, 34
BSCL2 124

CAV1 124
CD25 84, 87
CEL, maturity-onset diabetes of the young
    mutations 35
CIDEC 127
CTLA-4 88

DM, *see* Myotonic dystrophy
DMPK 183
Donahue syndrome (DS) 109–111
Down syndrome (DS)
    clinical features 160
    diabetes association
        age at onset 162
        epidemiology 160, 161
        genetic susceptibility 162, 163
        islet cell autoimmunity 163, 164
        management 164
        pancreas histopathology 161
        prospects for study 164, 165
DS, *see* Donahue syndrome; Down syndrome

EIF2AK3, neonatal diabetes mellitus
    mutations 12, 13

Familial partial lipodystrophy (FPLD) 125–127

FBN1 129
FOXP3
    IPEX mutations 2, 78, 80, 81, 85, 167
    T-regulatory cell function 79, 80
FPLD, *see* Familial partial lipodystrophy
Frataxin
    function 173, 174
    trinucleotide repeat expansion in Friedreich
        ataxia 173
FRDA, *see* Friedreich ataxia
Friedreich ataxia (FRDA)
    clinical features 172, 173
    diabetes
        management 178, 179
        mechanisms 174–177, 179
    epidemiology 172
    frataxin function 173, 174
    genetics 173
    genotype-phenotype correlations 177, 178

GAD65 92, 98.99, 163
GCK
    maturity-onset diabetes of the young
        mutations 30, 31, 36–39
    neonatal diabetes mellitus mutations 2, 3,
        12
GH, *see* Growth hormone
Growth hormone (GH)
    deficiency in Alström syndrome 139, 140
    therapy effects in Turner syndrome 169

Hashimoto's thyroiditis, Turner syndrome
    167
HNF1A, maturity-onset diabetes of the young
    mutations 31, 32, 36–40
HNF1B, maturity-onset diabetes of the young
    mutations 32, 37
HNF4A, maturity-onset diabetes of the young
    mutations 31, 32, 36, 39, 40
Hypogonadism, *see* Klinefelter syndrome

IL-10 88
IL-10R 88
Immune dysregulation, polyendocrinopathy,
    enteropathy, X-linked syndrome (IPEX)
    clinical features 81, 82
    diabetes features 83
    FOXP3 mutations 2, 78, 80, 81, 85,
        167
    IPEX-like syndromes and diabetes 84,
        86–88

INS
    maturity-onset diabetes of the young
        mutations 33
    neonatal diabetes mellitus mutations 3,
        8–12, 18
Insulin resistance, *see* Klinefelter syndrome;
    Severe insulin resistance
IPEX, *see* Immune dysregulation,
    polyendocrinopathy, enteropathy, X-linked
    syndrome
ITCH 87, 88

KCNJ11, neonatal diabetes mellitus
    mutations 3–6, 17, 18
KLF11, maturity-onset diabetes of the young
    mutations 32, 33
Klinefelter syndrome (KS)
    body composition and insulin
        resistance 154–157
    clinical features 152
    diabetes association 157, 158
    genetics 151, 152
    hypogonadism and insulin sensitivity 152,
        153
    testosterone replacement therapy 158
    visceral adiposity and insulin
        sensitivity 153, 154
KS, *see* Klinefelter syndrome

Leptin 154, 156
Lipodystrophies
    classification 120–122
    complex syndromes 128, 129
    complications 122, 123
    genetic subtypes
        congenital generalized
            lipodystrophies 123–125
        partial lipodystrophies 125–128
    obesity consequences 119, 120
LMNA 125–128
LRBA 88

Maturity-onset diabetes of the young
    (MODY)
    epidemiology 27
    genetic subtypes
        ABCC8 mutations 34
        BLK mutations 33, 34
        CEL mutations 35
        GCK mutations 30, 31, 36–39
        HNF1A mutations 31, 32, 36–40

HNF1B mutations 32, 37
HNF4A mutations 31, 32, 36,
  39, 40
INS mutations 33
KLF11 mutations 32, 33
NEUROD1 mutations 32, 33
overview 27–29
PAX4 mutations 32, 33
PDX1 mutations 32, 33
stem cell research and therapeutic
  prospects 42, 43
WFS1 mutations 34
molecular diagnosis
clinical relevance 38–40
next generation sequencing
  40–42
personalized pharmacogenomic
  treatment 35–38
prospects for study 43, 44
MDP syndrome 129
Mitochondrial diabetes
cardiac disease 62, 63
management 64–66
maternally inherited diabetes and
  deafness 55, 56, 58, 61
mitochondrial DNA features 56, 57
molecular diagnostics 63, 64
nephropathy 62
neuropathy 63
pathogenesis 57, 58
pattern recognition in diagnosis
  age at onset 61
  body mass index 61
  insulin requirement 61
  overview 60
phenotypes 58–60
retinopathy 61, 62
screening 64
stroke-like episodes 63
MODY, *see* Maturity-onset diabetes of the
  young
Myotonic dystrophy (DM)
clinical features
  DM1 183–185
  DM2 185
  overview 182
diabetes mechanisms 185, 186
genetics 182, 183

NALP5 92
NDM, *see* Neonatal diabetes mellitus

Neonatal diabetes mellitus (NDM)
clinical features 2
permanent form
  ABCC8 mutations 3–6
  EIF2AK3 mutations 12, 13
  GCK mutations 2, 3, 12
  INS mutations 3, 8–12
  KCNJ11 mutations 3–6
  mouse models
    insulin mutations 11, 12
    potassium channel mutations
      7, 8
  SLC2A2 mutations 12
  sulfonylurea treatment 6, 7
  transcription factor mutations 12
transient form
  clinical findings 16, 17
  etiology 14
  genetic counseling 17
  genomic imprinting defects 13, 14
  INS mutations 18
  KCNJ11 mutations 17, 18
  pathogenesis 15
  penetrance 17
  treatment 17
  uniparental disomy 15
NEUROD1, maturity-onset diabetes of the
  young mutations 32, 33

Obesity, *see* Alström syndrome; Klinefelter
  syndrome; Lipodystrophies; Prader-Willi
  syndrome

PAX4, maturity-onset diabetes of the young
  mutations 32, 33
PCYT1A 128
PDX1, maturity-onset diabetes of the young
  mutations 32, 33
PEO1 57
PIK3R1 113, 114, 128
PLIN1 127, 128
POLD1 129
POLG1 57, 60
Polycystic ovary syndrome 106, 107
PPARG 127
Prader-Willi syndrome (PWS)
clinical features 145–147
diabetic surveillance 148
treatment 147
PSMB8 129
PTPN22 167

PTRF 124, 125
PWS, *see* Prader-Willi syndrome

Rabson-Mendenhall syndrome (RMS)
    111
Resistin 154
RMS, *see* Rabson-Mendenhall syndrome
RRM2B 57

Severe insulin resistance
    biochemical diagnosis 105, 106
    clinical features 106, 107
    congenital insulin resistance without insulin
        mutations
        AKT2 mutation 114
        SHORT syndrome 113, 114
        TBC1D4 mutation 114, 115
        type A insulin resistance 112, 113
    Donahue syndrome 109–111
    insulin receptor mutations 107–109
    lipodystrophy association, *see*
        Lipodystrophies
    management 129, 130
    Rabson-Mendenhall syndrome 111
SHORT syndrome 113, 114, 128
SLC19A2, thiamine-responsive
    megaloblastic anemia syndrome
    mutations 49, 51, 52
SLC2A2, neonatal diabetes mellitus
    mutations 12
SOCS3 87
STAT1 87
STAT3 84, 86, 88
STAT5 79, 84, 87
Sulfonylurea, neonatal diabetes mellitus
    treatment 6, 7

TBC1D4 114, 115
Testosterone replacement therapy (TRT),
    Klinefelter syndrome and insulin
    sensitivity 158

Thiamine-responsive megaloblastic anemia
    (TRMA) syndrome
    clinical features
        anemia 50
        deafness 51
        diabetes 50, 51
        ocular manifestations 51
    SLC19A2 mutations 49, 51, 52
    thiamine metabolism 50
TRMA syndrome, *see* Thiamine-responsive
    megaloblastic anemia syndrome
TRT, *see* Testosterone replacement therapy
TS, *see* Turner syndrome
Turner syndrome (TS)
    autoimmunity 167, 168
    clinical features 166
    diabetes 168–170
    epidemiology 166
    glucose homeostasis 168
TWNK 60

Uniparental disomy (UPD), neonatal diabetes
    mellitus 15
UPD, *see* Uniparental disomy

WFS1, maturity-onset diabetes of the young
    mutations 34
WFS1, Wolfram syndrome mutations and
    function 34, 70, 72–75
WFS2, Wolfram syndrome mutations 75
Wolcott-Rallison syndrome 2, 12, 13
Wolfram syndrome (WS)
    clinical features 69–72
    linkage studies 72
    WFS1 mutations and function 34, 70,
        72–75
    WFS2 mutations 75
WS, *see* Wolfram syndrome

ZMPSTE24 129
ZNF9 183